D1267537

Myocardial Diseases

CLINICAL CARDIOLOGY MONOGRAPHS

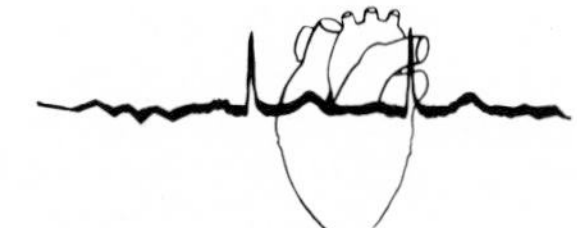

SERIES CONSULTANTS

J. Willis Hurst, M.D.
Professor and Chairman, Department of Medicine, Emory University School of Medicine, Atlanta, Georgia

and

Dean T. Mason, M.D.
Professor, Departments of Medicine and Physiology, and Chief, Section of Cardiovascular Medicine, University of California School of Medicine, Davis, California

Myocardial Diseases

Edited by

NOBLE O. FOWLER, M.D.

Professor of Medicine and Director, Division of Cardiology,
University of Cincinnati Medical Center,
Cincinnati, Ohio

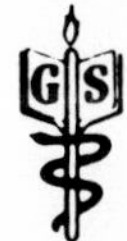

GRUNE & STRATTON New York and London
A Subsidiary of Harcourt Brace Jovanovich, Publishers

Library of Congress Cataloging in Publication Data

Fowler, Noble O
Myocardial diseases.

(Cardiovascular diseases, v. 2)
Includes bibliographical references.
1. Heart—Muscle—Diseases. I. Title. [DNLM:
1. Myocardial diseases, Primary. 2. Myocardial
diseases, Secondary. WG 280 M996 1963]
RC685.M9F68 616.1'24 73-1685
ISBN: 0-8089-0799-9

Grune & Stratton, Inc.
111 Fifth Avenue
New York, New York 10003

Library of Congress Catalog Card Number 73–1685
International Standard Book Number 0-8089-0799-9

Printed in the United States of America

Contents

Contributors vii

Preface xi

1. Some Historical Notes on the Development of the Present State of Knowledge of Diseases of the Myocardium
THOMAS W. MATTINGLY, M.D. 1

2. Classification and Diagnosis of Myocardial Diseases
NOBLE O. FOWLER, M.D. 25

3. Clinical Features and Natural History of Cardiomyopathy
JACK P. SEGAL, M.D., W. PROCTOR HARVEY, M.D., AND JOHN F. STAPLETON, M.D. 37

4. Morphologic Observations in the Cardiomyopathies
WILLIAM C. ROBERTS, M.D. AND VICTOR J. FERRANS, M.D., PH.D. 59

5. Hemodynamics and Myocardial Metabolism Studies and Their Application to Myocardial Diseases
JOHN W. VESTER, M.D. 117

6. Radiologic Features of Myocardial Diseases
HAROLD B. SPITZ, M.D. AND JOHN C. HOLMES, M.D. 167

7. Electrocardiographic and Vectorcardiographic Features of Myocardial Diseases
NANCY C. FLOWERS, M.D. AND LEO G. HORAN, M.D. 181

8. Heritable and Familial Aspects of Myocardial Diseases
RALPH SHABETAI, M.D. AND IAN SHINE, M.D.
WITH THE ASSISTANCE OF ROGER FREEMAN, WILLIAM SHUFFETT, LEE COLEMAN AND GRACE CARLSON, R.N. 213

9. Alcoholic Cardiomyopathy
TIMOTHY J. REGAN, M.D. 233

10. Clinical Aspects of Viral Cardiomyopathy
WALTER H. ABELMANN, M.D. 253

11. Immunologic Studies in Myocardial Diseases
EVELYN V. HESS, B.CH., B.A.O., M.D. AND ALAN KIRSNER, M.D. 281

12. Hypertrophic Obstructive Cardiomyopathy (Muscular or Hypertrophic Subaortic Stenosis)
E. DOUGLAS WIGLE, M.D., CLARENCE H. FELDERHOF, M.D., MALCOLM D. SILVER, M.D., AND ALLAN G. ADELMAN, M.D. 297

13. The Myocardial Disease of Heredofamilial Neuromyopathies
JOSEPH K. PERLOFF, M.D. 319

14. The Secondary Cardiomyopathies
NOBLE O. FOWLER, M.D. 337

15. The Treatment of Myocardial Diseases
NOBLE O. FOWLER, M.D. 361

Index 375

Contributors

WALTER H. ABELMANN, M.D., Associate Professor of Medicine, Harvard Medical School; Visiting Physician, Boston City Hospital; Consultant in Cardiology, Children's Medical Center, Boston, Massachusetts

ALLAN G. ADELMAN, M.D., F.R.C.P.(C), Division of Cardiology and Cardiovascular Unit, Toronto General Hospital; Assistant Professor, Department of Medicine, University of Toronto, Toronto, Ontario, Canada

CLARENCE H. FELDERHOF, M.D., F.R.C.P. (C), Research Fellow in Cardiology (Medical Research Council of Canada); Cardiovascular Unit, Toronto General Hospital, Toronto, Ontario, Canada

VICTOR J. FERRANS, M.D., PH.D., Senior Investigator, Section of Pathology, National Heart and Lung Institute, National Institutes of Health, Bethesda, Maryland

NANCY C. FLOWERS, M.D., Chief, Section of Cardiology, Medical Service, FHD, Veterans Administration Hospital; Professor of Medicine, Department of Medicine, Medical College of Georgia, Augusta, Georgia

NOBLE O. FOWLER, M.D., Professor of Medicine; Director, Division of Cardiology, University of Cincinnati Medical Center, Cincinnati, Ohio

W. PROCTOR HARVEY, M.D., Professor of Medicine, Department of Medicine, Georgetown University School of Medicine; Director, Division of Cardiology, Georgetown University Medical Center, Washington, D.C.

EVELYN V. HESS, M.D., F.A.C.P., McDonald Professor of Medicine; Director, Division of Immunology, Department of Medicine, University of Cincinnati Medical Center, Cincinnati, Ohio

JOHN C. HOLMES, M.D., Associate Professor of Medicine; Assistant Professor of Radiology, University of Cincinnati Medical Center; Director, Cardiac Catheterization Laboratory, Cincinnati General Hospital, Cincinnati, Ohio

LEO G. HORAN, M.D., Chief, Medical Service, FHD, Veterans Administration Hospital, and Professor of Medicine, Department of Medicine, Medical College of Georgia, Augusta, Georgia

ALAN KIRSNER, M.D., Assistant Clinical Professor of Medicine, Medical College of Ohio; Physician, Toledo Clinic, Toledo, Ohio

THOMAS W. MATTINGLY, M.D., Clinical Professor Emeritus, Georgetown University School of Medicine; Special Lecturer, George Washington University School of Medicine; Consultant in Cardiology to the Surgeon General, Department of the Army and to the Office of Medical Services, Department of State; formerly Chief of Medicine and Cardiology, Walter Reed General Hospital and the Washington Hospital Center, Washington, D.C.

JOSEPH K. PERLOFF, M.D., Professor of Medicine and Pediatrics; Chief, Section of Cardiology, University of Pennsylvania School of Medicine, Philadelphia, Pennsylvania

TIMOTHY J. REGAN, M.D., Professor of Medicine, Department of Medicine; Director, Division of Cardiovascular Disease, College of Medicine and Dentistry of New Jersey at Newark, Newark, New Jersey

WILLIAM C. ROBERTS, M.D., Chief, Section of Pathology, National Heart and Lung Institute, National Institutes of Health, Bethesda, Maryland; Clinical Associate Professor of Pathology and Medicine (Cardiology), Georgetown University School of Medicine, Washington, D.C.

JACK P. SEGAL, M.D., Clinical Associate Professor of Medicine, Department of Medicine, Division of Cardiology, Georgetown University Medical Center, Washington, D.C.

RALPH SHABETAI, M.D., Professor of Medicine, Director, Division of Cardiology, The University of Texas Medical School, at Houston, Houston, Texas

IAN SHINE, M.D., Geneticist, Hunt-Morgan Foundation, Lexington, Kentucky

MALCOLM D. SILVER, M.D., B.S., M.Sc., Ph.D., F.R.C.P.A. Senior Staff Pathologist, Cardiovascular Unit, Toronto General Hospital; Associate Professor, Department of Pathology, University of Toronto, Toronto, Ontario, Canada

HAROLD B. SPITZ, M.D., Professor of Radiology, Department of Radiology, University of Cincinnati Medical Center, Cincinnati, Ohio

JOHN F. STAPLETON, M.D., Professor of Medicine, Department of Medicine, Division of Cardiology, Georgetown University School of Medicine; Medical Director, Georgetown University Medical Center, Washington, D.C.

JOHN W. VESTER, M.D., Professor of Medicine and Associate Professor of Biochemistry, University of Cincinnati College of Medicine; Director of Research, Good Samaritan Hospital, Cincinnati, Ohio

E. DOUGLAS WIGLE, M.D., F.R.C.P.(C), F.A.C.P., Director, Division of Cardiology and Cardiovascular Unit, Toronto General Hospital; Professor and Co-ordinator of Cardiology, Department of Medicine, University of Toronto, Toronto, Ontario, Canada

Preface

Future Perspectives in Diseases of the Myocardium

The last 15 years have clearly established that the myocardial diseases represent a significant proportion of the circulatory disorders which may lead to cardiac enlargement, congestive heart failure, cardiac arrhythmias, and sudden death. Although formerly believed rare and largely limited to alcoholics and impoverished minority groups, myocardial diseases are now recognized in every stratum of society and in all age groups.

Although we have made much progress in the clinical recognition of the myocardial diseases, in many instances their background is not understood and thus, an informed search for appropriate preventive measures is not yet possible. One problem area lies in the gray zone between myocardial disease and hypertensive heart disease. Some authorities believe that many patients labeled as having myocardial disease actually have "burned-out" hypertensive heart disease. On the other hand, others believe that in many patients labeled as having hypertensive heart disease, the hypertension is of little significance, and that such patients actually have myocardial disease. It is well known that the cardiac response to hypertension is variable. Further, many patients without previous hypertension temporarily develop elevated diastolic blood pressures of 100 or 110 mm Hg during bouts of cardiac decompensation. In our own studies we have not considered such patients to have hypertensive heart disease. Progress in this area is limited by the lack of a specific test for myocardial disease; further, anatomic examination of the heart, including electron microscopy, does not allow the pathologist to distinguish between hypertensive heart disease and cardiomyopathy, once heart failure has occurred.

The role of alcoholism in the genesis of the myocardial diseases is difficult to quantify. There is little doubt, as Regan has shown, that acute alcoholism impairs left ventricular function in man; the step from these acute studies to the establishment of chronic alcoholic myocardial disease is a long one. It seems clear that most of the "idiopathic" congestive cardiomyopathies, the largest single group of the myocardial diseases, are not caused by alcoholism; the majority of our patients with myocardial diseases do not use alcohol. How can one tell, among those who drink, when alcohol is a factor? Why do some who drink get myocardial disease; others, liver diseases; a few, both, and most, neither? It seems clear that nutritional differences are not the only answer. Here too, we have been disappointed to learn that the electron microscopic picture of alcoholic cardiomyopathy, formerly believed specific, is, in fact, not.

Iatrogenic myocardial disease: As in other aspects of medicine, we are observing effects upon the myocardium of customs encouraged by our drug-oriented society. Procainamide, hydralazine, dilantin, and isoniazid may cause a lupus-like syndrome, with fever, arthralgia, pleuropericarditis, and myocardial involvement. Large doses of irradiation directed toward the mediastinum may cause irradiation-induced myocarditis and pericarditis. We have recently observed eight instances of cardiac dysfunction or arrhythmia, probably related to psychotropic drugs. Mellaril is a particular offender. Future studies of myocardial diseases must consider environmental factors, as well as the use of drugs and the role of nutrition.

Peripartal heart disease: A decade ago, it was commonly believed that unexplained heart failure in relation to the third trimester of pregnancy, or in the early postpartum period, was usually related to unrecognized toxemia or pulmonary embolism. It is now clear that this is usually not true; that there is, in fact, an unexplained relationship of myocardial disease to late pregnancy and to the postpartum period. Probably ten percent of our patients with myocardial disease are in this category. The explanation is unknown. Perhaps nutritional factors or undiagnosed viral infections are important in some instances.

Familial disease: The prevalence of familial myocardial disease needs further study. It is generally recognized that obstructive cardiomyopathy very commonly has an heredofamilial background. Familial factors, however, are often of importance in "idiopathic" congestive cardiomyopathy; Dr. Ralph Shabetai illustrates this relationship in his chapter of this book. This matter needs much more attention and study than it has received in the past. Hereditary factors may determine predisposition to myocardial disease when drugs, toxins, alcohol, pregnancy and other etiologic or precipitating agents appear.

Viral disease: It is now recognized that Coxsackie B viral myocarditis may, uncommonly, be followed by the syndrome of congestive cardiomyopathy. More studies are needed to evaluate both during life and at the postmortem table, the role of undetected viral disease in the genesis of what may emerge later as "idiopathic" cardiomyopathy.

Autoimmune disease: Studies made in our own medical school have failed to show a relationship between circulating antimyocardial antibodies and the course of idiopathic congestive cardiomyopathy. Dr. Evelyn Hess alludes to these investigations in her chapter of this book. Although our studies and those of others have not shown a consistent relationship, further studies of patients earlier in the disease, and by other methods, are needed. The interpretation to be placed upon evidence of antiheart antibodies in patients with myocardial disease is difficult, since myocardial damage produced by infarction, trauma, or infection may be followed by evidence of circulating antiheart antibodies as a secondary manifestation.

The author wishes to thank Mrs. Roberta Waltz and Mrs. Mary Roche for their assistance in retyping the manuscript.

Noble O. Fowler, M.D.

THOMAS W. MATTINGLY, M.D.

Some Historical Notes on the Development of the Present State of Knowledge of Diseases of the Myocardium

The history of the development of the concept of myocardial disease and of the recognition of its clinical and pathologic features is so closely interwoven with the development of the knowledge of heart disease in general, that one must begin with a brief historical outline of heart disease. In this outline, only key points which have an important relationship to the initial and current concepts of myocardial disease will be mentioned.

The development of the initial concepts of heart disease and later of myocardial disease, as well as subsequent progress, has been closely related to the availability of clinical and research tools, to periodic advancements in general scientific knowledge principally gained by the use of these tools, to the development of techniques whereby this new knowledge and these techniques could be applied to medicine, and finally to communication of this knowledge and these skills to others. Accordingly, it becomes appropriate to divide this historical presentation into eras that correspond to significant developments.

ERA OF LIMITATION OF TOOLS TO UNAIDED EYES, EARS, AND HANDS (B.C. to A.D. 1799)

Prior to the nineteenth century, the physician had only his unaided eyes, ears, and hands to aid him in the diagnosis and investigation of heart disease. Although the earlier physicians described symptoms and physical signs recognized today as evidence of myocardial dysfunction such as dyspnea, dropsy, and irregularities of the pulse, they did not relate the observed clinical features to disease of the heart or myocardium. During the first fourteen centuries A.D., little progress occurred and what did develop from the simple observations and deductions of individual physicians, recognized as brilliant in retrospect, was not effectively communicated before the development of printing in the midfifteenth century. The published observations and theoretic considerations made from patient observations and gross autopsy and anatomic studies, chiefly by Italian physicians during the period 1500-1600, began to relate specific symptoms to what were considered abnormalities in the heart, but actual diseases were not identified. Harvey's publication in 1628 provided proof of a circulatory system with the concept that the heart was the central pump, thus establishing a basis for the subsequent recognition of faults in function and structure of this central pump (myocardium) as a manifestation of myocardial disease. Even these deductions were slow in development. In 1618, Albertini's treatise on the heart contained an extensive description of the arterial pulse and its irregularities as well as descriptions of syncope and palpitation. However, his theoretical considerations did not give disease of the heart (or myocardium) as the cause but rather considered these manifestations either to result from reflex action on the heart or to develop directly from abnormalities in other organs. It was perhaps Lower and Bonetus, writing in the period 1600-1700, who first gave correlations of symptoms during life with gross abnormalities in the heart at autopsy, thereby establishing what later became recognized as disease of the heart and myocardium. Senac's publication, in 1749, represents the first of many publications by contemporaries of his time which was worthy of being titled a textbook on heart diseases. Although he made no mention of diseases of the myocardium, he referred to the use of quinidine for the treatment of "rebellious palpitation" which was the beginning of effective drug therapy of arrhythmias resulting from diseases of the myocardium.

Auenbrugger's introduction of the technique of percussion, combining the use of the hands, ears, and eyes, and its later perfection by Skoda, provided a new clinical technic that continues to be used today. Percussion permitted clinical recognition of cardiac enlargement and pleural and pericardial effusions which was helpful in the recognition of heart disease and myocardial failure.

DEVELOPMENTS RELATED TO THE INTRODUCTION AND USE OF THE STETHOSCOPE AND THE MICROSCOPE IN MEDICINE (1800-1900)

The introduction of the stethoscope by Laennec, in 1819, provided the first effective tool to aid the clinician in the recognition and study of heart disease and provided the basis for the first classification of heart diseases. The identification and correlation of certain auscultatory findings resulted in the concept that there were basically two types of heart disease: *valvular* and *nonvalvular*. Any concept of myocardial disease which might have existed at the time was included in the category of nonvalvular disease. In later years, the stethoscope proved to be an important tool in the recognition of myocardial disease, not by exclusion but by reliable auscultatory findings, Harvey and Perloff [1] and Mattingly [2].

The introduction of the monocular light microscope and later the Wenham prism (1861) with the development of the binocular microscope gave the early pathologist an important tool to aid his eyes in studying disease of the heart and especially the myocardium. The use of microscopes in the study of the cellular changes in organs and tissues and the widespread acceptance of Virchow's theory of cellular pathology established a firm basis for the concept of myocarditis, that is, the inflammatory phase of the cellular response of the myocardium to injury. Earlier clinical publications, especially those of Johnson [3] in 1826 had referred to "carditis," but the case reports clearly indicate that the clinical concept was vague and probably included instances of myocarditis, pericarditis, pleuritis, pneumonia, and likely, acute myocardial infarction. All were diagnosed as inflammation of the chest. The term "myocarditis" and the concept of myocarditis as an inflammatory reaction of the myocardium were first introduced by Sobernheim [4] in 1837. In his early concept and practice, it is apparent that he did not separate acute vascular lesions from acute inflammatory lesions associated with infections.

The introduction of the microscope likewise resulted in the development of a new science of bacteriology. This development led to the study of the myocardium in infections recognized at the time, with diphtheria as an early model. The publications of Ruhle [5], in 1878, provided excellent descriptions of diphtheritic myocarditis as well as of acute myocarditis in other infections, including localized as well as diffuse myocardial involvement. Pathologic changes were described which the pathologists considered as evidence of "chronic myocarditis." The recognized clinical manifestations of chronic myocarditis were "cardiac weakness and failure." "Chronic myocarditis," often unsupported by pathologic correlation, became a popular clinical diagnosis of the time. "Chronic myocarditis" became synonymous with "nonvalvular heart disease," which had come into usage earlier; the use of the two terms prevailed well into the first three decades of the twentieth century.

Failure to correlate changes in the myocardium at autopsy with the presence of an infectious disease, a state of sepsis, or a systemic disease soon resulted in new concepts of myocardial disease. In 1891, Krehl [6], an outstanding clinician and pathologist and perhaps the father of pathologic physiology, was one of the first to investigate and write about "idiopathic disease of the heart muscle." His clinical and pathologic descriptions, founded on a series of cases which he observed, fit well into what is described today as idiopathic cardiomyopathy or idiopathic myocardial hypertrophy. He considered the clinical disorders and the pathologic changes in the myocardium to have been the result of a preceding acute myocarditis. He believed that the pathologic changes were chronic and noninflammatory which eventually led to "myocardial failure even when all adverse influences of the initial disease had been eliminated." He referred to these residual changes in the myocardium which resulted in heart muscle failure as "interstitial changes." The term "interstitial" was later used by Fiedler [7] to describe acute interstitial myocarditis, and it continues in medical usage today. Krehl described "idiopathic myocardial hypertrophy" and referred to heart failure as having been caused by "anatomical disease of the tissues." He appears to have been the first to describe idiopathic heart muscle disease and idiopathic myocardial hypertrophy.

Shortly after the above reports by Krehl, observations and reports by Fiedler [7] in 1899 and by Josserand and Gallavardin [8], in 1901, resulted in the introduction of other new terms to describe forms of idiopathic myocardial disease. Fiedler's concepts were derived from clinical and pathologic studies of five young adults with a similar disease, fatal in four. The illness was characterized by a rapidly developing progressive biventricular failure without high fever or symptoms of sepsis. At autopsy, the heart was the chief site of disease where the predominant changes were localized to the interfibrillary tissues (interstitial) of the heart muscle, and there were only minimal parenchymal changes. He considered the changes as one of "acute interstitial myocarditis" not due to diphtheria, scarlet fever, nor a sepsis but to some microorganism or its toxin which directly localized its action to the heart muscle. This perhaps was the first suggestion that an invasive organism or its toxin might be cardiotrophic, with ability to localize to the myocardium. This concept of the inflammation limited to the myocardium led to reports by others of "isolated myocarditis" or "Fiedler's myocarditis" with varied concepts of the disease process. Josserand and Gallavardin [8] reported similar inflammatory processes limited to the myocardium in which the myocardial lesion was the only explanation for death from heart failure in young adults. They considered the disease as one primarily in the myocardium and used the terms "primary myocarditis" and "primary myocardial diseases." This is the first appearance of these terms in medical literature and the author was not aware of it when he introduced the latter term with a somewhat different concept in 1957 [9].

These important observations of Josserand and Gallavardin [8] were followed, in 1904, by those of Aschoff [10] who described peculiar myocardial lesions in the hearts of individuals dying of rheumatic fever. This peculiar constellation of cellular changes became known as "Aschoff bodies." Thus began the concept of identification of the nature of myocardial lesion by a specific type of cellular response, and the basis for the pathologic diagnosis of rheumatic myocarditis was established.

DEVELOPMENTS RELATED TO INTRODUCTION AND USE OF ELECTROCARDIOGRAM, SPHYGMOMANOMETER, AND ROENTGENOGRAM (1900-1950)

These diagnostic and research tools were introduced in medicine during the last decade of the nineteenth century and gradually came into clinical use during the early decades of the twentieth century. They became highly perfected and widely accepted by midcentury. Their use helped develop new concepts of cardiovascular disease and provided useful tools for recording specific information about myocardial function in health and disease.

Clinical Recognition of Occlusive Coronary Artery Disease and Hypertensive Cardiovascular Disease

Herrick's [11] recognition of the clinical features of acute infarction of the myocardium due to occlusive coronary disease was a milestone in the history of myocardial disease. It established the concept of vascular disease as an important cause of secondary myocardial damage and myocardial failure. Since then coronary artery disease has been recognized as the most important of all causes of myocardial disease in most areas of the world. It permitted the clinical and anatomic separation of myocardial damage from vascular disease from that resulting from an inflammatory myocarditis. Up to this time myocarditis was the only recognized myocardial disease. The electrocardiogram soon became an important tool in establishing objective evidence of the acute infarction. Later it became valuable in the recognition of residuals of previous damage, of early ischemic myocardial changes before the acute infarction occurred, as well as in the identification of arrhythmias and conduction abnormalities common to coronary artery disease and other types of myocardial impairment.

The clinical application of the sphygmomanometer provided a tool for the recognition and evaluation of systemic arterial hypertension, and the roentgenogram aided in the recognition of cardiac hypertrophy, cardiac dilation, and pulmonary vascular congestion. These conditions develop in the course of secondary work hypertrophy and failure of hypertensive cardiovascular disease. In subsequent years, further development of radiographic methods aided in the diagnosis of congenital and acquired cardiovascular lesions, many of which led to myocardial hypertrophy and failure secondary to such cardiac abnormalities.

The relatively poor medical communications of this period (1900-1930) resulted in slow recognition and acceptance of these new concepts of myocardial disease and retarded use of new techniques in the diagnosis and evaluation of coronary and hypertensive cardiovascular diseases. Advances in clinical medicine were slow. The clinical features of these new cardiovascular diseases, with their secondary myocardial changes, were frequently misidentified by the physician and diagnosed clinically as "chronic myocarditis" or simply as nonvalvular heart disease. Chronic myocarditis or nonvalvular heart disease was the most common cause of death appearing on death certificates unsupported by autopsy study. Outstanding pathologists such as Clawson [12] and Warren [13] were frankly stating that they could not confirm such clinical diagnoses. It is difficult to believe that such a disparity could exist between the clinician and the pathologist, even in the same academic area. For example, in Minneapolis, Fahr [14], an outstanding clinician, published a paper entitled "Hypertension heart. The most common form of so-called chronic myocarditis." At the same time, Clawson published on the subject of myocarditis [12], stating that such clinical diagnosis could not be confirmed at autopsy. In Boston, where Cabot [15] pioneered in publishing on the subject of hypertensive heart disease, Christian [16], in 1933, published a paper entitled "Diagnosis of chronic nonvalvular heart disease (chronic myocarditis)" in which he was obviously discussing problems of unrecognized coronary and hypertensive heart disease. Warren [13], publishing in the same issue of a popular journal, again emphasized that there were no pathologic findings to support the clinical diagnosis of chronic myocarditis as made by Christian. The indiscriminate clinical diagnosis of chronic myocarditis gradually fell into disrepute following strong rebukes from such outstanding cardiologists of the time as Lewis [17] and White [18]. The following pertinent paragraph is quoted from a two-page discussion of the subject of myocarditis in the 1932 edition of White's popular text *Heart Disease* [18].

> "The clinical diagnosis of "myocarditis," so freely used in the past, has wrongly included many other conditions, in particular the frequent instances of hypertensive heart disease in which there is cardiac hypertrophy and enlargement but no inflammatory reaction in the muscle; the term "myocarditis" has also wrongly included frequent instances of coronary disease, in which degenerative changes, fibrosis and atrophy may occur without actual inflammatory process. In the attempt to diagnose heart disease more accurately, the term myocarditis is being wisely abandoned in large part; we must remember nevertheless that there does exist occasionally such a condition as myocarditis."

This advice contained in a textbook of cardiology, which was widely used throughout the world, was so effective that in the decade following this, a clinical diagnosis of acute myocarditis was made only in instances of diphtheria when it was an occasional clinical complication and in rheumatic fever when it occurred as part of a carditis. Chronic myocarditis soon disappeared from death certificates as a cause of death.

Splintering of Idiopathic Myocardial Disease into Multiple Entities

With better utilization of diagnostic tools and with increasing clinical knowledge of heart disease—especially hypertensive, coronary, chronic valvular, and congenital lesions—both clinical and autopsy diagnosis of heart disease became more accurate. However, both the clinician and the pathologist observed instances of myocardial disease which did not fall into these common anatomic and etiologic classifications. Many of these were neither inflammatory nor vascular, leading to the diagnosis of idiopathic myocardial disease. Occasionally, a new specific etiologic agent was identified. Historically, it becomes important to list some of the entities as they were a continuation of the idiopathic myocardial disease initially described by Krehl in 1891 [6]. Many of the entities described during this period continue to be included as types of idiopathic disease in current classifications of myocardial diseases.

MYOCARDOSIS

Riseman [19], in 1928, writing on the popular subject of "acute and chronic weakness of the myocardium," called attention to the large number of deaths of patients in whom a diagnosis of chronic myocarditis was made but in whom the study of the myocardium presented degenerative changes, but not the changes of cellular proliferation—the hallmark of myocarditis. Comparing the situation to that of the noninflammatory changes in the kidney, which Epstein had earlier called nephrosis, he coined the term "myocardosis" to explain what he considered nonvascular and noninflammatory lesions in the myocardium. In all probability such lesions were, in part, chronic myocardial changes of coronary and hypertensive disease, but some may have been idiopathic disease. This concept as well as the term have continued in medicine, being revived from time to time without ever receiving general acceptance.

Idiopathic Hypertrophy and Idiopathic Cardiomegaly

Howland [20], in 1919, reported on young children in whom idiopathic myocardial hypertrophy and failure were the only findings at autopsy. Earlier reports had considered myocardial hypertrophy in infants and children to be congenital [21]. Other reports of similar hypertrophy followed but there were, in addition, variations in the form of myocardial degeneration and myocardial and endomyocardial fibrosis. Many of these were labeled as "congenital hypertrophy." Various concepts of etiology and pathogenesis developed with new terms such as "myocardial fibroelastosis," "endocardial sclerosis," or "endomyocardial sclerosis," depending on the extent and location of the predominant pathology. Concepts of etiology included those of a fetal myocarditis [22], strictly hereditary disease [23], or biochemical defects [24], or dietary deficiency alone or in association with some infectious disease. Similar types of idiopathic hypertrophy were soon reported in adults [25]. In the latter part of this period, idiopathic endomyocardial disease was reported in various parts of the world, especially Africa [26, 27] where it was considered the most common type of heart disease with a strong suggestion of being a deficiency disease. By the 1950s large series of idiopathic myocardial disease were reported in young adults and occasionally in older age groups [28]. The outstanding clinical features were cardiac hypertrophy and eventual myocardial failure but some presented features of myocardial restriction without predominant hypertrophy. A common etiologic basis or concept of pathogenesis has not developed; however, myocardial disease in the postpartal state and in alcoholism has received special attention.

Idiopathic Myocardial Disease of Pregnancy and the Puerperium (Postpartal Heart Disease)

History is somewhat vague as to the first observations of idiopathic myocardial disease associated with the postpartal state. Current writers [29] on the subject have credited Virchow as describing such disease, but the first reports with a specific concept of a postpartal disease were made in

1937 [30] and 1938 [31]. These early observers noted certain similarities to beriberi disease reported a few years earlier and, as is true today, considered nutritional deficiency as a possible factor. Musser and Soderman [32] were of the opinion that an endocrine disturbance related to pregnancy might be involved in the pathogenesis. Several reports were made under the title of "postpartal myocardosis," again emphasizing the noninflammatory character of the myocardial lesions [33]. Today, many classifications of idiopathic myocardial disease include postpartal disease related to pregnancy and puerperium.

Beriberi Heart Disease and Alcoholic Cardiomyopathy (Nutritional, Metabolic, or Toxic Myocardial Disease)

Historically, the concepts of these varieties of myocardial disease developed at two different periods, the latter after 1950, but they will be discussed together even though they may not have any relationship. Both varieties of myocardial disease were related to a large alcoholic intake and disturbances in nutritional and metabolic states. Beriberi heart disease was initially described in 1929 [34] and 1930 [35] and was considered the result of a combination of the effects of alcohol and the poor dietary intake in the alcoholic. The specific deficiency was later identified as thiamine deficiency and reversal of the myocardial dysfunction and circulatory disorders occurred with the administration of thiamine. Such observations revived interest in the earlier reports of deleterious effects of alcohol observed by Bollinger [36] in beer drinkers as early as 1884. Although the metabolic effects of acute thiamine deficiency are well accepted today, the possibilities of chronic myocardial disease as a result of this type of dietary deficiency has not gained general acceptance.

The subsequent designation of a form of chronic idiopathic myocardial disease as "alcoholic heart disease" [37] or "alcoholic cardiomyopathy" [38] simply because there were large numbers of alcoholics among those with idiopathic myocardial disease continues to leave many vital questions of specific etiology and pathogenesis unanswered. In spite of this questionable relationship, many of those currently reporting cardiomyopathies and primary myocardial disease include this category of idiopathic disease as an important component. An acceptable relationship has not been developed except in the isolated instances of the Quebec beer-drinkers' cardiomyopathy [39, 40] in which there is excellent circumstantial and laboratory evidence to incriminate the toxic effect of an additive, cobalt, either alone or in synergistic action with a direct effect of alcohol on the myocardium. Alcohol has been incriminated in the production of liver disease with or without cirrhosis but with dysproteinemia. A related alcoholic myocardosis of hepatogenous origin, postulated by Wuhrmann [41], remains debatable, especially so since most patients with so-called alcoholic cardiomyopathy do not have associated liver disease or dysproteinemia.

Fibroplastic Myocarditis

In 1936, Loeffler [42] introduced the entity of fibroplastic myocarditis and endomyocarditis with the concept that it represented an altered or hyperergic reaction to injury. This was the first concept of a hypersensitivity reaction of the myocardium. Earlier, Aschoff [10] had shown that myocardial reaction in rheumatic fever could be recognized by a specific type of cellular change. Application of these concepts resulted in the gradual recognition of patterns of vascular and myocardial changes in a variety of diseases, especially those classified as collagen or connective tissue diseases and granulomatous diseases. Recognition of myocardial changes in these diseases at autopsy, and the subsequent recognition of correlative clinical features of myocardial dysfunction, began in this period and continued after 1950. Their initial recognition in sarcoidosis and systemic sclerosis was followed by similar reports in systemic lupus erythematosus, polyarteritis nodosa, dermatomyositis, rheumatoid arthritis, and hypersensitivity and granulomatous myocarditis, especially that from sensitivity to drugs. Since the etiology of these diseases is unknown, there has been no uniform classification of the myocardial disease associated with them. Some have simply classified them as nonspecific myocarditis and thus a form of primary myocardial disease; others have classified them as secondary myocardial disease or a secondary form of cardiomyopathy.

Myocardial Disease and Failure Associated with Diseases of Other Systems

As pathologists began to report chronic myocardial changes accompanying diseases of systems other than the cardiovascular system, clinicians found clinical manifestations of myocardial dysfunction in many noncardiac diseases. These manifestations included electrocardiographic abnormalities, arrhythmias, and cardiac enlargement. Cabot's [43] description of cardiac and myocardial hypertrophy in pernicious anemia, in 1919, was one of the earlier reports; later myocardial dysfunction, including fatal heart failure, was documented in thyroid diseases. These reports were followed by similar descriptions of myocardial dysfunction and pathologic changes in a variety of endocrine and metabolic diseases. Pulmonary hypertensive cardiovascular disease, usually related to chronic lung disease, was firmly established as a serious form of heart disease even though it was masked under the syndrome of "cor pulmonale." Although varying degrees of myocardial involvement occur with many noncardiac diseases, the historical development of such relationships cannot be given in this brief chapter. A few are mentioned because of their importance in the differential diagnosis of cardiomyopathies. That certain diseases might produce infiltrating lesions in the myocardium with disturbance of function was recognized during this period, some years after the basic disease entities were recognized. Important in this group are amyloidosis, both primary and secondary types, hemochromatosis, and primary and metastatic neoplasms. The unexpected myocardial involvement in neuromuscular and neurologic diseases was either recognized in the early clinical and pathological observations or, as in the case of Friedreich's ataxia, were so well documented that retrospective review of the earliest case reports clearly indicated myocardial involvement [44]. The demonstration, in recent years, that certain viruses are both neurotrophic and cardiotrophic supports possible pathogenesis of combined organ involvement in the initial stages of a disease.

Revival of Interest in, and the Development of, Additional Knowledge About Specific Types of Acute and Chronic Myocarditis

The earlier loss of interest in the clinical diagnosis of acute and chronic myocarditis in this period did not prevent the bacteriologist and the virologist from establishing that specific etiologic agents might produce myocarditis. Although both pathologists and clinicians reported sporadic cases or series of cases of myocarditis under such titles as Fiedler's myocarditis, isolated myocarditis, or interstitial myocarditis, the establishment of syphilis and tuberculosis of the myocardium were recognized as specific types. Cardiac involvement was described in the early pathology of Chagas' disease, and after a long period of clinical observation and experimental animal studies, the clinical and pathologic features of chronic Chagasic myocarditis or cardiomyopathy were finally established around 1950 [45]. Today, it is recognized as the most important type of myocardial disease in certain areas of South America.

Since this period includes World War II, interest revived in myocardial involvement accompanying both common and exotic infectious diseases. Previously, opportunities and facilities had not existed to study such diseases. Electrocardiography, chest radiography, and facilities for bacteriologic, serologic, and postmortem studies followed troops into many areas where these diseases were endemic. The result was identification of myocarditis in a great variety of diseases and the etiologic spectrum of myocarditis was greatly extended. Most fatal cases were subjected to postmortem study with multiple sections of the myocardium, thus permitting the recognition of localized as well as diffuse myocarditis. Gore and Saphir [46, 47] and later Manion [48], pathologists in the Armed Forces Institute of Pathology where much of this material was assessed for careful study, attested to the frequency of myocardial disease as well as the diversity of etiological agents. A broader view of the etiology and pathogenesis of myocarditis developed. The concept was extended to include many bacterial, mycotic, protozoal, and rickettsial infectious diseases and parasitic infestations. In addition, toxins produced by these organisms, toxic chemicals administered in the therapy of these infections, and various forms of physical injury were involved in the etiology of myocarditis. The virus of poliomyelitis was suspected of producing myocarditis long before proof was established. Myocarditis was suspected of accompanying influenza in the pandemic of World War I, but it was not until 1945 that Finland et al. [49] successfully isolated influenza virus A from fatal cases of myocarditis. This achievement was followed by reports by other investigators of successful recoveries of other viruses in myocarditis. Coxsackie viral myocarditis became established as the most common variety of fatal myocarditis of the newborn but remains an uncommon cause of acute severe myocarditis in the adult. Whether or not antecedent Coxsackie virus infection is responsible for chronic idiopathic myocardial disease is uncertain.*

This renewed interest in specific etiologic types of myocarditis also revived interest in the clinical diagnosis of myocarditis. Several reports [50, 51] in the early 1950s constitute the first renewed attempts to make a diagnosis of myocarditis during life since the clinical diagnosis of myocarditis fell into disrepute following the admonitions of White [18] in the late 1930s.

DEVELOPMENTS RELATED TO INTRODUCTION AND UTILIZATION OF MODERN TOOLS AND METHODS IN DIAGNOSIS AND RESEARCH. (1950-1972)

This period has seen great progress in the development of techniques for the study of myocardial function in health and disease. As a result, there has been great progress in clinical recognition and in the hemo-

* *Editorial Note:* In occasional instances, chronic myocardial disease has been observed to follow Coxsackie B viral myocarditis. Sainini, G. L. et al., Medicine 47:133, 1968.

dynamic, biochemical, histochemical, and immunologic evaluation of many diseases previously identified by postmortem study. This progress has been made by contributions from many investigators and clinicians, often working as teams. Perhaps future historians will identify the great contributors; it is unwise to do so at the present. However, a few will be mentioned who provided new concepts or contributed to the development of old ones.

Although the techniques of cardiac catheterization and angiocardiography were introduced at an earlier period, they were not developed as practical diagnostic and research tools until the late 1940s. When funds became available to provide equipment, to train personnel, and to provide laboratory space, such basic tools were developed rapidly, and other techniques were designed to study myocardial function in health as well as in many disease states.

Recognition of Clinical and Hemodynamic Types of Myocardial Disease

Cardiac catheterization and ancillary techniques were first used by accident in the diagnostic investigation of myocardial disease since, in error, the patients were thought to have valvular disease. Later, by design, the hemodynamic features of myocardial diseases were studied by these methods. Cardiac catheterization and angiocardiography served to identify congestive, restrictive, and obstructive types of myocardial disease and permitted the distinction of myocardial disease and acquired valvular disease, congenital lesions, pericardial disease, and myocardial disease secondary to coronary artery disease.

The recognition of the hemodynamic and pharmacodynamic features of idiopatic hypertrophic muscular cardiopathy is of historical interest because information was obtained about this form of myocardial disease in a very short period by individuals and groups working in many areas of the world. A short chronological history of the observations and development of concepts is given along with historical documentation that this is an old disease which only recently attracted attention. In 1957, Sir Russell Brock [52] made his initial publication on an acquired form of aortic subvalvular stenosis which he considered to result from a functional obstruction of the outflow tract of the left ventricle by hypertrophy of the myocardium. One year later, Teare [53] described a peculiar type of myocardial hypertrophy in young adults who died with a clinical diagnosis of idiopathic hypertrophy. A bulging mass of hypertrophic myocardial tissue simulating a myocardial tumor mass was found in the outflow tracts of the ventricles. He called the unusual type of cardiac hypertrophy "asymmetrical hypertrophy." In the same year and later in 1959, several additional important observations were made by clinical and hemodynamic studies of individuals with clinical findings suggestive of aortic stenosis: Bercu et al. [54] and Morrow and Braunwald [55] both demonstrated physiologic obstruction or resistance to left ventricular outflow but no anatomical obstruction. Bercu et al. [54] described the finding as pseudoaortic stenosis, produced by hypertrophy of the ventricular myocardium; Morrow and Braunwald [55] simply called it "functional aortic stenosis." In 1960, Goodwin et al. [56] studied patients with idiopathic asymmetrical hypertrophy like that previously reported by Teare and observed similar hemodynamic findings. He concluded that ventricular septal hypertrophy produced a functional obstruction to the outflow of one or both ventricles. They called the condition one of "obstructive cardiomyopathy" to differentiate it from congestive and constrictive forms of cardiomyopathy. Brachfeld and Gorlin [57] likewise noted similar obstructive features but added an additional observation that there was no obstruction to flow early in systole, suggesting that the obstruction developed as the muscle mass contracted later in systole. They used the term "functional subaortic stenosis." Brent et al. [58] in reporting their findings in a group of patients with marked familial characteristics, introduced the term "familial muscular subaortic stenosis." Wigle et al. [59] reported such cases chiefly as "muscular subaortic stenosis." In 1960, Braunwald et al. [60] presented the clinical, hemodynamic, and angiographic manifestations in a sizeable group of patients; and in 1962 broadened their concept of the disease [61] and suggested the term "idiopathic hypertrophic subaortic stenosis." This term and Wigle's "muscular subaortic stenosis" remain the most frequently used terms in the USA today, whereas Goodwin's term of "obstructive cardiomyopathy" or "hypertrophic obstructive cardiomyopathy" is more generally used throughout the rest of the world. In a very short time it was realized that this disease presented, in its fully developed state, distinctive features that were readily identified clinically and easily confirmed by hemodynamic, angiographic, and pharmacodynamic studies. These findings resulted in the application of specific surgical and pharmacologic therapies which are still under evaluation. In 1964 [62], a monograph was prepared on the basis of a 7-year experience with this entity at the National Heart Institute, Bethesda. Later that year a symposium on cardiomyopathies (Ciba Foundation, London, 1964) [63] devoted most of its time to this type of cardiomyopathy. A similar symposium in London in 1971 [64] was devoted entirely to this subject. It was learned that there is a group with a familial history and a group without such history. Although this worldwide interest and effort accumulated much information during the past 14 years, neither the etiology nor the pathogenesis of the myocardial derangement have been clarified completely.

In review, it appears probable that this type of myocardial disease has been observed in the past and that some of its features, including the functional nature of the muscular obstruction, were recognized earlier. In describing idiopathic cardiac hypertrophy in 1891, Krehl [6] indicated that heart failure in these patients was due to "anatomical disease of the tissue." In 1907, Schmincke [65] reported on adults with diffuse hyperplasia of the left ventricular outflow tract which he considered to be of congenital origin. He hypothesized that this large muscle mass obstructed the outflow tract. In 1910, Bernheim [66] described obstruction of the outflow tract of the right side of the heart caused by idiopathic hypertrophy of the left ventricle. Later, there were reports of so-called Bernheim's syndrome which included instances of severe left ventricular hypertrophy in patients with hypertensive cardiovascular disease and right-sided failure. Right-sided heart failure was considered to be produced by the hypertrophied interventricular septum. It is of interest that one of the two subjects of Brock's original observation of functional ventricular outflow-tract obstruction was described to have severe arterial hypertension. Glycogen-storage disease of the heart with outflow tract obstruction was reported by Ehlers et al. [67], in 1962. Although the earlier cases of Garrett et al. [68] in 1959 and Davies [69] in 1952 of familial cardiomyopathy were not studied hemodynamically, there were clinical features that suggested the possibility of obstructive cardiomyopathy. The familial features of cases with well-substantiated ventricular outflow tract obstruction have been well documented in recent reports as well as in those studied at NIH [62].

Advances in Knowledge of Myocardial Function in Health and Disease

During this period (1950-1972), further developments in the study of the physiology of the myocardium have provided much additional information about myocardial function, the phenomena of myocardial contraction, functions of specialized conduction tissues within the myocardium, and of specialized muscle such as the papillary muscles. The demonstration of papillary muscle dysfunction as a complication of myocardial infarction or endomyocardial disease provides additional understanding of the myocardial failure in these lesions. Invasive and noninvasive studies of myocardial function have greatly aided in the diagnosis of diffuse aneurysm formation as well as in regional asynergy in myocardial disease of both coronary and noncoronary origin.

The symptom complex of angina pectoris no longer remains the sole evidence of myocardial ischemia. Recognition of reliable auscultatory and palpatory signs of myocardial dysfunction on clinical examination, specific changes in the resting and exercise electrocardiogram and techniques of selective angiographic examination of the coronary arteries have provided both early and accurate diagnosis of ischemic myocardial disease. Development of techniques of His bundle electrocardiography and continuous electrocardiographic monitoring have aided in the recognition and management of arrhythmias and conduction abnormalities, common manifestations of both coronary and noncoronary myocardial disease. Paradoxically, angiographic techniques have demonstrated that occlusive coronary artery disease may produce a clinical cardiomyopathy indistinguishable from noncoronary cardiomyopathy. Gross myocardial necrosis (infarction), clinically indistinguishable from that commonly seen in atherosclerotic occlusive coronary disease, may occur despite a normal arterial system on angiographic study. Thus, the coronary and noncoronary myocardial diseases are brought closer together and the difficulties in clinical recognition are emphasized.

The application of information derived from hemodynamic studies and of the knowledge of the laws of physics in evaluating the dilated failing heart of myocardial disease have provided a better concept and understanding of the pathologic physiology of cardiac dilation. Burch and Walsh [70] developed the therapeutic concept of prolonged bedrest in the effort to overcome the mechanical disadvantages of the dilated heart of myocardial disease in failure.

Advancements in general scientific knowledge during this latter period, especially those in general chemistry, both biochemical and immunochemistry, in immunology, and genetic and molecular biology have greatly influenced the history of myocardial diseases. The introduction of galvanometric and, later, spectrophotometric methods into general chemistry and medicine confirmed earlier concepts that certain electrolytes, especially sodium, potassium, calcium, and magnesium had an important role in normal myocardial function. It was shown that quantitative alterations in intracellular and extracellular content of these electrolytes resulted in disorders of myocardial function and, if severe, caused irreparable damage or dysfunction. Various concepts of pathogenesis of myocardial dysfunction and disease have developed from these observations such as current concepts of arrhythmias and conduction disorders which may be produced by hypokalemia and hyperkalemia. Therapeutic applications in the management of cardiac arrest and ventricular fibrillation have resulted, and this information has enabled the production of transient chemical myocardial paralysis during open heart surgery.

In his concept of multiple etiologies of the cardiomyopathies, Selye [71] visualized many structurally distinct myocardial lesions as being produced or prevented by varying combinations of electrolytes, steroids, hormones, and stress. His concept provided a basis for understanding the physiologic and pathologic changes in the myocardium related to normal and abnormal functional states of the endocrine system. If the abnormal function is prolonged, metabolic cardiomyopathies develop eventually. Investigative studies of the effects of catecholamines on myocardial function have permitted more intelligent use of these substances as therapeutic agents. Other drugs which enhance, block, or deplete catecholamine myocardial activity can also be used more effectively. Diagnostic angiographic studies during life have failed to show occlusive coronary disease in some instances of overt myocardial necrosis and infarction, especially in young females [72]. This demonstration has suggested the possible importance of exogenous hormonal products administered in birth control in producing myocardial necrosis.

Advances in histochemistry, enzyme chemistry, isotope labeling, and electron microscopy have been applied to the study of the structure and function of the myocardium in health and disease. Electron microscopy in myocardial disease will be discussed in another chapter. It is hoped that these new techniques will provide more knowledge about idiopathic diseases of the myocardium. An example of the application of these techniques was the rapidity with which a solution was found to the cause of the Quebec beer-drinkers' cardiomyopathy [40].

Molecular biology has developed in this period so that it is now regarded as a distinct discipline. Myocardial disease may now be considered a molecular disease, that is, a disease in which important cellular proteins or other basic substances are lacking altogether, or impaired, or lost by acquired disease. This concept has increased our knowledge of glycogen-storage disease and may eventually provide better understanding of idiopathic myocardial disease such as the postpartal and alcoholic cardiomyopathies. Knowledge obtained from detailed study of the chemistry and physiology of muscle function is bringing investigators nearer to an understanding of defects in energy production, contractility, impulse formation, and conduction which are key functional defects in myocardial disease.

Developments in the field of immunology and immunochemistry have provided additional methods for the recognition of potential etiologic agents such as the viruses; likewise, new concepts tend to incriminate viral infections and subsequent immunologic responses in the myocardium as a mechanism for the pathogenesis of idiopathic cardiomyopathies. A subsequent chapter is devoted to these immunologic studies which are distinctly a part of this period.

Advances in Clinical Recognition and Classification of Myocardial Diseases

The clinical and hemodynamic features of the various noncoronary and nonvalvular myocardial diseases became better understood during the mid-1950s. It was apparent that the myocardial diseases have certain features which should enable the clinician to identify them as a form of heart disease distinct from valvular disease, pericardial disease, congenital, coronary, and hypertensive heart disease. Cardiomegaly and myocardial failure are features common to each group. In 1950, Christian [73] polarized thinking in this respect when he published his paper entitled, "Clinically the myocardium." He called attention to the important functions of the myocardium and enumerated the clinical features one should expect when faults in these normal functions occur as the result of disease. Burchell [74, 75] emphasized the possibilities of identification and separation when he listed many of the splintered diseases in his publications "Unusual forms of heart disease" and "Unusual causes of heart failure." Pathologists had repeatedly prodded clinicians over the years to make appropriate clinical antemortem diagnoses of myocardial disease. It was prodding from Manion that caused the author [9] to develop the concept of "primary myocardial disease" in 1957, not as a pathological nor etiological term but as a clinical concept and communication tool to aid in the clinical recognition of these splintered diseases. Myocardial dysfunction and failure developing in other common and easily recognized cardiovascular diseases, such as valvular, pericardial, congenital, coronary, and hypertensive diseases, were considered secondary types of myocardial diseases. Primary myocardial diseases were defined as those diseases involving primarily the heart muscle and either spared or only minimally involved other structures of the heart and cardiovascular system. These primary myocardial diseases, by the above definition, include specific and nonspecific types of acute and chronic myocarditis, myocardial dysfunction associated with diseases of systems other than the cardiovascular system itself, and myocardial disease of unknown etiology (idiopathic). The clinical and hemodynamic features of these primary diseases often permit a positive bedside diagnosis. These features were given in the initial publication [9] and subsequent publications by the author [76, 77]. Many subsequent contributors [78, 79, 80] have written about this subject; some have modified the initial definition of primary myocardial disease or have presented new terms and classifications. Others developed independent concepts as well as terminology and classifications for lumping together these splintered diseases. Notably, Brigden [81] described essentially the same clinical grouping and features under the label of *noncoronary cardiomyopathies*. Burch and

De Pasquale [82] preferred a general classification of *heart muscle disease* which they divided into primary and secondary types with the idiopathic types under primary and all others under secondary. Goodwin et al. [83] followed Brigden's terminology with the simple term of *cardiomyopathies* and added a very useful clinical division into congestive, constrictive, and obstructive types, based on the mechanism for the type of myocardial dysfunction and failure. Burch and De Pasquale [82] added a fourth clinical type of ischemic cardiomyopathy which would complete an ideal clinical or mechanistic classification. A current classification and discussion will be presented in another chapter of this book, but these historical notes may enlighten those who are constantly confused by terminology and classifications that may hinder as well as improve communication. Most of the confusion lies in the use of the terms primary, secondary, and idiopathic. To some, idiopathic has meant primary and all other myocardial disease is called secondary myocardial disease. There are other variations. The general terms primary myocardial disease, cardiomyopathy and heart muscle disease are used rather interchangeably in medicine today, even though they have different degrees of inclusiveness. Classifications developed under these headings have much the same entities, arranged according to the particular author's experience and concepts; consequently, communication is not greatly disturbed. Fowler [84] in a recent publication recommends for purposes of clarity that the term "primary myocardial disease," which he had also used earlier, be dropped. The term cardiomyopathy has currently developed worldwide usage and the term primary myocardial disease, having served its purpose of encouraging better clinical recognition, will perhaps become a little historical note as it did when first used by Josserand and Gallavardin in 1901 [8]. Future historians may describe an overdiagnosis of cardiomyopathy in the last decades of this century; chronic myocarditis was overdiagnosed by clinicians in the first decades of this century. Furthermore, they may record that cardiomyopathy is essentially chronic myocarditis if one defines myocarditis as a residual of previous reaction of the myocardium to some form of injury.

The pathologists have adopted the clinical terminology but with subclassifications of their own which are encyclopedic in scope, especially those provided by Manion [85] and by Hudson [86]. A clinician's viewpoint of Hudson's classification has been given [87]. It is hoped that future historians may record that all myocardial disease has been identified by etiology and those not prevented are easily recognized, clinically. The pathologist will be left with an empty court of last judgment on the mistakes of clinicians and no new entities to classify. Until that perfection is reached, there will always be healthy differences of opinion between splinterers and lumpers and between clinicians and pathologists. These differences will produce a provocative and stimulating atmosphere in which progress will continue.

REFERENCES

1. Harvey, W.P. and Perloff, J.K.: The auscultatory findings in primary myocardial disease. Amer Heart J 61:199, 1961.
2. Mattingly, T.W.: Auscultatory findings in primary myocardial diseases (myocardiopathies). In, The theory and practice of auscultation (Segal, B.L., Ed.). Philadelphia, Davis, 1964, p. 318.
3. Johnson, J. A.: A Treatise on Derangement of The Liver, Internal Organs, and Nervous System. Pathological and Therapeutical, 2nd ed., Philadelphia, L.B. Clark, 1826, p. 132 (revised and improved from 3rd London ed.).
4. Sobernheim, J.F.: Praktische diagnostik der inneren krankheiten mit vorzueglischer ruecksicht auf pathologische anatomie. Berlin: Hirschwald, 1837, p. 117.
5. Ruhle, H.: Zur diagnose der myokarditis. Dtsch Arch Klin Med 22:82, 1878.
6. Krehl, L.: Idiopathic diseases of the heart muscle. Dtsch Arch Klin Med 48:414, 1891.
7. Fiedler, A.: Ueber akute interstielle myokarditis. Zentralbl Inn Med 21: 212, 1900 (abst., W. Baensch).
8. Josserand, E. and Gallavardin, L.: De l'asystolie progressive des jeunes subjets par myocardite subaique primitive. Arch Gen Med 6:513, 1901.
9. Mattingly, T. W.: The clinical and hemodynamic features of primary myocardial disease. Trans Am Clin Climatol A. 70:132, 1958.
10. Aschoff, L.: Zur myokarditisfrage verh. Dtsch Ges Pathol 8:46, 1905.
11. Herrick, J.B.: Clinical features of sudden obstruction of the coronary arteries. JAMA 59: 2015, 1912.
12. Clawson, B.J.: Myocarditis. Am Heart J 4:1, 1928.
13. Warren, S.: The pathology of chronic myocarditis. New Engl J Med 208:573, 1933.
14. Fahr, G.E.: Hypertension heart. The most common form of so-called chronic myocarditis. JAMA 80:981, 1923.
15. Cabot, R.C.: Hypertensive heart disease. Case Records of the Massachusetts General Hospital. Boston Med Surg J 192:312, 1925.
16. Christian, H. A.: Diagnosis of chronic non-valvular cardiac diseases (Chronic Myocarditis). New Eng J Med 208:574, 1933.
17. Lewis T.: Disease of the Heart. Macmillan, London, 1933. Vol. 2, p. 254.
18. White, P.D.: Heart Disease. Macmillan, New York, 1932, p. 471.
19. Riesman, D.: Diagnosis and treatment of acute and chronic myocardial weakness. Med Clin. North Am 10:261, 1926.
20. Howland, J.: Idiopathic hypertrophy of the heart in young children. Contrib Med Biol Res. New York, Sir W. Osler, 1919, Vol. I, pp. 584-599.
21. Sinmonds: So-called primary congenital hypertrophy. Muench Med Wochschr 46:108, 1899. Quoted by Abbot, M.E.: Atlas of congenital heart disease. New York, American Heart Assn, 1936, p. 26.

22. Farber, S. and Hubbard, J.: Fetal endomyocarditis: Intrauterine infection as the cause of congenital cardiac anomalies. Am J Med Sc. 186:705, 1933.
23. Evans, W.: Familial cardiomegaly. Br. Heart J 11:68, 1949.
24. Putschar, W.: Ueber angeborene glykogenspeicherkaukhert des herzens thesauresmosis glycogenica (von Gierke) Beitr Pathol An 90:222, 1932.
25. Levy, R.L. and Rousellot, L.M.: Cardiac hypertrophy of unknown etiology in young adults: A clinical and pathological study of three cases. Am. Heart J 9:178, 1933.
26. Bedford, D.E., and Kostam, G.L.S.: Heart failure of unknown aetiology in Africans. Br Heart J 8:236, 1946.
27. Davies, J.N.P.: Endocardial fibrosis in Uganda. E African Med J 25:10, 1948.
28. Elster, K.S., Tuckmann, L.R., and Horn, H.: Cardiac hypertrophy and insufficiency of unknown origin. Am J Med 18:900, 1955.
29. Meadows, W.R.: Postpartum heart disease. Am J Cardiol 6:788, 1960.
30. Gouley, B.A., McMillan, T.M., and Bellet, S.: Idiopathic myocardial degeneration associated with pregnancy and especially the puerperium. Am J Med Sci 194:185, 1937.
31. Hull, E. and Hafkesbring, E.: "Toxic" postpartal heart disease. New Orleans Med Surg J, 89:550, 1937.
32. Musser, J.H. and Soderman, W.A.: Heart changes of unusual etiology in pregnancy. Trans Assoc Am Physicians 54:181, 1939.
33. Vilter, R.W. and McKee, E.E. Postpartum myocardosis. Ohio Med J 39:142, 1943.
34. Aalsmeer, W.C. and Wenckenbach, K.F.: Herz und kreislauf bei den beri-beri krancheit. Wein Arch Intern Med 16:193, 1929.
35. Keifer, C.S.: The beriberi heart. Arch Intern Med 45:1, 1930.
36. Bollinger, O. Von: Ueber die Haugfigkeit und Ursachen der idiopathischen Herzhypertrophie in Munchen. Dtsch Med Wochschr 10:180, 1884.
37. Brigden, W. and Robinson, J., Alcoholic heart disease. Br Med J 2:128, 1954.
38. Evans, W.: Alcoholic cardiomyopathy. Am Heart J 61:556, 1961.
39. Morin, Y. and Daniel, P.: "Quebec beer-drinkers" cardiomyopathy. Etiological considerations. Can Med Assoc J 97:926, 1967.
40. Mohiuddin, S.M., Taskar, P.K., Rheault, M., Paul, E.R., Chenard, J., and Morin Y.: Experimental cobalt cardiomyopathy. Am Heart J 80:532, 1970.
41. Wuhrmann, F.: Hepatogenic myocardosis. Scand J. Gastroenterol Suppl 7:97, 1970.
42. Loeffler, W.: Endocarditis parietalis mit blutoeosinophile schweiz. Med Wochschr 66:817, 1936.
43. Cabot, R.C. and Richardson, O.: Cardiac hypertrophy in pernicious anemia. JAMA 72:991, 1919.
44. Nadas, A.S., Alimuring, M.M., and Sieracki, L.A.: Cardiac manifestations of Friedreick's ataxia. New Engl J Med 244: 239, 1951.
45. Laranja, F.S., Dias, E., Norbega, G., and Miranda, A.: Chagas disease. A clinical epidemologic and pathologic study. Circulation 14:1035, 1956.
46. Gore, I. and Saphir, O.: Myocarditis, a classification of 1402 cases. Am Heart J 34:827, 1947.
47. Saphir, O.: Myocarditis: A general review with an analysis of 240 cases. Arch Pathol 32:1000, 1951.
48. Manion, W.C.: Myocarditis—A frequent complication of systemic disease. Am J Pathol 61:329, 1956.

49. Finland, M., Parker, F., Barnes, M.W., and Joliffe, L.S.: Acute myocarditis in influenza A infections. Am J Med Sci 209:455, 1945.
50. Fine, I., Brainerd, H., and Sokolow, M.: Myocarditis in acute infectious diseases: Clinical and electrocardiographic study. Circulation 2:859, 1950.
51. de la Chapelle, C.E. and Kossmann, C.E.: Myocarditis. Circulation 10:747, 1954.
52. Brock, R.: Functional obstruction of the left ventricle. Guys Hosp Rep 106:221, 1957. Ibid 108:126, 1959.
53. Teare, D.: Asymmetrical hypertrophy of the heart in young adults. Br Heart J 20:1, 1958.
54. Bercu, B.A., Diettert, G.A., Danforth, W.H., Pund, E.E., Ahlvin, R.C., and Belliveau, R.R.: Pseudoaortic stenosis produced by ventricular hypertrophy. Am J Med 25:814, 1958.
55. Morrow, A.G. and Braunwald, E.: Functional aortic stenosis: A malformation characterized by resistance to left ventricular outflow without anatomic obstruction. Circulation 20:181, 1959.
56. Goodwin, J.F., Hollman A., Cleland, W.P., and Teare, D.: Obstructive cardiomyopathy simulating aortic stenosis. Br Heart J 22:403, 1960.
57. Brachfeld N. and Gorlin, R.: Subaortic stenosis: A revised concept of the disease. Medicine 38:415, 1959.
58. Brent, L.B., Aburano, A., Fisher, D.L., Moran, T.J., Myers, J.D., and Taylor, W.J.: Familial muscular subaortic stenosis: An unrecognized form of "idiopathic heart disease" with clinical and autopsy observations. Circulation 21:167, 1960.
59. Wigle, E.D., Heimbecker, R.O., and Gunton, R.W.: Muscular subaortic stenosis. Circulation 26:325, 1962.
60. Braunwald, E., Morrow, A.G., Cornell, W.P., Aygen, M.M., and Hilbish, T.F.: Idiopathic hypertrophic subaortic stenosis: Clinical, hemodynamic, and angiographic manifestations. Am J Med 29:924, 1960.
61. Braunwald, E., Brockenbrough, E.D., and Morrow, A.G.: Hypertrophic subaortic stenosis: A broadened concept. Circulation 26:161, 1962.
62. Braunwald, D., Lambrew, C.T., Rockoff, S.D., Ross, J., Jr., and Morrow, G.M.: Idiopathic hypertrophic subaortic stenosis: 1. Description of the disease based upon an analysis of 64 patients. In, American Heart Association, Monograph No. 10. New York, American Heart Assn., 1964.
63. In, Wolstenholme, G.E.W. (Ed.): Ciba Foundation Symposium Cardiomyopathies. Boston, Little, Brown, 1964.
64. Hypertrophic obstructive cardiomyopathy. In, (Wolstenholme G.E.W. and O'Conner, M. Eds.): Ciba Foundation Study Group No. 37 London, Churchill, 1971.
65. Schmincke, A.: Ueber linkseitige muskulose conusstenosen. Dtsch Med Schnschr. 33:2082, 1907.
66. Bernheim, P.I.: De L'asystole veineuse dans l'hypertrophe du coeur gauche par stenose concomitante du ventricle droit. Rev Med 30:785, 1910.
67. Ehlers, K.H., Redo, S.F., and Engle, M.A.: Glycogen-storage disease of the myocardium with obstruction to left ventricular outflow. Circulation 25:96, 1962.
68. Garrett, G., Hay, W.J. and Richards, A.G.: Familial cardiomegaly. J Clin Pathol 12:355, 1959.
69. Davies, L.G.: A familial heart disease. Br Heart J 14:206, 1952.
70. Burch, G.E. and Walsh, J.J.: Cardiac enlargement due to myocardial degener-

ation of unknown cause: Preliminary report on effect of prolonged bed rest. JAMA 172:207, 1960.
71. Selye, H.: The pluricausal cardiopathies. Springfield, Charles C Thomas, 1961, p. 315.
72. Glancy, D.L., Marcus, M.L., and Epstein, S.E.: Myocardial infarction in young women with normal coronary arteriograms. Circulation 44:495, 1971.
73. Christian, H.A.: Clinically the myocardium. Arch Intern Med 86:491, 1950.
74. Burchell, H.B.: Unusual forms of heart disease. Circulation 10:574, 1954.
75. Burchell, M.B.: Unusual causes of heart failure. Circulation 21:436, 1960.
76. Mattingly, T.W.: Clinical features and diagnosis of primary myocardial disease. Mod Conc Cardiovasc Dis 30:677, 1961.
77. Mattingly, T.W.: Primary myocardial disease. In, Encyclopedia of Medicine, Vol. 3. Philadelphia, Davis, 1964, p 1073.
78. Fowler, N.O., Gueron M., and Rowlands, D.T., Jr.: Primary myocardial disease. Circulation 23:498, 1961.
79. Harvey, W.P., Segal, J.P., and Gurel, T.: The clinical spectrum of primary myocardial disease. Prog Cardiovasc Dis 7:1, 1964.
80. Theodori, M.I.: On so-called primary diseases of the myocardium—idiopathic myocarditis and idiopathic hypertrophy of the myocardium: Problems in clinical manifestations, diagnosis and therapy. Kardiologia 2:3, 1962.
81. Brigden, W.: Uncommon myocardial diseases: Noncoronary cardiomyopathies. Lancet 273:1179, 1243, 1957.
82. Burch, G.E. and De Pasquale, N.P.: Recognition and prevention of cardiomyopathy. Circulation 42:A47, 1970.
83. Goodwin, J.F., Gordon, H., Hollman, A., and Bishop, M.B.: Clinical aspects of cardiomyopathy. Br Med J 1:69, 1961.
84. Fowler, N.O.: Differential diagnosis of cardiomyopathies. Progr Cardiovasc Dis 14:113, 1971.
85. Manion, W.C.: Conferencia las cardiomiopatias, in memorias XXV anniversario Instituto de Cardiologia Mexico, 1944-69. Mexico City, Mundez-Oteo, 1970, p. 637.
86. Hudson, R.E.B.: The cardiomyopathies: Order from chaos. Am J Cardiol 25:70, 1970.
87. Mattingly, T.W.: Diseases of the myocardium (cardiomyopathies): The viewpoint of a clinical cardiologist. Am J Cardiol 25: 79, 1970.

NOBLE O. FOWLER, M.D.

Classification and Diagnosis of Myocardial Diseases

General clinical recognition of the importance and prevalence of myocardial diseases has taken place almost entirely within the last 10 to 15 years. However, medical knowledge of myocardial disease is much older than this statement might suggest. Beer-drinkers' myocardosis [1] was recognized in Germany in the 1880s and Saphir [2] wrote of myocarditis in the 1940s. In 1950, Henry Christian [3] discussed the clinical importance of myocardial dysfunction. In Cincinnati in 1956, Blankenhorn and Gall [4] wrote of the anatomic changes found at postmortem examination of patients with several varieties of myocardial disease. Despite these important publications, there was little correlation between the anatomic features of the myocardial diseases and their clinical counterparts until Brigden [5], in 1957, and Mattingly [6], in 1958, wrote their important contributions to this subject. In 1961, Goodwin described 66 patients with cardiomyopathy [7], Harvey discussed the auscultatory findings in patients with myocardial diseases [8], and Fowler and Gueron [9] wrote a description of their experience with the natural history of the idiopathic myocardial diseases in a series of patients who came to autopsy. Alexander estimated that patients with myocardial disease comprised only 2.4 percent of all his patients with heart disease [10], but in our experience the disease is more common. Harvey's clinic in Washington, D.C., under the guidance of Dr. Jack Segal, now has more than 600 patients with myocardial disease. Often at the Cincinnati General Hospital, several patients with heart failure resulting from cardiomyopathy are in the hospital at the same time. Each year, we examine 10 to 20 heart specimens from patients who have died of myocardial disease.

Nomenclature. A discussion of the myocardial diseases is attended by considerable semantic difficulty. The myocardial diseases have been called by a number of other names: myocardosis [4] (noninflammatory, nonneoplastic myocardial diseases), idiopathic myocardial hypertrophy [11], myocardopathy, cardiomyopathy [7], noncoronary myocardopathy, and idiopathic left ventricular hypertrophy. In addition to the problem of a label for this group of diseases, there is also the question of their classification. The cardiomyopathies may be divided in accordance with either an etiologic classification or a functional classification. The etiologic classification that we recommend has two large groupings: the idiopathic or "primary" cardiomyopathies and the secondary cardiomyopathies. In this system, the secondary cardiomyopathies are those in which the myocardial involvement results from some identifiable disease which is usually also manifested outside the heart, for example, malignant neoplasm, connective tissue disease, neuromuscular disease, metabolic disease, or granulomatous disease. Here, we must insert a note of admonition. The Washington, D.C. group, led by Harvey [8, 12] and Mattingly [6], use the term "primary myocardial disease" in a different sense. These investigators use this term to indicate any myocardial disease, whether idiopathic or secondary, in which the heart involvement is the principal clinical feature. Thus, scleroderma of the heart might be labeled "primary myocardial disease" in their classification if heart failure or arrhythmia is the principal clinical feature. In this chapter, we shall attempt to avoid ambiguity by referring to myocardial disease of unknown cause as *idiopathic cardiomyopathy*, and to that of known cause as *secondary cardiomyopathy*.

The myocardial diseases may also be divided by a physiologic classification into congestive or nonobstructive, obstructive, and restrictive (constrictive) types [7]. Of these, the nonobstructive (congestive) cardiomyopathies are the most common; nearly all of the secondary and most of the primary cardiomyopathies belong in this group, and it is with the nonobstructive group that this presentation will principally be concerned. Classification of the myocardial diseases is given in the following outline:

I. Idiopathic cardiomyopathy
  A. Nonobstructive
    1. Familial
    2. Hypertrophic without obstruction
    3. Peripartal (postpartal)
    4. Postinfectious (infectious agent not identified)
    5. Those with unknown antecedent
    6. Endocardial fibroelastosis
    7. Endomyocardial fibrosis

- B. Obstructive
  1. Familial
  2. Nonfamilial
- II. Secondary cardiomyopathy
  - A. Neuromuscular disease
    1. Friedreich's ataxia
    2. Myotonic muscular dystrophy
    3. Duchenne muscular dystrophy
    4. Facioscapulohumeral muscular dystrophy
    5. Limb-girdle muscular dystrophy
  - B. Connective tissue diseases
    1. Scleroderma
    2. Dermatomyositis
    3. Rheumatoid heart disease
    4. Rheumatic myocardial disease
    5. Disseminated lupus erythematosus
    6. Ankylosing spondylitis
  - C. Neoplastic heart disease: primary and metastatic neoplasm, lymphoma, leukemia
  - D. Metabolic disease
    1. Thyrotoxicosis
    2. Hemochromatosis
    3. Myxedema
    4. Glycogen-storage disease (Pompe's disease)
    5. Infiltrative diseases, e.g., Refsum's disease, mucopolysaccharidosis, Hunter's syndrome, Hurler's syndrome, the lipidoses
    6. Pheochromocytoma
    7. Acromegaly
  - E. Nutritional disease
    1. Beriberi
    2. Kwashiorkor
  - F. Myocarditis
    1. Viral: Coxsackie B, Coxsackie A, echovirus, influenza virus, infectious mononucleosis, poliovirus, mumps, measles, chickenpox, smallpox, vaccinia, psittacosis, lymphogranuloma venereum, herpes simplex, cytomegalovirus, infectious hepatitis, German measles; rabies, yellow fever
    2. Parasitic: trichinosis
    3. Protozoal: trypanosomiasis cruzi (Chagas' disease), syphilis, toxoplasmosis, amebiasis, Borrelia recurrentis
    4. Bacterial: bacterial endocarditis, septicemia, diphtheria
    5. Unknown or allergic: drug reaction (e.g., penicillin) Loeffler's parietal endocarditis, serum sickness
  - G. Granulomatous cardiomyopathy: sarcoidosis

H. Amyloidosis
   1. Primary
      a. Senile
      b. Familial
      c. Nonfamilial
   2. Secondary

I. Posttraumatic cardiomyopathy: following penetrating or nonpenetrating trauma or surgical procedures

J. Toxic cardiomyopathy
   1. Uremia
   2. Alcoholism
   3. Carbon monoxide poisoning
   4. Phenothiazine and related drugs
   5. Cobalt
   6. Physical agents: radiation therapy, heatstroke [13], lightning [14]
   7. Other drugs and chemical agents

Segal et al. [15] found that the idiopathic myocardial diseases were approximately three times as common as those associated with an identifiable illness. This proportion is approximately in accord with our own experience. Alternative systems of classification are used by other investigators [12, 16, 17, 18].

A few words should be said in explanation and amplification of some portions of the foregoing classification. If one examines an unselected group of patients with cardiomyopathy, most will be found in the group classified as I, A, that is, idiopathic nonobstructive cardiomyopathy, and most of those have biventricular failure as their presenting problem. A small percentage of these patients have a family background of a similar disease. In 3 families, we have observed that siblings of the propositus with idiopathic nonobstructive cardiomyopathy died of the same illness at a similar age. During the past few years, it has been recognized that there are patients who display some of the features of idiopathic hypertrophic subaortic stenosis (IHSS) but without evidence of left ventricular outflow tract obstruction when studied carefully by left heart catherization. Such patients may have relatives with IHSS and evidence of obstruction to left ventricular outflow [19]. They may have electrocardiograms with abnormal Q waves or preexcitation (Wolff-Parkinson-White) syndrome. Such patients may show intraventricular pressure gradients caused by entrapment of the cardiac catheter tip within the apex of the left ventricular cavity rather than true outflow tract obstruction. Whether or not such patients may develop outflow tract obstruction is unknown. We have classified this group as hypertrophic cardiomyopathy without obstruction.

Peripartal Cardiomyopathy

Peripartal or postpartal cardiomyopathy has not been assigned a separate section of this book and some discussion is needed here. Some pregnant women develop clinical evidence of myocardopathy during the last trimester of pregnancy, usually the last month) rather than after delivery. Thus, the term "peripartal cardiomyopathy" seems preferable to "postpartum cardiomyopathy." Possibly 5 to 10 percent of our patients with idiopathic, nonobstructive cardiomyopathy first became ill either during the last trimester of pregnancy or during the first several weeks after delivery. Although some physicians have questioned the existence of a variety of cardiomyopathies related to pregnancy, we are very much convinced that the relationship is more than coincidental. Some have suggested that toxemia, pulmonary embolism, or unrecognized viral myocarditis will explain nearly all instances of peripartal cardiomyopathy. Others have attributed it to poor nutrition or alcoholism. However, these features are absent in most of our patients. Demakis and associates found no evidence of viral disease, alcoholism, or malnutrition in their 27 patients with peripartal cardiomyopathy [20, 21]. In 3 of our patients, heart failure began before childbirth rather than afterward. The course of peripartal cardiomyopathy shows great variation. One of our patients now shows no evidence of cardiac disease several years after a bout of peripartal heart failure; this course has taken place with no further pregnancies, which has been our recommendation to these women. Another patient suffered from constant cardiac enlargement and died of progressive heart failure 7 years after her last pregnancy. Another patient, a 19-year-old woman who developed heart failure a few weeks after the birth of twins, died of constant and intractable heart failure a year later. Demakis, Rahimtoola, and their associates found that those women whose hearts returned to normal size following peripartal heart failure were less likely to develop heart failure with later pregnancies [20, 21].

In at least 6 patients, we have observed the syndrome of chronic congestive heart failure caused by cardiomyopathy which followed soon after acute febrile idiopathic pericarditis. It is known that chronic myocardopathy may follow acute Coxsackie B myocarditis [22], and we suspect that this may have occurred in some of our patients, but we have no proof of this hypothesis either by viral isolation or by serial serological studies for evidence of viral disease in these patients. Hence, we prefer to place these patients within the idiopathic cardiomyopathy group without confirmation of an infectious illness. Dr. Walter Abelmann will deal with the topic of specific viral myocarditis in Chapter 10 of this book. The category of idiopathic, nonobstructive cardiomyopathy with an unknown antecedent is an extremely important one, and is undoubtedly the largest single category in our experience.

Obstructive cardiomyopathies are not uncommon, but certainly are considerably less common in a general hospital population than nonobstructive cardiomyopathies are. About one-third of these patients with obstructive cardiomyopathy have a family history of a similar illness, as reported by Braunwald et al. [23]. Dr. Wigle and associates deal with this population in Chapter 12 of this book.

Restrictive cardiomyopathy. Burwell and Robin [24] pointed out that some patients with myocardial fibrosis have a hemodynamic pattern similar to that found in constrictive pericarditis. In these patients, the neck veins show a prominent *y* descent, and there is an early diastolic dip in the right ventricular pressure trace. The right ventricular systolic pressure is not greatly elevated. There is a diastolic pressure plateau: systemic venous pressure, right atrial pressure, right ventricular and pulmonary artery diastolic pressure, and the mean pulmonary arterial wedge pressure tend to be equal. Goodwin et al. [7] described a number of such patients with cardiomyopathy. Scleroderma, hemochromatosis [25], amyloid disease [26], endocardial fibroelastosis [27], and endomyocardial fibrosis seem especially prone to produce patterns of restrictive cardiomyopathy. However, restrictive cardiomyopathy may occur in idiopathic cardiomyopathy [7].

Endocardial Fibroelastosis

Endocardial fibroelastosis is discussed here because it has not been assigned to a separate section of this book. This discussion deals with *primary* endocardial fibroelastosis (EFE) rather than with that secondary to another congenital defect, such as aortic stenosis, coarctation of the aorta, or pulmonic stenosis. A decade or two ago, endocardial fibroelastosis was one of the commonest causes of congestive heart failure during the first year of life. At present, the disease seems to be distinctly less common; only a few instances are now seen each year at the Cincinnati Children's Hospital. The cause of endocardial fibroelastosis (EFE) is unknown, and some have doubted that it is an entity to be separated from the group of patients with idiopathic cardiomyopathy [28]. It is also true that the diffuse fibroelastic whitish thickening of the heart's endocardial surface seen in infants is extremely rare in adults. I have never seen an example in an adult, but a sizable series of such patients has been reported [29]. Undoubtedly, we would have classified some of the patients in this series as having idiopathic cardiomyopathy in the more general sense. We have commonly observed patchy endocardial fibrosis, especially over the convex surfaces of the papillary muscles of the left ventricle, in patients who died of idiopathic myocardial disease [30]. Black-Shaffer postulated that this thickening was caused by the increased tension in the wall of the dilated heart [28]. On the other hand, diffuse endocardial elastosis may be found in the heart at birth, and involvement of the mitral and aortic valves by this process is common. Rarely, the pulmonary and tricuspid valves are involved.

The presenting feature of EFE is usually that of congestive heart failure with tachypnea, tachycardia, enlarged heart, and gallop rhythm appearing in a child between 6 and 18 months of age. Systolic murmurs, usually caused by relative mitral insufficiency, are common. Occasionally, a familial occurrence of the disease is found. The course is usually slowly downhill and death often takes place within a few months or years, but the disease may be observed in teenagers and adults, as well. At times, mitral insufficiency is of such severity that mitral valve replacement is warranted. Radiologic studies tend to show cardiac dilation, left atrial enlargement and, when there is heart failure, pulmonary congestion. Angiocardiography shows a limited excursion of the ventricular walls and prolonged opacification of the left ventricular cavity [31]. Occasionally, the left heart is not greatly dilated and constrictive pericarditis is simulated.

Endocardial fibroelastosis must be considered in the differential diagnosis of congestive heart failure accompanied by predominant left ventricular enlargement in children. Other common causes of this picture are aortic stenosis, coarctation of the aorta, ventricular septal defect, patent ductus arteriosus, viral myocarditis, aberrant left coronary artery, glycogen-storage disease, and idiopathic myocardiopathy without known antecedent. In 90 percent of instances of EFE, heart failure begins within the first 2 years of life, and death occurs by the age of 6. Involvement of the aortic valve or the mitral valve by this process may be a major feature. Severe mitral insufficiency, at times requiring the insertion of a prosthetic valve, may result. Both the electrocardiogram and cardiac fluoroscopy may show evidence of left atrial enlargement. At the bedside, the distinction between idiopathic cardiomyopathy without antecedent and EFE may be difficult. Sellers et al. pointed out two important features that may be useful in the distinction [32]. With EFE, the onset of heart failure tends to be earlier in life: In his review of this disease, heart failure began before 8 months of age in 85 percent of the patients, and seldom began after the age of 18 months. In "myocarditis" (presumably idiopathic cardiomyopathy), only 30 percent demonstrated an onset before 8 months of age. In EFE, pronounced electrocardiographic signs of left ventricular hypertrophy were more common than in idiopathic cardiomyopathy. When the S wave in lead V_1 or the R wave in lead V_6 exceeded 20 mm in amplitude, EFE was more likely. Uncommonly, the ECG pattern in EFE is that of right ventricular hypertrophy rather than left ventricular hypertrophy.

Endomyocardial Fibrosis

Endomyocardial fibrosis is not assigned to a separate section of this book, therefore it is briefly described here. Endomyocardial fibrosis may be classified as one of the idiopathic cardiomyopathies. It is one of the most common causes of heart failure among Africans in Uganda, being responsible for 15 percent of the deaths from cardiac failure in one study [33]. Although probably widespread in Africa, being reported in Southern and Northern Rhodesia, Gambia, Nigeria, West Africa [34], and the Sudan, it is rarely reported in Europe [35] and the United States [36]. Cases have also been reported from Brazil [37]. The cause of the disease is unknown; malnutrition, viral disease, and autoimmune disease have been suspected. The anatomic findings include cardiac enlargement with marked fibrous thickening of the endocardium which may involve the inner third or half of the myocardium. Thickening and shortening of the mitral chordae tendineae may result. The fibrotic process tends to decrease the volume of the ventricular cavity and to cause AV-valve insufficiency, or less commonly, AV-valve stenosis [38]. Rarely, the aortic valve is thickened. The hemodynamic changes may resemble those of constrictive pericarditis; pulsus paradoxus may be present [38]. Mural thrombi may occur and systemic and pulmonary emboli are common. Unlike the histologic picture of endocardial fibroelastosis, there is no proliferation of elastic tissue.

The clinical features are similar to those of the other varieties of cardiomyopathy; cardiomegaly and congestive heart failure are the common manifestations. Cerebral, peripheral, or visceral infarction may dominate the clinical picture [39]. Death may result from heart failure, bacterial endocarditis, or from superimposed infection.

Aging. Burch and Giles have suggested that the effects of aging alone may be responsible for otherwise unexplained heart failure in the elderly [40]. Until we have more specific tests for idiopathic cardiomyopathy and have solved the riddle of its etiologic background, this concept will be difficult to evaluate.

SECONDARY CARDIOMYOPATHIES

The secondary cardiomyopathies are those which represent myocardial involvement of a generalized illness, such as a connective tissue disease, a neoplasm, or a metabolic disease. Myocardial diseases which may accompany the neuromuscular disease are described in Chapter 13, written by Dr. Joseph Perloff. The remaining secondary myocardial diseases are discussed in Chapter 14 by Dr. Noble Fowler.

A few comments might be made about some of the other varieties of secondary cardiomyopathy. Uremia is believed to be associated, at times, with myocarditis [41] which comprises cardiac function and which along with anemia, hypertension, water overload, and electrolyte imbalance contributes to the heart failure so common in uremic patients. Glycogen-storage disease involving the heart muscle (Pompe's disease) is virtually limited to infants and very young children since it is compatible with only a greatly abbreviated life span [42]. In the United States, beriberi heart disease is largely limited to alcoholics and to a few patients in charity hospitals in large cities [43]. Kwashiorkor is largely restricted to Africa. With a few possible exceptions, Chagas' disease has been seen primarily in South America [44], and it is essentially unknown in the United States. Diphtheritic myocarditis was seldom seen in recent times until a few years ago; however, recent outbreaks of this disease in the impoverished minority groups in southwestern cities of the United States have once again made diphtheria a disease to be reckoned with [45]. Treatment with penicillin, procainamide, diphenylhydantoin, isoniazid, and hydralazine may cause a lupus-like syndrome which may include myocardial or pericardial involvement [46]. In addition, the use of penicillin may cause an acute allergic myocarditis. The inhalation of carbon monoxide may lead to fatal hemorrhagic myocardial necrosis. It has been suspected that less severe but more extended exposures may cause chronic myocardial disease. It is generally recognized that surgical operations on the thorax and penetrating cardiac trauma may be followed by febrile pleuropericarditis [47]; myocardial involvement may accompany this syndrome. Similar symptoms may occur following myocardial infarction (Dressler's postmyocardial-infarction syndrome). In addition, recurrent febrile pleural, pericardial, and myocardial disease may follow nonpenetrating trauma; we have observed this syndrome following a chest injury from a steering wheel in an auto accident.

Our classification must deal with the relationship between cardiomyopathy and alcoholism. The question is a complex one. Some writers have maintained the position that nearly all instances of nonobstructive idiopathic cardiomyopathy are related to alcoholism [10]. However, in our first postmortem study of 19 patients with idiopathic nonobstructive cardiomyopathy, only one-third had a history of alcoholism and not all of this one-third could be clearly indicted of alcoholic cardiomyopathy [9]. Alcoholics may develop thiamine deficiency; and alcoholic cardiomyopathy must be distinguished from beriberi heart disease. Beer drinkers may develop cardiomyopathy which, in some instances, has been suspected of being related to cobalt toxicity [48]. However, there is clear evidence that alcohol may exert an acute and probably a chronic toxic effect on the myocardium aside from the question of thiamine deficiency or cobalt toxicity [49]. Dr. Timothy Regan will deal with this topic in Chapter 9 in this book.

In our classification and the accompanying discussion in this book, we have not used the term "coronary cardiomyopathy." Occasionally, in patients with occlusive coronary disease, there is no evidence of either angina pectoris or myocardial infarction. Rather, at times, the course is that of chronic, apparently idiopathic, heart failure in a young adult or a middle-aged person. In our opinion, such cases should be considered as examples of coronary artery disease and not examples of cardiomyopathy.

REFERENCES

1. Bollinger, O.: Ueber die Haufigkeit und Ursachen der Idiopathischen Herzhypertrophie in Munchen. Dtsch Med Wochschr (Berl) (X): 180, 1884.
2. Saphir, O.: Myocarditis. Arch Pathol 33:88, 1942.
3. Christian, H.A.: Clinically the myocardium. Trans Assoc Am Physicians 63: 255, 1950.
4. Blankenhorn, M.A. and Gall, E.A.: Myocarditis and myocardosis. Circulation 13:217, 1956.
5. Brigden, W.: Uncommon myocardial diseases. The non-coronary cardiomyopathies. Lancet 2:1179, 1243, 1957.
6. Mattingly, T.W.: The clinical and hemodynamic features of primary myocardial disease. Trans Am Clin Climatol Assoc 70:132, 1958.
7. Goodwin, J.F., Gordon, H., Hollman, A., and Bishop, M.B.: Clinical aspects of cardiomyopathy. Br Med J 1:69, 1961.
8. Harvey, W.P. and Perloff, J.K.: The auscultatory findings in primary myocardial disease. Am Heart J 61:199, 1961.
9. Fowler, N.O., Gueron, M., and Rowlands, D.T., Jr.: Primary myocardial disease. Circulation 23:498, 1961.
10. Alexander, C.S.: Idiopathic heart disease. I Analysis of 100 cases, with special reference to chronic alcoholism. Am J Med 41:213, 1966.
11. Spodick, D.H. and Littmann, D.: Idiopathic myocardial hypertrophy. Am J Cardiol 1:610, 1968.
12. Harvey, W.P., Segal, J.P., and Gurel, T.: The clinical spectrum of primary myocardial disease. Progr Cardiovasc Dis 7:17, 1964.

13. Kew, M.C., Tucker, R.B.K., Bersohn, I., and Seftel, H.C.: The heart in heatstroke. Am Heart J 77:324, 1969.
14. Barda, C.D.: Electrocardiographic changes in lightning stroke. Am Heart J 72:521, 1966.
15. Segal, N.P., Harvey, W.P., and Gurel, T.: Diagnosis and treatment of primary myocardial disease. Circulation 32:837, 1965.
16. Perloff, J.K.: The cardiomyopathies—current perspectives. Circulation 44:942, 1971.
17. Mattingly, T.W.: Diseases of the myocardium (cardiomyopathies). The viewpoint of a clinical cardiologist. Am J Cardiol 25:79, 1970.
18. Hudson, R.E.B.: The cardiomyopathies: Order from chaos. Am J Cardiol 25:70, 1970.
19. Kariv, I., Kreisler, B., Sherf, L. Feldman, S., and Rosenthal, T.: Familial cardiomyopathy. A review of 11 families. Am J Cardiol 28:693, 1971.
20. Demakis, J.G. and Rahimtoola, S.H.: Peripartum cardiomyopathy. Circulation 44:964, 1971.
21. Demakis, J.G., Rahimtoola, S.H., Sutton, G.C., Meadows, W.R., Szanto, P.B., Tobin, J.R., and Gunnar, R.M.: Natural course of peripartum cardiomyopathy. Circulation 44:1053, 1971.
22. Lerner, A.M.: Virus myopericarditis. Ann Intern Med 69:1068, 1968.
23. Braunwald, E., Lambrew, C.T., Rockoff, S.D., Ross, J., Jr., and Morrow, A.G.: Idiopathic hypertrophic subaortic stenosis: I. A. description of the disease based upon an analysis of 64 patients. Circulation 30 (Suppl IV): 3-119, 1964.
24. Burwell, C.S. and Robin, E.D.: Some points in the diagnosis of myocardial fibrosis. Trans Assoc Am. Physicians 67:67, 1954.
25. Wasserman, A.J., Baird, C.L., Richardson, D.W., and Wyso, E.M.: Cardiac hemochromatosis simulating constrictive pericarditis. Am J Med 32:316, 1962.
26. Gunnar, R.M., Dillon, R.F., Wallyn, R.J., and Elisberg, E.I.: The physiologic and clinical similarity between primary amyloid of the heart and constrictive pericarditis. Circulation 12:827, 1955.
27. Clark, G.M., Valentine, E., and Blount, S.G.: Endocardial fibrosis simulating constrictive pericarditis. New Engl J Med 254:349, 1956.
28. Black-Shaffer, B.: Infantile endocardial fibroelastosis: A suggested etiology. Arch Pathol 63:281, 1957.
29. Thomas, W.A.: Endocardial fibroelastosis: A factor in heart disease of obscure etiology. A study of 20 autopsied cases in children and adults. New Eng J. Med 251:327, 1954.
30. Fowler, N.O., Gueron, M., and Rowlands, D.T.: Primary myocardial disease. Circulation 23:498, 1961.
31. Linde, L.M., Adams, F.H., and O'Loughlin, B.J.: Endocardial fibroelastosis. Angiocardiographic studies. Circulation 17:40, 1968.
32. Sellers, F.J., Keith, J.D., and Manning, J.A.: The diagnosis of primary endocardial fibroelastosis. Circulation 29:49, 1964.
33. Davies, J.N.P. and Ball, J.D.: The pathology of endomyocardial fibrosis in Uganda. Br Heart J 17:337, 1955.
34. Abrahams, D. and Brigden, W.: Syndrome of mitral incompetence, myocarditis, and pulmonary hypertension in Nigeria. Br Med J 2:134, 1961.
35. Faruque, A.A.: Adult endomyocardial fibrosis in Britain. Lancet 2:331, 1963.

36. Smith, J.J. and Furth, J.: Fibrosis of the endocardium and the myocardium with mural thrombosis. Arch Intern Med 71:602, 1943.
37. Andradi, A.Z. and Guimaraes, A.C.: Endomyocardial fibrosis in Bahia, Brazil. Br Heart J 26:813, 1964.
38. Parry, E.H. and Abrahams, D.G.: The function of the heart in endomyocardial fibrosis of the right ventricle. Br Heart J 25:619, 1963.
39. Shaper, A.G. and Wright, D.H.: Intracardiac thromboses and embolism in endomyocardial fibrosis in Uganda. Br Heart J 25:502, 1963.
40. Burch, G. and Giles, T.: Editorial. Senile cardiomyopathy. J Chronic Dis 24:1, 1971.
41. Comty, C.M., Cohen, S.L., and Shapiro, F.L.: Pericarditis in chronic uremia and its sequels. Ann Intern Med 75:173, 1971.
42. diSant'Agnese, P.A., Andersen, D.H., and Mason, H.H.: Glycogen-storage disease of the heart. II. Critical review of the literature. Pediatrics 6:607, 1950.
43. Blakenhorn, M.A., Vilter, C.F., Scheinker, I.M., and Austin, R.S.: Occidental beriberi heart disease. JAMA 131:717, 1946.
44. Burchell, H.B.: Unusual causes of heart failure. Circulation 21:436, 1960.
45. Zalma, V.M., Older, J.J., and Brooks, G.F.: The Austin, Texas diphtheria outbreak. Clinical and epidemiological aspects. JAMA 211:2125, 1970.
46. Alarcon-Segovia, D.: Drug-induced lupus syndromes. Mayo Clin Proc 44:664, 1969.
47. Robinson, J. and Brigden, N.: Immunological studies in the postcardiotomy syndrome. Br Med J 2:706, 1963.
48. Sullivan, J.F., George, R., Bluvas, R., and Egan, J.D.: Myocardiopathy of beer drinkers: Subsequent course. Ann Intern Med 70:277, 1969.
49. Regan, T.J.: Ethyl alcohol and the heart. Circulation 44:957, 1971.

JACK P. SEGAL, M.D.,
W. PROCTOR HARVEY, M.D.,
and JOHN F. STAPLETON, M.D.

Clinical Features and Natural History of Cardiomyopathy

The recognition of cardiomyopathy has become increasingly common in the past two decades [1-7]. The severity and location of the myocardial involvement is determined by the specific symptoms, and physical and laboratory findings in each patient. Although, by definition, the myocardium is predominantly affected, there is often significant involvement of pericardium and endocardium which may influence the clinical picture and course.

The classification in Table I divides cardiomyopathy patients into two groups: unknown etiology (idiopathic) (primary) and specific etiology (secondary). As noted, many disease processes may cause cardiomyopathy. Although in the majority of patients the classification is "idiopathic," a "specific" etiology may subsequently be found in approximately one-fourth [5, 6]. However, with few exceptions the clinical picture is similar whether the etiology is specific or unknown and depends on the extent and location of the myocardial involvement.

Initial evaluation of the patient must include a detailed history, complete physical examination, and pertinent laboratory studies. The diagnosis depends on both positive characteristic features and on the exclusion of other common types of heart disease [3, 4-7, 9]. The history should include specific questions related to recent respiratory infections and febrile ill-

From the Department of Medicine, Division of Cardiology, Georgetown University Medical Center, Washington, D.C.
This study was supported in part by the Benjamin May Memorial Fund and the Metropolitan Heart Guild.

Table I
Etiology of Cardiomyopathy

I. Unknown etiology (idiopathic) (primary)
II. Specific etiology (secondary)
   A. Infectious (viral, bacterial, mycotic, parasitic, protozoal, rickettsial)
   B. Connective tissue diseases
   C. Metabolic (hyperthyroidism, hypothyroidism, pheochromocytoma, nutritional, electrolyte imbalance)
   D. Toxic (emetine, carbon tetrachloride, bacterial toxins, cobalt)
   E. Alcoholic cardiomyopathy
   F. Infiltrative (malignancy, sarcoidosis, hemochromatosis, amyloidosis, glycogen-storage disease)
   G. Neuromuscular disorders (progressive muscular dystrophy, dystrophia myotonia, Friedreich's ataxia, pseudohypertrophic and facioscapulohumeral muscular dystrophy)
   H. Hypertrophic muscular outflow tract obstruction (obstructive cardiomyopathy)
   I. Pregnancy and postpartum state
   J. Congenital or familial myocardial disease
   K. Miscellaneous
      1. Endocardial fibroelastosis
      2. Endomyocardial fibrosis
      3. Hypersensitivity

nesses, nutritional deficiency, high intake of alcohol, or ingestion of toxic substances such as emetine or carbon tetrachloride. In addition, the physician should carefully search for symptoms suggestive of systemic involvement with connective tissue diseases, malignancy, or metabolic disturbances [4, 9, 10]. A history of classic angina pectoris, particularly in a patient with coronary risk factors, strongly suggests arteriosclerotic heart disease rather than cardiomyopathy. The diagnosis of cardiomyopathy should be suspected in a cardiac patient with a family history of cardiomyopathy or sudden death. A positive family history is more prevalent in patients with obstructive cardiomyopathy than in patients with nonobstructive cardiomyopathy [9]. Cardiomyopathy is a likely possibility when a woman without a previous history of heart disease develops congestive heart failure in the third trimester of pregnancy or during the first several weeks postpartum, particularly if there is no evidence for toxemia, pulmonary infarction, rheumatic heart disease, or hypertension [11]. The appearance of unexplained heart disease in patients who have had a recent viral illness, especially those with pleurisy, pericarditis, diarrhea, fever, or skin rash is also suggestive of cardiomyopathy [16, 19].

The physical examination affords immediate clues, and one must carefully search for findings indicative of a myocardial disease as well as any specific etiologic factor. Other varieties of heart disease, such as rheumatic or hypertensive disease, can usually be excluded by a careful complete

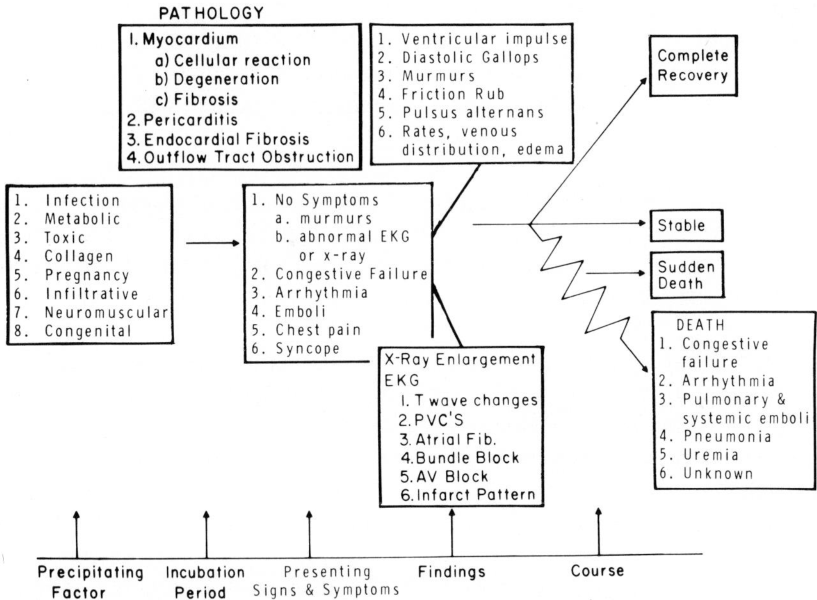

Figure 1. Cardiomyopathy. Profile history following myocardial injury of many etiologies. Presenting symptoms developed after a variable incubation period. Wide spectrum of symptoms and physical findings occur. Clinical course may vary from complete recovery to death.

cardiovascular examination. Detailed laboratory studies must be obtained in order to complete the search for specific causes of myocardial disease such as hyperthyroidism, pheochromocytoma, malignancy, connective tissue disease, infiltrative disease, chronic alcoholic ingestion, or other toxic substances. Of the specific group, collagen vascular disease has been the most common identifiable etiology (30 percent), and bacterial infections and hyperthyroidism have each been present in approximately 10 percent [5-7].

To best understand cardiomyopathy, one should remember that there is a wide spectrum of symptoms and signs; there is an equally wide spectrum for the clinical course and pathology (Fig. 1) [5-7]. Symptoms of cardiomyopathy also often mimic other diseases. A thorough understanding and an acute awareness of the possibilities of this disease enable the physician to diagnose the mild or early cases.

This can be accomplished by focusing attention on the symptoms and physical findings which will be discussed in this chapter. It is extremely important that the mild cases be recognized early in the course of the disease since the prompt institution of appropriate therapy may favorably alter the clinical course, possibly preventing death in some [3, 5, 6]. In fact, with a benign course there may be no residual signs or symptoms [14, 15, 17]. Occasionally cardiomyopathy coexists with other forms of heart disease, and although the clinical picture may be confusing, a correct diagnosis can usually be established if the spectrum of findings associated with this disease is carefully analyzed [8].

Mode of onset. Although the majority of patients have symptoms, a number are without symptoms. As a rule, the asymptomatic patients have milder degrees of myocardial involvement; they are usually referred for evaluation of extrasystoles, cardiac enlargement, an abnormal electrocardiogram, or a murmur—abnormalities discovered for the first time on routine examination. Most patients, however, are symptomatic when their condition is first diagnosed. Congestive heart failure, usually left ventricular, is by far the most frequent presenting symptom complex [5, 6, 7, 8, 12]. Cardiac arrhythmias cause symptoms in approximately one-third of patients. Other symptoms include pleuritic chest pain, syncope, coronary type of chest pain, and clinical features related to systemic or pulmonary emboli. Rarely sudden death is the initial event in a patient with no previously known heart disease. Cardiomyopathy is most often first diagnosed in patients between the ages of 30 and 50, but the disease is found in the newborn and in infancy as well as in the very elderly [5-7]. In some series, men predominate over women, although this may be related to case selection.

SYMPTOMS AND PHYSICAL FINDINGS

Congestive failure. As illustrated in Figure 2, the most common manifestations of cardiomyopathy are related to congestive heart failure [4-7]. Symptoms of left-sided failure such as dyspnea, orthopnea, and paroxysmal nocturnal dyspnea occur earlier and more frequently than those of right-sided congestive heart failure, such as edema. Weakness and fatigue, presumably related to reduced cardiac output, are common complaints. Physical findings confirmatory of left ventricular failure include pulmonary congestion, pulsus alternans, and gallop rhythm. On examination of the precordium, the physician may palpate a ventricular impulse—either apical or parasternal, or both; and an accentuated closure of the pulmonic second sound may be felt which is indicative of elevated pulmonary artery pressure. Frequently, gallop rhythm, both atrial and ventricular, can also be detected by palpation as abnormal outward ventricular movements. A ventricular gallop is frequently heard in early diastole, and an atrial gallop, in presystole, or both. Palpation may disclose either left or right ventricular

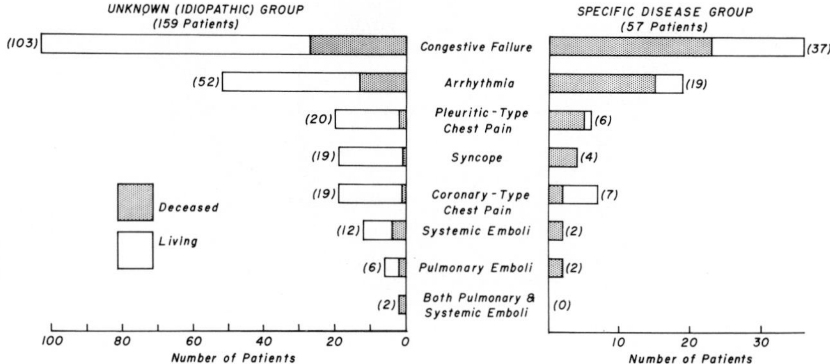

Figure 2. Myocardial Disease Symptoms. Common clinical symptoms and features occurring with cardiomyopathy. (From Harvey, W.P. and Segal, J.P.: Progr Cardiovasc Dis 7:17, 1964.)

enlargement, or both. Right ventricular failure, when present, is often secondary to left ventricular failure, and thus is associated with pulmonary hypertension. Right ventricular failure is manifested by hepatomegaly, by peripheral edema, and also by distention of the neck veins. A prominent jugular venous "a" wave may be observed, particularly when there is an element of pulmonary hypertension [13]. A prominent "v" wave may be present when there is tricuspid insufficiency.

Cardiac enlargement is found in most patients with cardiomyopathy. At times cardiac enlargement cannot be demonstrated, particularly in those patients whose disease is early or mild, and in those first seen because of arrhythmias or other electrocardiographic abnormalities. The spectrum concept of cardiomyopathy is emphasized by the observation that a patient with a heart of normal size may have a serious or even fatal arrhythmia.

The prognosis and clinical course of patients with congestive heart failure is variable, depending on the duration of symptoms, specific etiologic factors, and heart size. For example, congestive heart failure secondary to acute viral myocarditis might be completely reversible [17]. A favorable prognosis can result, particularly when the heart is of normal size or only slightly enlarged, if the diagnosis is established early, and if therapy (particularly restriction of activities) is instituted promptly [3]. On the other hand, the prognosis is poor in patients with long-standing congestive heart failure, associated with moderate or marked cardiac enlargement. Figure 3 represents a 24-year-old woman with a 2-year history of slowly progressive congestive heart failure and cardiomegaly. Frequent ventricular premature beats and atrial and ventricular gallops were present. In spite of prolonged

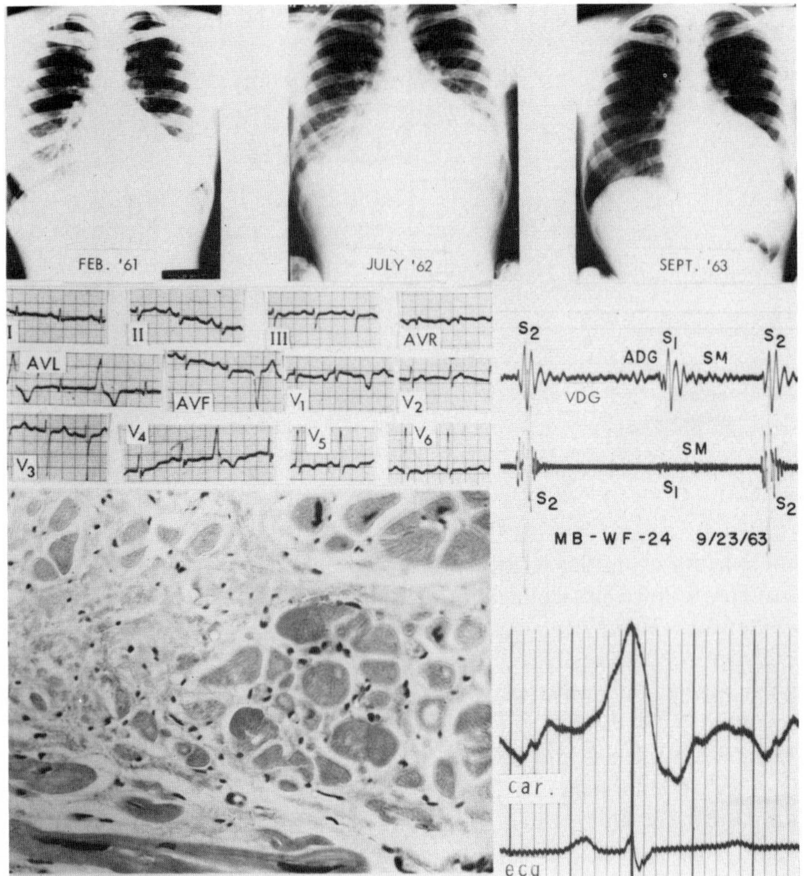

Figure 3. Idiopathic Cardiomyopathy. Twenty-four-year-old woman, incapacitated despite all known forms of therapy. Note persistence of extreme cardiomegaly on x-rays. Electrocardiogram shows ventricular extrasystoles and nonspecific S-T and T-wave changes.

bed rest, many periods of hospitalization, digitalis, diuretics, and antiarrhythmic drugs, she died suddenly at home on the day following discharge from the hospital. The microscopic section shows extensive fibrotic replacement of the myocardium.

In many cardiomyopathy patients with a poor prognosis, a specific etiology cannot be identified; however, in retrospect, it is evident that symptoms have been slowly progressive over months, or even years. In general, right ventricular failure associated with left ventricular failure implies a worse prognosis than left ventricular failure alone. The prognosis

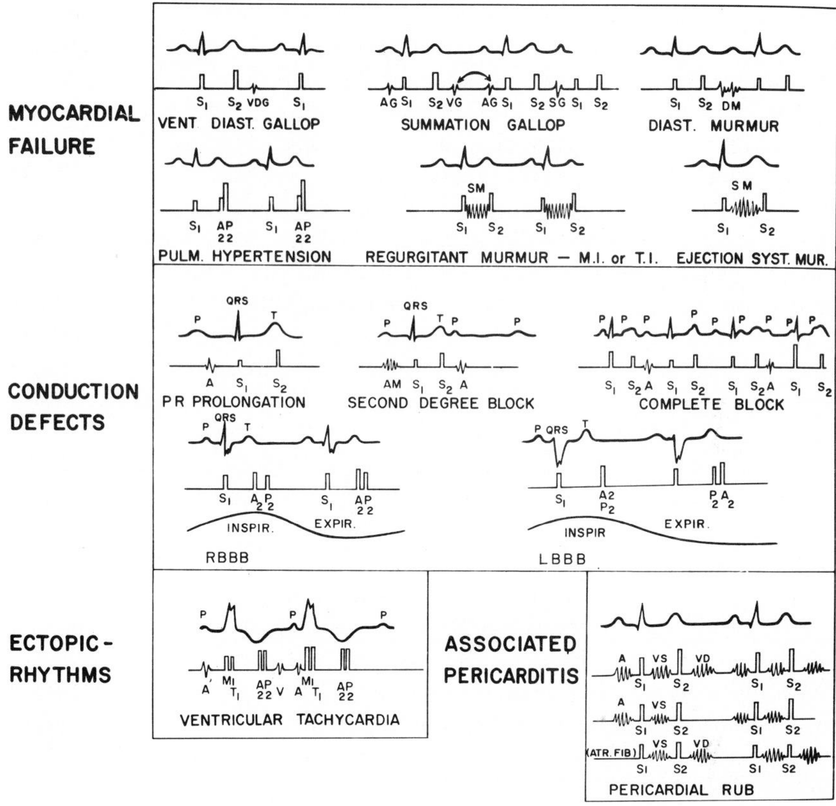

Figure 4. Myocardial Disease. Composite of Most Frequent Myocardial Abnormalities on Auscultation. S_1 =first sound; S_2 =second sound; VDG =ventricular gallop; AG =atrial gallop; A_2 =aortic valve closure of second sound; P_2 =pulmonic valve closure of second sound; M_1 =mitral valve closure of first sound; T_1 =tricuspid valve closure of first sound; SM =systolic murmur; DM =diastolic murmur; A =atrial sound. (From Harvey, W.P. and Perloff, J.K.: Am Heart J 61:199-205, 1961, and from Harvey, W.P. and Segal, J.P.: Progr Cardiovasc Dis 7:17, 1964.)

is grave if, in addition to congestive heart failure, there are associated rhythm disturbances such as atrial fibrillation, frequent premature ventricular contractions (particularly when multifocal), or major conduction disturbances in the electrocardiogram (second- and third-degree AV block and bundle branch block).

Auscultation. The findings by auscultation of the heart represent a most important aspect in recognition of cardiomyopathy, and these will be discussed in detail (Fig. 4) [6, 18]. As one might predict, *gallop rhythm* is a hallmark of cardiomyopathy and represents one of the more common findings. A careful search for the presence of gallop rhythm will be rewarding; atrial or ventricular gallops, or both, are almost always present. In all patients with an element of cardiac decompensation, a ventricular diastolic gallop was heard. An atrial gallop is also a frequent finding when there is normal sinus rhythm. In still others who did not have congestive heart failure, the finding of an atrial gallop in presystole represents an early clue to the presence of myocardial disease. At times, atrial and ventricular diastolic gallops occur in diastole at exactly the same time, producing a summation gallop. At other times, close proximity of an atrial and a ventricular gallop without superimposition simulates a rumbling diastolic murmur (Fig. 4). Because of this, the diagnosis of mitral stenosis is sometimes erroneously made. Gallop rhythm, therefore, is a significant feature of cardiomyopathy and occurs in the majority of patients.

At times, there is a diastolic sound occurring slightly later than the expected timing of an opening snap of tight mitral stenosis. This sound is generally earlier than a ventricular diastolic gallop or normal physiologic third sound; it resembles and corresponds in timing to the pericardial knock sound of constrictive pericarditis. It represents a ventricular filling sound, probably resulting in this instance from a restrictive type of cardiomyopathy rather than from constrictive pericarditis. The differential diagnosis is sometimes difficult even after complete clinical and hemodynamic studies have been performed. Postmortem examination in these cases usually demonstrates extensive fibrosis or infiltrate or both, to have replaced the normal cardiac musculature.

Alternation of intensity of heart sounds or murmurs. This alternation is also common in patients with cardiomyopathy who have some element of cardiac decompensation. If carefully searched for, *pulsus alternans* and a ventricular diastolic gallop can also usually be detected.

With increasing degrees of pulmonary hypertension, the *second heart sound* usually becomes more accentuated and closely split, although there is slight widening with inspiration. With complete right bundle branch block the second heart sound is widely split on expiration, and the degree of splitting increases slightly with inspiration. In myocardial disease, left bundle branch block occurs more frequently than right bundle branch block. Hence, paradoxical splitting of the second sound is heard more often—the second sound is widely split on expiration and becomes closely split or single with inspiration. A bedside clue as to the presence of complete left bundle branch block is thereby available even before the electrocardiogram is taken.

Various *arrhythmias* are readily detected on auscultation, ranging from extrasystoles to paroxysmal or sustained tachycardia. Ventricular tachycardia represents a serious complication which might be recognized at the bedside by a changing intensity of the first sound, multiple sounds in each cardiac cycle, and lack of response of the arrhythmia to carotid sinus pressure. Patients with pleuritic chest pain may also have pericarditis, as documented by hearing a 2- or 3-component pericardial friction rub. When a differential diagnosis between myopericarditis and myocardial infarction is being considered in a patient with a pericardial friction rub, a friction rub persisting over several days favors the diagnosis of myopericarditis (discussed in more detail later).

Systolic *murmurs* occur frequently [4, 8, 18, 20] in patients with myocardial disease. They are most common over the mitral area, but may also be heard over the pulmonary area, and less commonly over the aortic area. A tricuspid systolic murmur due to tricuspid insufficiency is more likely to occur when there are more advanced degrees of cardiac decompensation; the murmur is generally pansystolic, increasing in intensity on inspiration. A diastolic rumbling murmur heard at the cardiac apex is interpreted, at times, as the rumble of mitral stenosis. As already mentioned, and worthy of reemphasis, the combination of atrial and ventricular gallops in close proximity can result in sounds similar to the diastolic rumble of mitral stenosis. In our experience, the presence of an early blowing aortic diastolic murmur is unusual in cardiomyopathy; if present, this murmur should lead one to suspect a different or superimposed disease [13].*

Patients with hypertrophic subaortic stenosis present a unique and specific group of physical signs and symptoms [8, 9, 21]. In the great majority, the following sequence of events has transpired, thus affording a clue to the diagnosis: Palpation of the radial pulse (or other arterial pulses) reveals a quick rise, suggesting possibility of aortic insufficiency. However, on examining the patient—making a careful effort to detect the murmur of aortic insufficiency—it has rarely been present. Instead there is a systolic murmur, loudest along the lower left sternal border and cardiac apex, which becomes fainter over the aortic area and neck. One then thinks of the possibility of mitral insufficiency. At this point the diagnosis of idiopathic hypertrophic subaortic stenosis should be considered and ruled in or out. Although there are numerous bedside aids in making a differential diagnosis between obstructive cardiomyopathy and mitral in-

* *Editorial Note:* We have observed 2 patients with congestive, nonobstructive cardiomyopathy who had aortic insufficiency with no other cause demonstrated at autopsy. We agree that aortic insufficiency is uncommon in cardiomyopathy.

sufficiency, such as the Valsalva maneuver or use of amyl nitrite and vasopressor drugs, squatting has proved quite practical and helpful. With squatting, the murmur of idiopathic hypertrophic subaortic stenosis generally decreases, whereas the murmur of mitral insufficiency increases.

In some patients with cardiomyopathy, the murmur of left ventricular papillary muscle dysfunction is present due to pathologic involvement of the papillary muscles or left ventricular wall in the region of the papillary muscle attachment or both [20]. This murmur may be early, mid-, or late systolic and sometimes is associated with one or more systolic clicks.

Arrhythmias. Symptoms related to arrhythmias are next in prevalence to symptoms of congestive heart failure. Tachycardias or extrasystoles may be noted by the patient; light-headedness may be a complaint. With more serious arrhythmias resulting in decreased cardiac output, syncope may occur. Premature beats, particularly those of ventricular origin, are quite common. Atrial arrhythmias also may occur: atrial and AV junctional premature contractions, atrial fibrillation or flutter, and paroxysmal tachycardia with AV block. Ventricular arrhythmias represent a serious complication of cardiomyopathy. As mentioned, premature ventricular contractions are commonplace, and at times there are short paroxysms or multifocal ventricular beats. Ventricular tachycardia or ventricular fibrillation or both represent more serious complications; occasionally a patient is first seen by his physician because of ventricular tachycardia. Both atrioventricular and intraventricular conduction defects are not unusual. Careful inspection of the neck veins combined with auscultation of the heart can be helpful in diagnosis of the arrhythmia (see section on auscultation). Sudden death is a dreaded, too frequent complication of cardiomyopathy and is most likely to occur in those having ventricular ectopic beats or in those having atrioventricular conduction defects, particularly complete heart block with Stokes-Adams syncope. A particularly serious finding is that of frequent multifocal premature beats, especially if associated with congestive heart failure and significant cardiomegaly. In general, patients with arrhythmias that are detected early and who receive prompt treatment (including rest) have a more favorable prognosis than those whose disease is chronic and associated with moderate to advanced cardiomegaly. Occasionally, a patient with ventricular ectopic beats without cardiac enlargement or congestive failure will die suddenly. However, in others, with appropriate therapy, the ventricular ectopic beats disappear over a period of several weeks to several months or longer.

Some patients with cardiomyopathy are sensitive to digitalis preparations; at times, smaller than usual doses produce serious arrhythmias or conduction disturbances or both [5, 6]. Most commonly, these occur in patients having advanced myocardial disease characterized by congestive failure and cardiac enlargement. However, serious (even fatal) arrhythmias may occur in patients without cardiac enlargement or congestive failure, particularly if the "predigitalis" electrocardiogram reveals premature ventricular contractions, especially of the multifocal variety.

Chest discomfort. Chest pain of the pleuritic type may be observed in those patients with pleural or pericardial involvement; usually a viral infection is the cause. Careful physical examination often reveals a pericardial or pleural friction rub or both, indicative of acute pericarditis, pleuritis, or a combination of these. Patients have been observed in the initial stage of the disease to have clinical features of acute "benign" pericarditis with or without associated signs of myocarditis. In many, the friction rub, pericardial effusion, and signs of myocarditis completely disappear over a period of several weeks, and there are no apparent residual effects. However, in some, at a later date (usually after months to years) the features of myocardial disease become a chronic and serious manifestation of their illness [22, 23]. If one did not have the opportunity of examining such a patient initially, there would be no indication that the first signs and symptoms were those of pericarditis. Months later, the symptoms and signs become those of myocardial disease with decompensation.

In a few patients, another type of chest discomfort of the "coronary insufficiency type" may occur. This will be discussed in the section dealing with differential diagnosis of arteriosclerotic heart disease.

Embolic phenomena. Both pulmonary and peripheral arterial emboli have been common features of this disease, sometimes representing the initial manifestation [5, 6]. For example, a few patients have been admitted to the hospital with a diagnosis of cerebrovascular accident in whom the diagnosis of cardiomyopathy was overlooked initially. Systemic emboli may originate from mural thrombi in the left ventricle and left atrium. Factors favoring embolization are cardiac enlargement, congestive failure, and atrial fibrillation. Also, as in patients with right-sided congestive failure of any cause, emboli may originate in the venous system, particularly in the calf or in the pelvic veins. Embolization, whether pulmonary or systemic, is always a serious prognostic sign. However, we have seen several patients who, after a single embolic episode, have progressed quite satisfactorily. As noted previously, the prognosis depends not only on the size and location of the emboli but also on the clinical response of other features of the

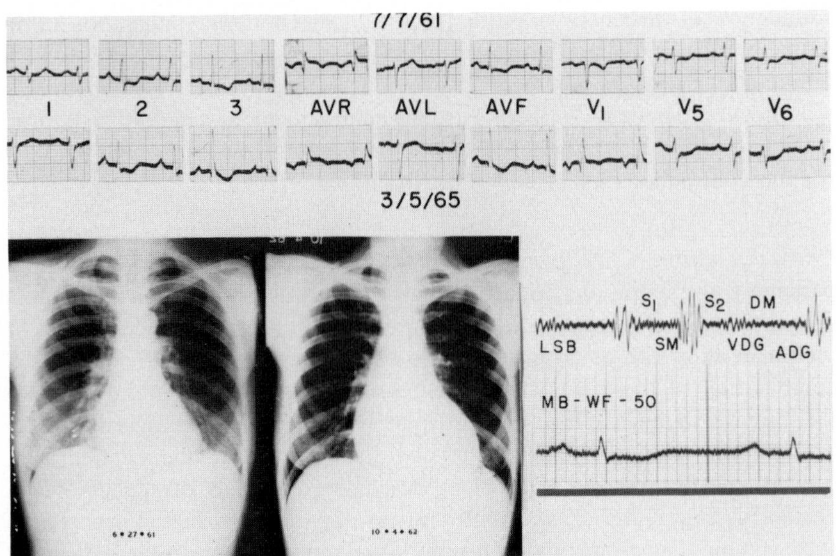

Figure 5. In 1961, this 50-year old woman presented with mild left heart failure, atrial and ventricular gallop sounds, and slight cardiac enlargement. Four years later, she developed pulmonary hypertension with dominant right ventricular failure and right ventricular hypertrophy on the ECG. Notice the atrial and ventricular diastolic gallops and the cardiac enlargement.

disease, such as congestive heart failure, arrhythmia, and heart size. Long-term treatment with anticoagulants may reduce the incidence of embolization and would appear to be appropriate (in the absence of contraindications) as part of the treatment.

Pulmonary hypertension. Patients with cardiomyopathy may eventually develop clinical features of severe pulmonary hypertension [5, 6]. If one had not observed the patient through the earlier stages of the disease, the diagnosis of primary pulmonary hypertension might be made. However, a patient with left ventricular myocardial disease may eventually develop the picture of pulmonary hypertension secondary to long-standing severe left ventricular failure. Figure 5 represents such a patient. Initially, this 50-year-old-woman had mild left heart failure, atrial and ventricular gallop sounds, and slight cardiac enlargement. Over a 4-year period, she developed progressive left ventricular failure terminating in pulmonary hypertension and right ventricular failure. Prior to her death, the electrocardiogram indicated right ventricular hypertrophy; in addition, prominent "a" waves were present in the jugular venous pulse. In a few patients, severe pulmonary hypertension followed pulmonary embolism.

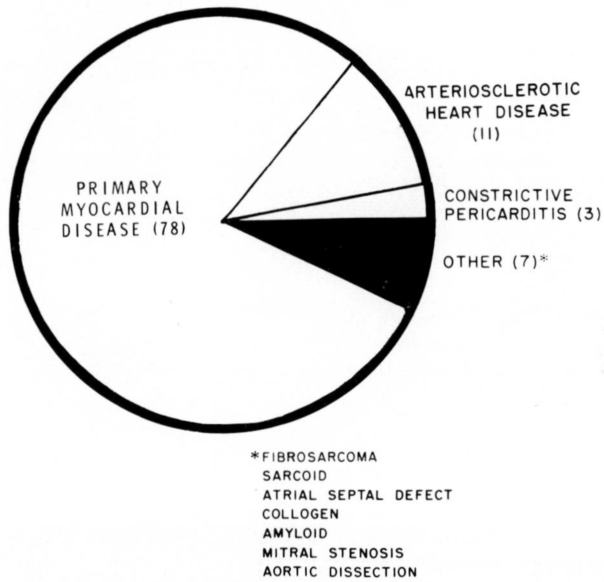

Figure 6. Cardiomyopathy. In a study of 99 patients initially believed to have primary myocardial disease, diagnosis of cardiomyopathy was established in 78 patients. (From Harvey, W.P. and Segal, J.P.: Postgrad Med 42: 145, 1967, copyright by McGraw Hill, Inc.)

DIFFERENTIAL DIAGNOSIS

Cardiomyopathy may at times be confused with other types of heart disease, including arteriosclerotic heart disease, hypertensive heart disease, acquired valvular disease, congenital heart disease, primary pulmonary hypertension, constrictive pericarditis, or pericardial effusion [5, 6, 8, 9, 24]. Figure 6 graphically presents some of the diagnostic pitfalls. Autopsies were performed on 99 patients initially thought to have cardiomyopathy; the diagnosis was correct in 78.

Arteriosclerotic heart disease. This disease has been the most common diagnostic error, particularly in male patients over the age of 40 [8, 9]. Some of the features differentiating cardiomyopathy and arteriosclerotic heart disease are listed in Table II. As previously mentioned, some patients with advanced cardiomyopathy may describe "coronary-type" chest dis-

Table II
Differentiating Features between Cardiomyopathy and Arteriosclerotic Heart Disease

Feature	*Cardiomyopathy**	*Arteriosclerotic Heart Disease*
Age	Any age	Over 40
Sex	Equal	Males predominate
"Angina pectoris"	Occasional	Frequent
"Angina pectoris" without CHF	Rare	Frequent
EKG infarction pattern	Occasional	Frequent
Infarction Pattern with normal or slightly enlarged heart	Rare	Frequent
Elevation of blood sugar, cholesterol, or blood pressure	Rare	Frequent

* Excluding obstructive cardiomyopathy.

comfort. Often, this discomfort can be distinguished from classic coronary insufficiency in that it usually occurs at the end of a fatiguing experience (rather than during effort); it may last from 30 to 60 minutes, and is frequently not completely relieved by nitroglycerin. These patients almost invariably have diffuse and extensive myocardial involvement resulting in marked cardiac enlargement, congestive failure, and serious arrhythmias. In some, the electrocardiogram may show QS deflections or small R waves, suggesting arteriosclerotic heart disease with old myocardial infarction [6, 13, 25]. These also are patients with extensive myocardial degeneration and fibrosis. A history of long-standing congestive heart failure, without definite clinical or electrocardiographic evidence of infarction would favor the diagnosis of cardiomyopathy [9]. On the other hand, if one excludes the obstructive cardiomyopathy group, a history of coronary insufficiency in a patient without congestive heart failure and with slight cardiac enlargement would favor the diagnosis of arteriosclerotic heart disease. As a practical point, the presence of any "coronary risk factor," such as hypertension, diabetes, hypercholesterolemia, or strong family history of coronary disease, would favor the diagnosis of arteriosclerotic heart disease [5, 6, 9, 10]. It must be remembered, however, that hypertension is often present in patients with cardiomyopathy in the presence of congestive heart failure, and after treatment for cardiac failure the blood pressure falls to more normal levels [9]. This sequence, at times, may be misinterpreted as evidence of chronic hypertension and may lead to the false diagnosis of hypertensive

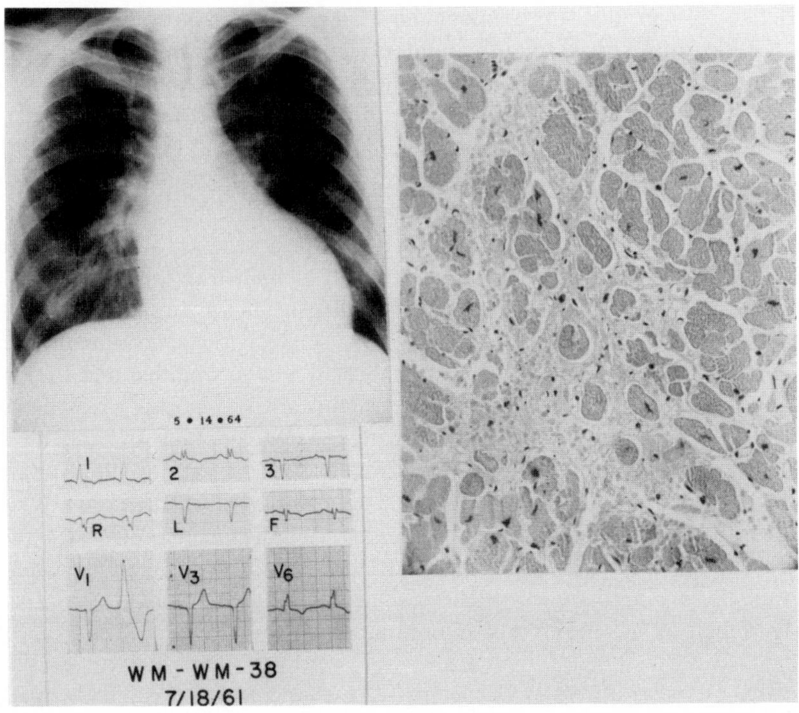

Figure 7. Congestive Failure. Thirty-eight-year-old man with no chest discomfort. Postmortem examination showed normal coronary arteries although previous coronary arteriogram reported significant narrowing. Note the left ventricular hypertrophy, left bundle branch block, and diffuse myocardial fibrosis.

heart disease. In the small minority of patients (approximately 10 percent) even after careful clinical evaluation, the differential diagnosis may still be in doubt and can only be resolved by coronary arteriography or postmortem examination. Figure 7 represents a 38-year-old man with cardiomyopathy proved at autopsy. This patient was completely evaluated at another hospital (including coronary angiography), and his condition had been diagnosed incorrectly as arteriosclerotic heart disease. His chief complaints were fatigue and dyspnea, and he gave no history of coronary insufficiency. Left ventricular enlargement was present, and the electrocardiogram showed premature ventricular contractions and left bundle branch block. Autopsy revealed diffuse myocardial fibrosis and normally patent coronary arteries.

Pericardial disease. Some patients with a "restrictive" type of cardiomyopathy have clinical features that cannot be differentiated from constrictive pericarditis. A prominent third heart sound may be misinterpreted as a pericardial knock sound, commonly heard in constrictive pericarditis. Cardiac catheterization and other laboratory procedures, including echocardiography, may be helpful in the differential diagnosis. However, in occasional instances hemodynamic findings are identical in restrictive myocardial disease and constrictive pericarditis. In patients with constrictive pericarditis, angiocardiography or echocardiography may settle the diagnosis by showing increased thickness of the pericardium; also in constrictive pericarditis, angiocardiography typically demonstrates straightening of the lateral border of the right atrium. In other instances, a definite diagnosis can be made only by surgical exploration. Acute pericarditis can progress to constrictive pericarditis over a period of weeks to months, and in some instances there may also be associated significant myocardial involvement.

At times, the heart may be greatly dilated, creating a problem by suggesting pericardial effusion. In fact, many patients with cardiomyopathy are first thought to have a pericardial effusion because of a greatly enlarged and dilated heart. In such patients, attempted pericardial aspiration yields blood from the ventricle rather than pericardial fluid. Echocardiography or angiography with radiopaque contrast medium or carbon dioxide may be helpful in settling this differential diagnosis.*

Rheumatic heart disease. Occasionally, the diagnosis of cardiomyopathy may be erroneously made in a patient with severe mitral stenosis, particularly with a calcified valve, pulmonary hypertension, and advanced heart failure (in which the opening snap is absent and apical diastolic rumble not readily discernable).

Figure 8 represents such a patient. However, the finding of broad-notched P waves on the electrocardiogram, a rightward axis deviation, and right ventricular hypertrophy, should alert the physician to the diagnosis of mitral stenosis rather than the diagnosis of cardiomyopathy. Also, because of the frequency of systolic murmurs in patients with cardiomyopathy, and atrial and ventricular gallops simulating a diastolic rumble (as already discussed), the diagnosis of rheumatic heart disease with mitral insufficiency, tricuspid insufficiency, or mitral stenosis or all three is sometimes incorrectly made. In rheumatic mitral insufficiency the murmurs generally increase in intensity as compensation occurs, whereas in cardiomyopathy the opposite may occur [8].

* *Editorial Note:* Patients with cardiomyopathy and advanced heart failure may have pericardial effusion unrelated to significant pericardial disease. In these instances echocardiography or angiography will usually show enlargement of the left ventricle and an increased end-systolic volume, but in cardiac tamponade, the ventricular end-diastolic and end-systolic volumes are small.

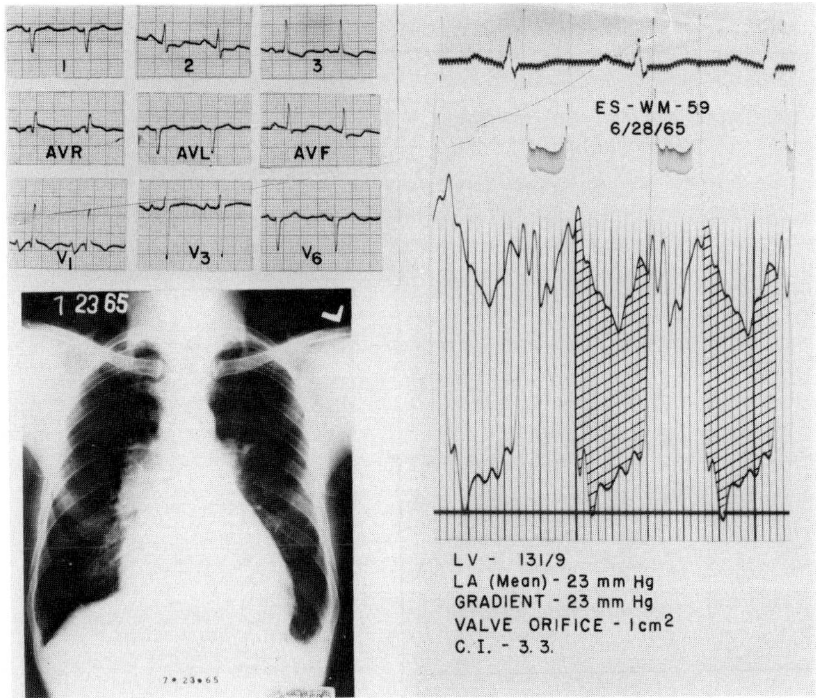

Figure 8. Tight Mitral Stenosis. Fifty-nine-year-old man initially thought to have cardiomyopathy but proved to have tight mitral stenosis. Note right ventricular hypertrophy, cardiac enlargement, and significant mitral diastolic pressure gradient (shaded area).

Congenital heart disease. Occasionally, due to misinterpretation of auscultatory findings, confusion between certain types of congenital heart disease and cardiomyopathy will occur. Figure 9 represents a patient whose condition was incorrectly diagnosed as cardiomyopathy when actually he had an atrial septal defect. The slight cardiac enlargement, increased pulmonary vascularity, and basal ejection murmur were accepted initially as evidence for cardiomyopathy. However, the presence of right bundle branch block and wide splitting of the second heart sound, together with a pulmonic ejection murmur, directed the clinical diagnosis to atrial septal defect. With improved clinical diagnostic techniques, congenital heart disease can be diagnosed correctly in the great majority of patients.

Hypertensive heart disease. Occasionally, confusion exists between cardiomyopathy and hypertensive heart disease because the blood pressure may be elevated on admission to the hospital when a patient is in congestive

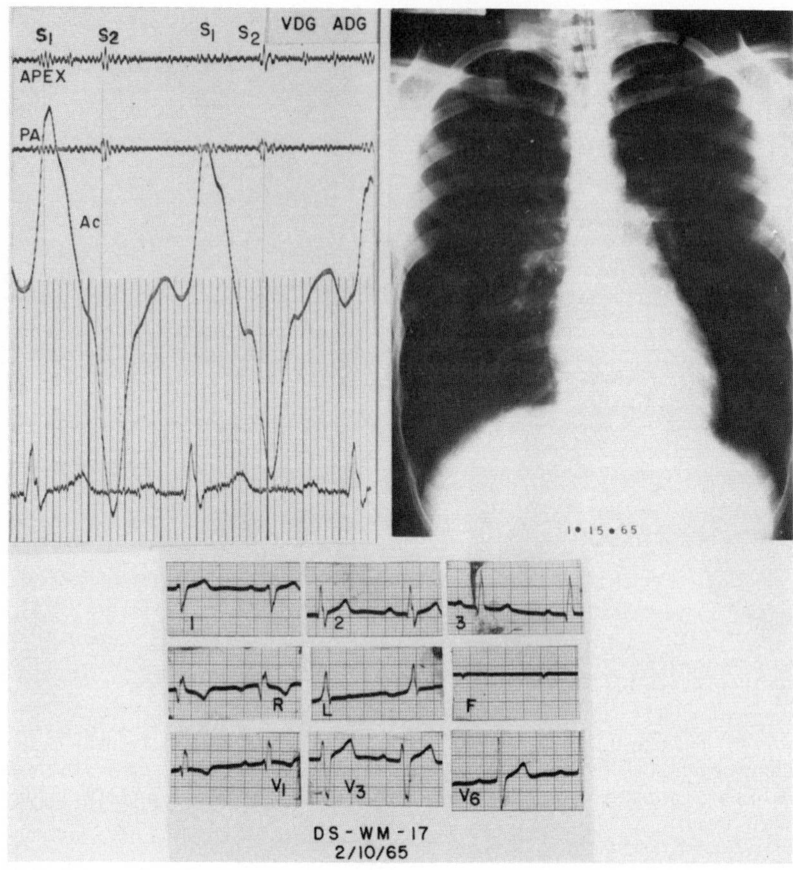

Figure 9. Atrial Septal Defect. Seventeen-year-old boy referred for cardiomyopathy but proved to have an atrial septal defect. Note atrial and ventricular diastolic gallops and right intraventricular conduction defect. A pulmonic ejection systolic murmur was heard.

heart failure [6, 9]. However, as previously mentioned, following treatment the blood pressure falls to normal levels in the patient with cardiomyopathy, whereas it is more likely to be sustained if true hypertension is present.

Occasionally, patients with cardiomyopathy will present clinical features which erroneously suggest the diagnosis of bacterial endocarditis (fever, emboli), pneumonia (pulmonary emboli), brain tumor (cerebral emboli), or even dissecting aneurysm of the aorta. Pulmonary or systemic emboli or both related to the cardiomyopathy are often responsible for producing a clinical picture that contributes to this confusion in diagnosis.

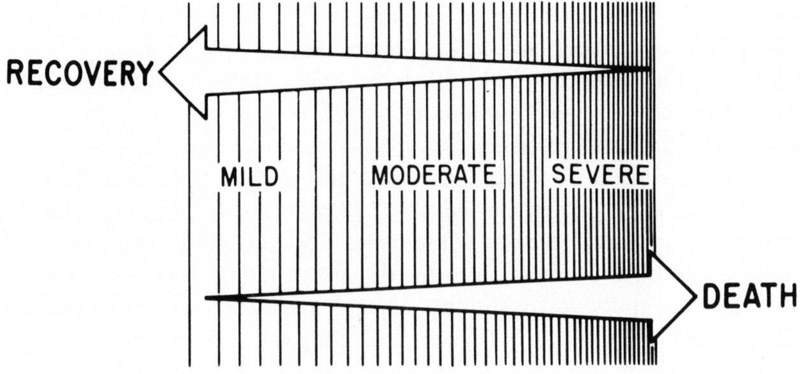

Figure 10. Spectrum of Cardiomyopathy. (From Harvey, W.P. and Segal, J.P.: Progr Cardiovasc Dis 7:17, 1964.)

Clinical suspicion and careful evaluation including appropriate laboratory tests will enable the physician to make an accurate differential diagnosis in most cases.

SPECTRUM

It should be emphasized that cardiomyopathy represents a spectrum (Fig. 10). The pathologic findings, and therefore the symptoms and signs, vary from mild to severe. Likewise, the course of the patient's disease may be mild, moderate, or severe. With mild myocardial involvement, there is more likelihood of regression of the symptoms and of recovery. On the other hand, the more severe involvement is more likely to result in death or chronic disability (Fig. 1). Frequently, intercurrent infections (even upper respiratory infections), surgical procedures, and emotional and physical stresses may precipitate exacerbation of congestive failure or arrhythmia. Some patients appear to have mild residual damage, others moderately severe or severe. It is probable, and clinically evident, that the present and subsequent symptoms and clinical features are dependent on the amount of residual damage to the myocardium. Prognosis, likewise, is also directly related. Sudden death is not rare in patients with cardiomyopathy, particularly those with many ventricular ectopic beats. Signs of a poor prognosis are chronic congestive heart failure, advanced cardiac enlargement, pulmonary hypertension, and ventricular ectopic beats (particularly multifocal premature ventricular beats, and ventricular tachycardia). If the aforementioned signs and symptoms persist in spite of adequate medical therapy, the prognosis is poor.

The "spectrum" concept has stood the test of time and should be reemphasized. The patient can have a mild myocarditis or cardiac involvement and eventually recover completely. On the other hand, the same patient might have progression of his disease resulting in significant pathologic changes in the myocardium; chronic residual signs and symptoms such as cardiomegaly, arrhythmias, and congestive heart failure may be irreversible. Those patients having severe initial involvement are more likely to have a rapid and serious clinical course. In our experience, the largest group lies between the two extremes. They demonstrate signs and symptoms of a chronically diseased myocardium, as evidenced by cardiac enlargement, congestive heart failure, and arrhythmias. However, many of these patients have been able to perform their usual occupational duties, although with some restrictions.

In patients with myocardial disease, early suspicion and early diagnosis with prompt institution of therapy may minimize myocardial damage, particularly in those with recent injury to the myocardium as occurs with acute viral myocarditis.

ACKNOWLEDGMENTS

The authors express their appreciation to Miss Jonnie Morrow, Administrative Assistant, Division of Cardiology, Miss Ruth A. Weinmann, Research Assistant, Division of Cardiology, and Mr. Bernard Salb, Medical Photographer, Department of Medical-Dental Communications, for their valuable assistance in the preparation of this manuscript.

REFERENCES

1. Blankenhorn, M.A. and Gall, E.A.: Myocarditis and myocardosis. Circulation 13:217, 1956.
2. Mattingly, T.W.: The clinical and hemodynamic features of primary myocardial disease. Trans Am Clin Climatol Assoc 70:132, 1958.
3. Mattingly, T.W.: The clinical concept of primary myocardial disease. Circulation 32:845, 1965.
4. Goodwin, J.F., Gordon, H., Hallman, A., and Bishop, M.B.: Clinical aspects of cardiomyopathy. Br Med J 1:69, 1961.

5. Segal, J.P., Harvey, W.P., and Gurel, T.: Diagnosis and treatment of primary myocardial disease. Circulation 32:837, 1965.
6. Harvey, W.P., Segal, J.P., and Gurel, T.: The clinical spectrum of primary myocardial disease. Progr Cardiovasc Dis 7:17, 1964.
7. Harvey, W.P. and Segal, J.P.: Primary myocardial disease. Postgrad Med 42:145, 1967.
8. Friedberg, C.K.: Symposium: Cardiomyopathy. Circulation 64, 935, 1971.
9. Fowler, N.O.: Differential diagnosis of cardiomyopathies. Progr Cardiovasc Dis 14:113, 1971.
10. Fowler, N.O.: Classification and differential diagnosis of the myocardiopathies. Progr Cardiovasc Dis 7:1, 1964.
11. Woolford, R.M., Postpartum myocarditis. Ohio State Med J 48:924, 1952.
12. Burchell, H.B.: Unusual causes of heart failure. Circulation 21:436, 1960.
13. Massumi, R.A., Rios, J.C., Gooch, A.S., Nutter, D., DeVita, V.T., and Datlow, D.W.: Primary myocardial disease: Report of fifty cases and review of the subject. Circulation 31:19, 1965.
14. Bengtsson, E. and Lamberger, B.: Five-year follow-up study of cases suggestive of acute myocarditis. Am Heart J 72:751, 1966.
15. Editorial: Mumps of the heart. Br Med J 1:187, 1966.
16. Ablemann, W.H.: Current concepts: Myocarditis. New Engl J Med 275:832, 1966.
17. Silber, Earl, N.: Respiratory viruses and heart disease. Ann Intern Med 48:228, 1958.
18. Harvey, W.P. and Perloff, J.K.: The auscultatory findings in primary myocardial disease. Am Heart J 61:199, 1961.
19. Editorial: Myocarditis. Lancet 1:883, 1967.
20. Rafferty, E.B., Banks, I.C., and Oram, S.: Occlusive disease of the coronary arteries presenting as primary congestive cardiomyopathy. Lancet 2:1147, 1969.
21. Harvey, W.P.: Auscultation is obvious—Or is it? Med Times 99(3):48, 1971.
22. Woodward, T.E., Yasuski, T., Yu-Chen, L., and Hornick, R.B.: Specific microbial infections of the myocardium and pericardium. Arch Intern Med 120:270, 1967.
23. Editorial: Nonrheumatic myopericarditis. Br Med J 2:544, 1971.
24. Fowler, N.O., Gueron, M., and Rowlands, D.T.: Primary myocardial disease. Circulation 13:498, 1961.
25. Stapleton, J.F., Segal, J.P., and Harvey, W.P.: The electrocardiogram of myocardopathy. Progr Cardiovasc Dis 8:217, 1970.

WILLIAM C. ROBERTS, M.D.
and VICTOR J. FERRANS, M.D., PH.D.

Morphologic Observations in the Cardiomyopathies

If "cardiomyopathy" is defined as any disease affecting myocardium, then coronary arterial narrowing from atherosclerosis is the most common cause of myocardial disease, with systemic hypertension (causing hypertrophy of the myocardial fibers) second, and rheumatic heart disease third. Obviously, nothing is gained by defining "cardiomyopathy" so broadly because practically every cardiac disease affects the function or structure of myocardium. Therefore, *cardiomyopathy* is defined herein as a condition affecting primarily the myocardium unassociated with significant narrowing of the extramural coronary arteries, or systemic hypertension, or anatomic valvular heart disease, or congenital malformation of the heart and vessels, or intrinsic pulmonary parenchymal, or vascular disease. Although differentiation between cardiomyopathy and coronary heart disease—at least at necropsy—would appear easy, most adults in the Western Hemisphere have some atherosclerotic plaquing of the coronary arteries. To what degree may the lumens of the extramural coronary arteries be narrowed and the diagnosis of cardiomyopathy still be appropriate? Mild degrees of systemic hypertension may occur in some patients with cardiomyopathy. To what level may the blood pressure be elevated, and for how long, and the diagnosis of cardiomyopathy still be appropriate? Although anatomic valvular disease may disallow a diagnosis of cardiomyopathy, valvular dysfunction may dominate the clinical course of a patient with cardiomyopathy and may

From The Section of Pathology, National Heart and Lung Institute, National Institutes of Health, Bethesda, Maryland.

prevent proper diagnosis. With these reservations and limitations in mind, the anatomic features of a number of the cardiomyopathies will be presented, as outlined in Table I.

Table I
Cardiomyopathies

I. Idiopathic
  A. Dilated type
    1. With alcoholism
    2. Without alcoholism
  B. Hypertrophic type
    1. With subaortic stenosis
    2. Without subaortic stenosis
II. Endomyocardial disease
  A. With eosinophilia
    1. Eosinophilic leukemia
    2. Löffler's fibroplastic parietal endocarditis
  B. Without eosinophilia: endomyocardial fibrosis of Davies
III. Infiltrative
  A. Amyloid
  B. Fibrous tissue
  C. Granuloma
    1. Sarcoid
    2. Unknown giant cell
  D. Calcium
  E. Iron
  F. Neoplasm
    1. Primary
    2. Secondary
  G. Glycogen
  H. Lipids and mucopolysaccharides
IV. Secondary or known associated condition
  A. Generalized infection
    1. Bacteria
    2. Viruses
    3. Parasites
    4. Rickettsiae
    5. Spirochetes and treponemata
    6. Fungi
    7. Type unknown

Table I (continued)
Cardiomyopathies

- B. Collagen disease
  1. Acute rheumatic fever
  2. Rheumatoid arthritis
  3. Systemic lupus erythematosus
  4. Scleroderma
  5. Dermatomyositis
  6. Polyarteritis nodosa
- C. Endocrine disorders
  1. Hyperthyroidism
  2. Acromegaly
  3. Cushing's syndrome
  4. Aldosteronism
  5. Pheochromocytoma
- D. Metabolic disorders
  1. Protein deficiency (Kwashiorkor)
  2. Vitamin deficiency
  3. Anemia
  4. Hypokalemia and hypomagnesemia
- E. Physical forces, drugs, and metals
  1. Toxins
  2. Trauma
  3. Radiation
- F. Neurologic disorder
  1. Friedreich's ataxia
  2. Progressive muscular dystrophy
  3. Myotonic muscular dystrophy

IDIOPATHIC CARDIOMYOPATHY

Dilated-type idiopathic cardiomyopathy (Congestive Type, Primary Myocardial Disease)

At necropsy, we have studied 34 patients with unequivocal idiopathic cardiomegaly of the dilated type (Figs. 1-3). In each the ventricles were dilated, the coronary arteries were free of significant luminal narrowing, the valves were normal except for possible focal thickening of the atrioventricular valve leaflets, and there was no clinical evidence at any time

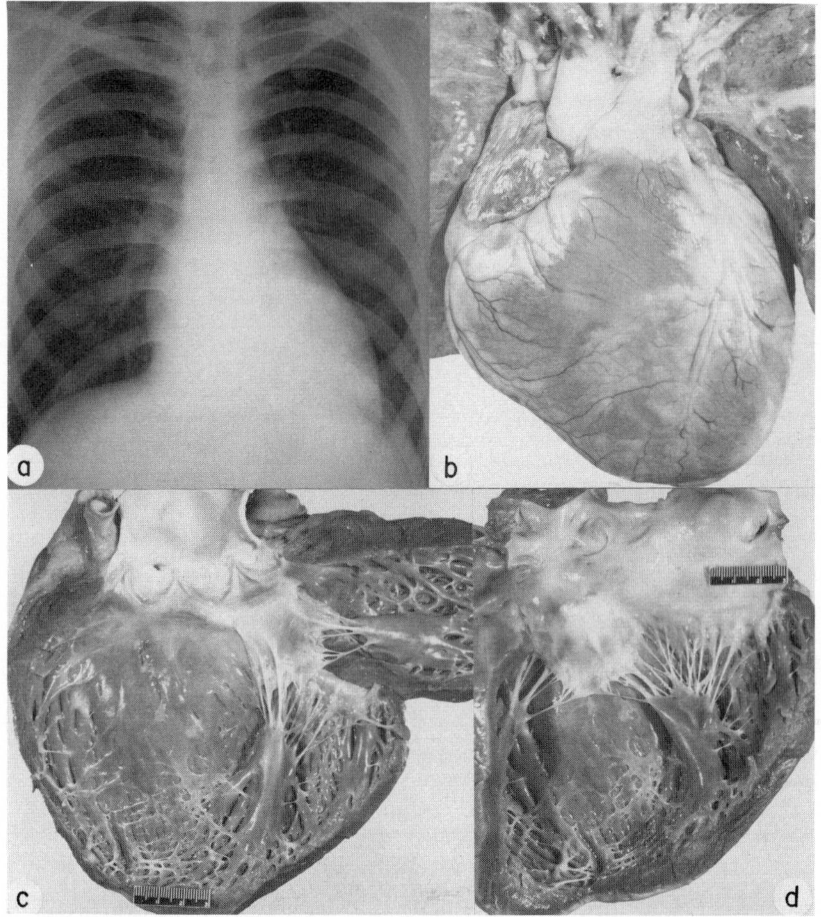

Figure 1. Idiopathic Cardiomegaly of the Dilated Type. This 22-year-old white man (A61-56) had been well until age 17 (5 years before death) when he had the onset of left inframammary pleuritic-type pain followed soon after by congestive cardiac failure. Electrocardiogram showed nonspecific T wave changes. After a 4-month hospitalization, he was entirely well with no limitation of activities until 2 months before death when an upper respiratory infection prompted overt congestive heart failure. During the next 2 months, the heart failure grew progressively worse and the heart enlarged. A grade II/VI apical systolic murmur appeared. At necropsy, the heart weighed 570 gms and both ventricles were very dilated (a-d). The valves and coronary arteries were normal. Histologic sections of left ventricular wall showed only mild interstitial fibrosis and no inflammatory cells. a. Chest radiograph during last week of life. b. Anterior aspect of heart. The pericardial sac contained 50 ml of serous fluid. c. Opened left ventricle, aortic valve, and aorta. Small focal endocardial thickenings are present. d. Opened left atrium, mitral valve, and left ventricle. The mitral annulus is not dilated.

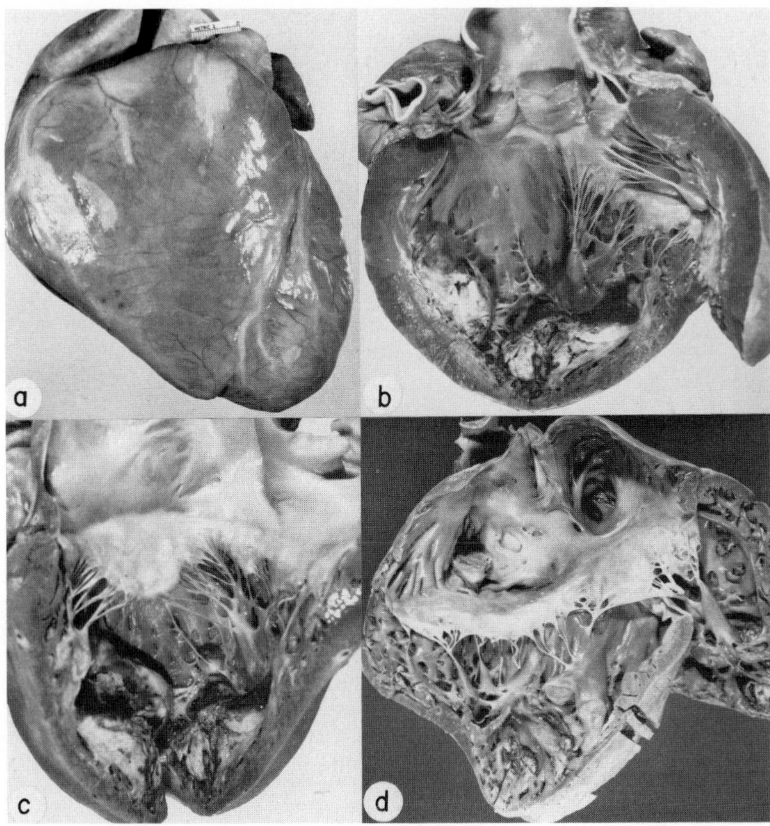

Figure 2. Idiopathic Cardiomegaly of the Dilated Type. This 36-year-old black man (A69-199) had been well until 2 years before death when evidence of congestive cardiac failure appeared. The latter gradually worsenend and various arrhythmias also appeared. He was a chronic alcoholic. Finally, pulmonary infiltrates, which proved to be secondary to pulmonary emboli, precipitated death. Radiographically, the heart was markedly enlarged. Electrocardiogram showed low-voltage, Q and T wave changes, suggesting old infarction, and intraventricular conduction defect. He never had chest pain, elevated blood pressure, or a precordial murmur. At necropsy, the heart plus the intracardiac thrombi, weighed 750 gm. "Milk spots" were present over the anterior surface of the right ventricle and at the left ventricular apex (a). Thrombi were present in the apex of both ventricles (b, c, d) and in the right atrial appendage (d). Histologically, large foci of replacement and interstitial fibrosis were seen in the left ventricular wall. Both left ventricular papillary muscles were atrophied and severely scarred. a. Heart as viewed anteriorly. The notch present at the junction of the right and left ventricular apices was considered at one time to be diagnostic of the African condition, endomyocardial fibrosis, but this is not so in this patient. b. Opened left ventricle, aortic valve, and aorta showing the large apical thrombus. c. Opened left atrium, mitral valve, and left ventricle. The mitral annulus is not dilated. d. Opened right atrium, tricuspid valve, and right ventricle showing a thrombus at the apex of the ventricle.

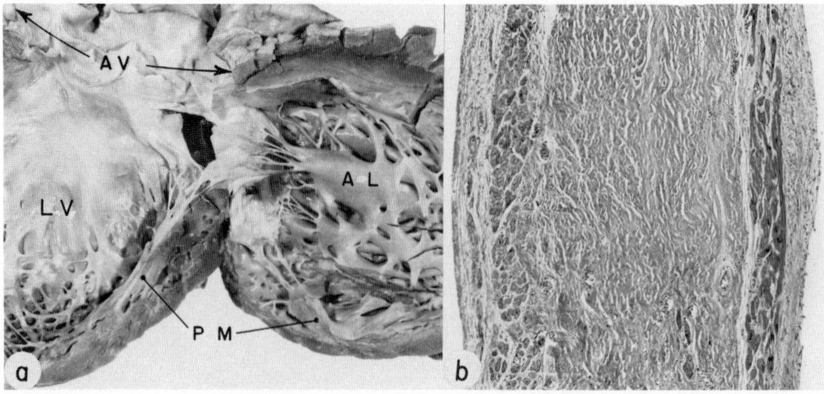

Figure 3. Idiopathic Cardiomegaly, Dilated Type. This 43-year-old black woman (A67-143) had been well until 2 years earlier when she had the sudden onset of acute pulmonary edema. Thereafter, she had repeated episodes of congestive heart failure. Although she had no precordial murmur when examined at age 39, during her last 2 years she developed a grade IV/VI pansystolic precordial murmur, loudest over the cardiac apex. She had been a chronic alcoholic for many years. Electrocardiograms showed sinus rhythm, left axis deviation, and an intraventricular conduction defect. At necropsy, the heart weighed 350 gm. Both ventricles were dilated. a. The posteromedial (PM) papillarly muscle and a portion of the left ventricular free wall beneath it were severely scarred. The anterolateral (AL) papillary muscle was normal except for being hypertrophied. b. Section through a portion of the scarred (PM) papillary muscle. This case illustrates severe papillary muscle fibrosis causing mitral regurgitation in a patient with primary myocardial disease. The coronary arteries were entirely normal.

of systemic hypertension (defined as systolic blood pressure > 140 mm Hg or diastolic blood pressure > 100 mm Hg or both). The ages of the 34 patients ranged from 15-63 years (avg. 41): The 27 male patients averaged 41 years, and the 7 women, 41 years. Nineteen patients were white and 15 were black. Twelve patients were known to be chronic alcoholics. Other family members of 4 patients had a similar cardiac condition (familial heart disease). Five patients had diabetes mellitus. Eight patients had episodic chest pains, 3 of whom clinically were believed to have had acute myocardial infarcts in the past. At necropsy, however, only 4 of the 8 had left ventricular scars and each was small. One patient, a 30-year-old man, died suddenly and unexpectedly without previous symptoms of cardiac dysfunction. His heart, known to have been enlarged for 16 years, weighed 780 gm. All of the remaining 33 patients had evidence of congestive cardiac failure, ranging from 1 to 168 months (avg. 46); 8 patients had evidence of congestive cardiac failure for more than 60 months, and 12 patients for more than 24 months. Nine patients had atrial fibrillation and 7 patients had left bundle branch block. Death in most patients was the result of progressive congestive cardiac failure, but at least 13 patients died suddenly without apparent worsening of congestive cardiac failure.

At necropsy, the hearts ranged in weight from 340 to 860 gm (avg. 586 gm): The hearts of the 7 women ranged from 340 to 860 gm (avg. 523 gm), and those of the 27 men, from 400 to 830 (avg. 602 gm). All 4 cardiac chambers were dilated in all 34 patients. The atria were less dilated than the ventricles. In some patients the left ventricular walls were thickened (> 1.5 cm), but in others the walls were of normal thickness. The greater the left ventricular dilatation, the less likely were the walls to be thickened. By histologic examination, however, the myocardial fibers were hypertrophied in all patients regardless of whether or not the left ventricular walls exceeded 1.5 cm in thickness. Intracardiac mural fibrin-platelet thrombi were found in 17 patients (50 percent). The most common location was the left ventricle (13 patients). The right ventricle contained thrombi in 5 patients, the right atrial appendage in 5, and the left atrial appendage in 1. Six patients had thrombi in more than 1 cardiac chamber. The apical portions of the ventricles, the areas between trabeculae carneae, were the locations of most ventricular thrombi, which usually were multiple. Huge thrombi were present in the left ventricle in 2 patients, and in 1 patient left ventricular outflow obstruction (24 mm Hg peak systolic pressure gradient) appeared to result from extension of the thrombus into the outflow tract. In all patients thrombus was absent in the body of each atrium. The myoendocardium beneath some ventricular thrombi was scarred. In several patients, focal endocardial thickening without superimposed thrombus was observed in the apices of the ventricles or in the atrial appendages. These lesions may have resulted from organization of fibrin-platelet thrombi. Many patients had diffuse uniform endocardial thickening of the left ventricle, usually of minimal degree, and occasionally also of the right ventricle. Foci of fibrosis were observed at gross examination in the left ventricular walls in only 11 of the 34 patients. The foci of scarring were most frequent in one or both left ventricular papillary muscles and, next, in the subendocardial portions of the free wall. In only 4 patients was there transmural scarring. By histologic examination, however, foci of fibrosis, mainly interstitial and perivascular in location rather than replacement fibrosis, were observed in the walls of the cardiac chambers of virtually every heart. Foci of necrosis and inflammatory cells were absent in the cardiac walls. Except for focal fibrous thickening of one or more leaflets of the tricuspid or mitral valves, or both, the valves were normal. The minimal focal scarring was of no functional significance. In most patients the circumferences of the tricuspid and mitral annuli were normal (< 11 cm). In patients with severe right ventricular dilatation, the tricuspid

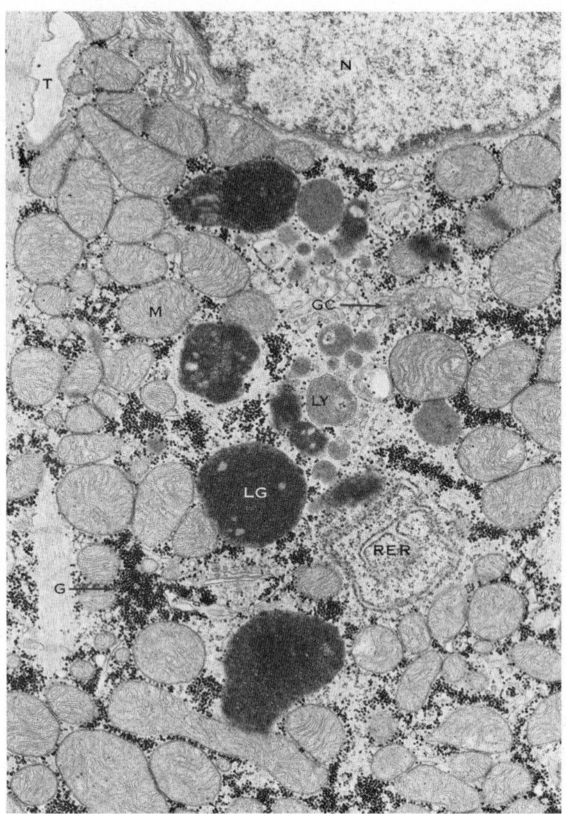

Figure 4. Idiopathic-Dilated Type Cardiomyopathy. Perinuclear area of cardiac muscle cell from a 40-year-old woman showing part of the nucleus (N), glycogen particles (G), rough-surfaced endoplasmic reticulum (RER), numerous lysosomes (LY) and lipofuscin granules (LG), Golgi elements (GC), a T tubule (T), and mitochondria (M) which vary considerably in size but are not damaged (X20,500).

valve annuli were dilated. The aorta and pulmonary trunk were usually normal in size. In most patients the extramural coronary arteries were grossly free of atherosclerotic plaques or other lesions. In the few patients in whom some atherosclerotic plaques were observed, the lumens were not narrowed more than 50 percent. No significant abnormality of intramural coronary arteries was observed in any of the 34 patients.

In addition to studying 34 necropsy patients with idiopathic cardiomegaly of the dilated type, we have examined by electron microscopy biopsies of ventricular myocardium (obtained either with a Konno catheter

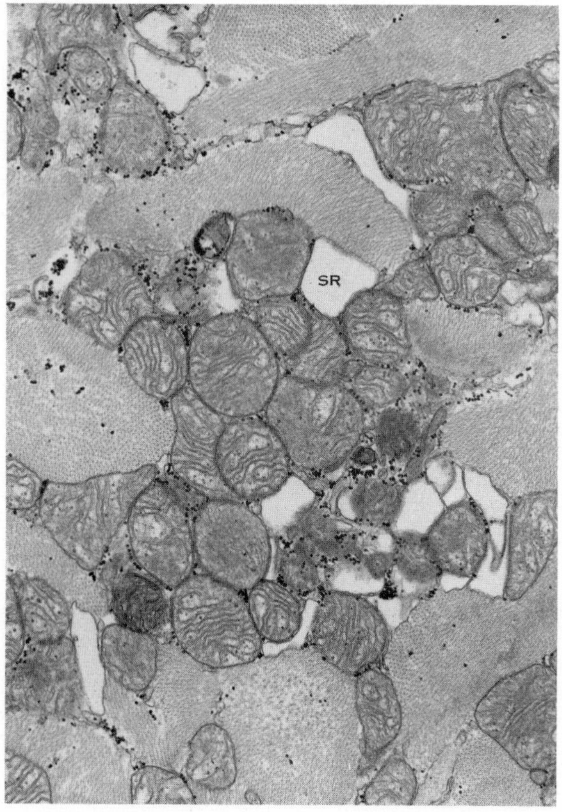

Figure 5. Cardiac Muscle Cell. This 56-year-old man had polymyositis, chronic alcoholism, and congestive cardiac failure. Specimen shows marked dilatation of sarcoplasmic reticulum tubules (SR) (×25,500).

or with a Menghini needle [1]) from 31 living patients with the same condition [2]. These biopsies showed three main types of morphologic findings (Figures 4 to 7): (1) Changes of interstitial fibrosis, that is, increased numbers of mature and developing collagen fibrils in interstitial spaces; (2) Changes of cellular hypertrophy, which consisted of increased transverse diameters of the muscle cells, increased size of nuclei and Golgi complexes, and increased numbers of mitochondria, myofibrils, glycogen granules, and free and membrane-bound ribosomes; and (3) Changes considered as probably degenerative, such as cellular edema; increased numbers of lipid droplets, lysosomes, and lipofuscin granules; dilatation of tubules of the sarcoplasmic reticulum and the T system; myofibrillar damage, and various mitochondrial alterations including mitochondrial

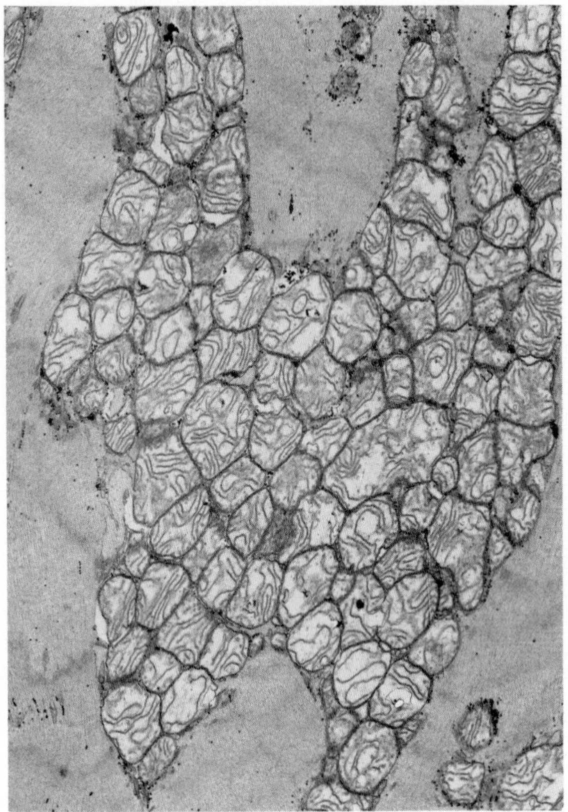

Figure 6. Idiopathic Dilated Type Cardiomyopathy. Area of myocardial biopsy from a 40-year-old man shows moderately severe mitochondrial damage, characterized by swelling, clearing of the matrices and loss of cristae (X19,000).

swelling, intramitochondrial concentric lamellae, and loss of mitochondrial cristae. In addition to these changes, the mitochondria in most patients showed a wide range of size, frequently with a predominance of mitochondria that were smaller than normal. No viral particles were found in any biopsy. Minimal abnomalities of myofibrillar orientation were observed in biopsies from only 3 of the 31 patients. Edematous and damaged myocardial capillaries were observed in biopsies from 9 patients. Morphologic findings in patients with histories of chronic alcoholism were indistinguishable from those of patients without chronic alcoholism. The degree to which degenerative changes occurred in individual biopsies generally correlated with the duration and severity of symptoms of cardiac dysfunction.

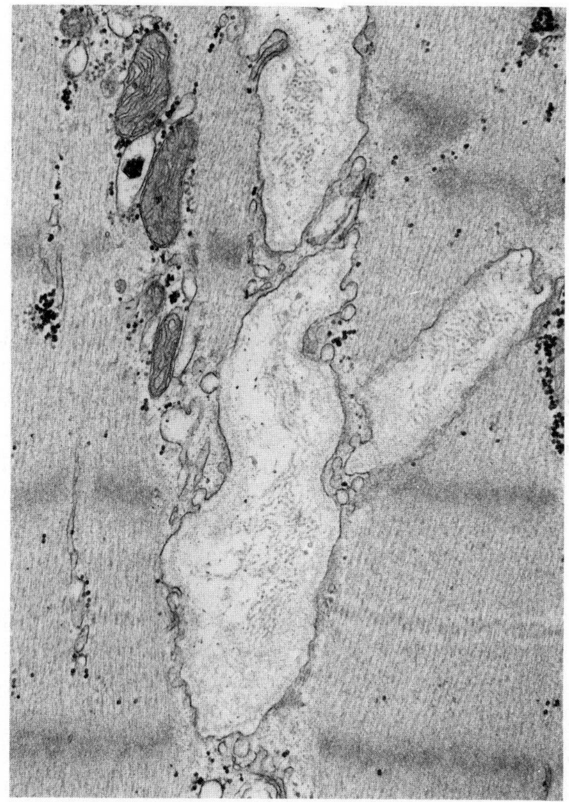

Figure 7. Idiopathic-Dilated-Type Cardiomyopathy. Markedly dilated T tubules filled with 100 to 200 Å fibrils are seen in muscle cell from chronic alcoholic 56-year-old man (X46,000).

Comments on Idiopathic Cardiomegaly of the Dilated Type

By definition, the cause of this cardiomyopathy is uncertain. If a viral or other etiology is established as the cause, the cardiomyopathy will no longer be "idiopathic," and with time it is hoped that the number of cases in the idiopathic category will decrease. This diagnosis is made by exclusion both clinically and at necropsy. Although valvular regurgitation (either tricuspid or mitral, or both) may occur, the valvular leaflets and chordae are normal except for occasional minimal focal thickening. Furthermore, although chest pain and electrocardiographic changes consistent with healed myocardial infarction may occur in this cardiomyopathy, the extramural coronary arteries must be free of "significant" luminal narrowing. But how much coronary arterial luminal narrowing is permissible before a diagnosis of idiopathic cardiomegaly is permitted? We have chosen 50 percent luminal narrowing as the upper limit. Our necropsy series would have been larger than 34 patients had we not excluded several cases because of coronary narrowing, even though at only one site, above this percentage. We also excluded from our series patients beyond the age of 65. We suspect that a number of patients included in other reported series of "idiopathic cardiomegaly" (primary myocardial disease), particularly those in the older age group, have significant narrowing of the extramural coronary arteries that was overlooked at necropsy examination.

The level of the systemic blood pressure is obviously an essential piece of information. At necropsy the heart of a hypertensive patient who had chronic congestive cardiac failure may be identical to the heart of a patient with idiopathic cardiomegaly of the dilated type. It seems probable to us that a number of patients considered to have idiopathic cardiomegaly, particularly those in the older age group, may have been normotensive during their symptomatic illness and yet may have had hypertension many years earlier. We initially had included 5 additional patients in our series of "idiopathic cardiomegaly of the dilated type," but on further examination of their older medical records found that elevated blood pressures had been recorded. Although minor elevations of blood pressure may occur in patients with idiopathic cardiomegaly and may be of little importance in its pathogenesis, we believe it better, at this stage, to exclude these cases. Other reasons for excluding patients from our idiopathic-dilated-cardiomegaly series included a previous history of poliomyelitis with cardiomegaly thereafter (1 patient), associated pulmonary parenchymal disease (excluding pulmonary emboli and infarcts) (3 patients), and congenital anomaly of the coronary sinus (1 patient). The latter patient, a 63-year-old man, was observed for several years with the diagnosis of primary myocardial disease [3]. The blood pressure had always been normal. At necropsy, the heart weighed 800 gm, the coronary arteries were virtually clean, and the valves were normal. On examination of the heart at necropsy, the ostium of the coronary sinus in the right atrium was atretic, and no drainage exit for coronary sinus blood was definitely identified. The coronary sinus and the cardiac veins draining into it were enormously dilated (varicosities of the heart). Although we are not aware of a coronary sinus anomaly of this type causing a clinical picture compatible with primary myocardial disease, this possibility cannot be excluded and, therefore, we did not include this case among our 34 patients.

Study of the myocardium in these patients either by light microscope or by electron microscope discloses only nonspecific findings. From a diagnostic standpoint, it is disappointing that the electron microscope has not been more useful in this condition. However, electron microscopic observations in idiopathic dilated-type cardiomegaly have been limited, and therefore it is possible that more specific findings will be demonstrated from further study. Our knowledge of myocardial pathology in the early stages of this disease is very limited. It is now evident, however, that once myocardial degeneration occurs, it can lead to a vicious circle of further cardiac failure and further degeneration. Progression of degenerative changes in cardiac muscle may be responsible for the clinical deterioration and therapeutic unresponsiveness of patients with advanced stages of idiopathic cardiomegaly of the dilated type. Certainly there is not enough fibrous scarring in the walls of these hearts to account for the poor cardiac function.

The intracardiac mural thrombi in idiopathic dilated-type cardiomyopathy are probably simply anatomic manifestations of relative stasis of blood within the heart as a result of extremely depressed cardiac output. The areas of greatest stasis appear to be the apices of the ventricles and the atrial appendages. On rare occasions, the left ventricular thrombi may be large enough to obstruct bloodflow within this chamber.

Although the typical heart of idiopathic dilated-type cardiomyopathy may have greatly dilated ventricles and ventricular walls of normal thickness, some patients with this condition may have relatively mild dilatation of the ventricular walls. It should be remembered, however, that some patients with pure aortic regurgitation have very thick left ventricular walls and proportionally smaller cavities. The size of the left ventricular cavity is probably proportional to the severity and duration of symptomatic congestive heart failure; the larger the cavity, the longer the symptoms and vice versa.

The dilated type of cardiomyopathy that occurs in the puerperium appears to represent a definite clinical entity [4, 5]. With the exception of fatty change in the cardiac muscle cells, which is common in patients with dilated cardiomyopathy and chronic alcoholism [6, 7] but not in puerperal cardiomyopathy, pathologic studies of the latter disorder have not revealed any changes that differ from those in patients with dilated cardiomyopathies of other causes.

HYPERTROPHIC (ASYMMETRIC) CARDIOMYOPATHY WITH OR WITHOUT SUBAORTIC STENOSIS (IDIOPATHIC HYPERTROPHIC SUBAORTIC STENOSIS (IHSS)

This section will summarize observations in 32 patients with hypertrophic cardiomyopathy studied at necropsy by the authors (Figs. 8-14). The 32 patients ranged in age from 12 to 78 years (avg. 46): twenty were

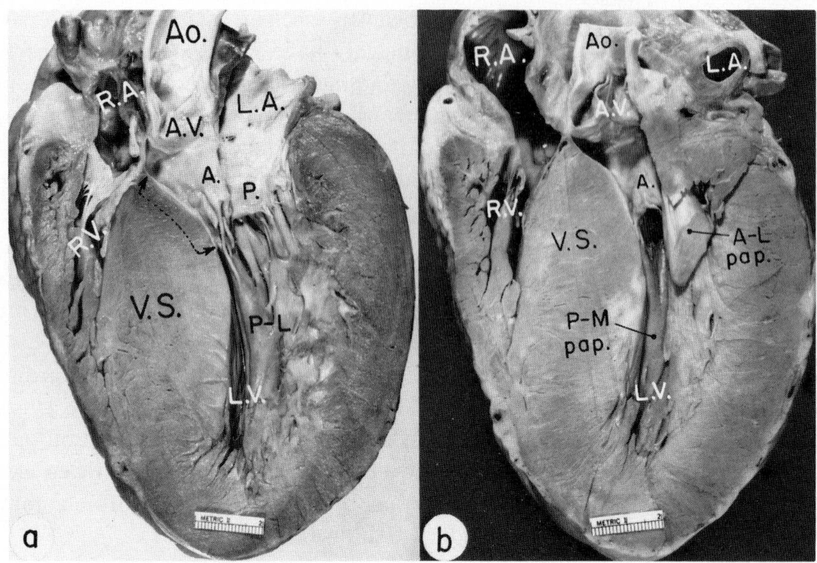

Figure 8. Hypertrophic Cardiomyopathy. a. Subaortic Stenosis. b. Without subaortic stenosis. The anterior half of each heart has been removed. In each, the ventricular septum (VS) is thicker than the left ventricular (LV) free wall. The ventricular cavities are small and slitlike. The mitral leaflets are thickened as is the mural endocardium in the left ventricular outflow tract. The aortic valve (AV) cusps are normal. RA = right atrium, RV = right ventricle, LA = left atrium, A = anterior mitral leaflet, P = posterior mitral leaflet, Ao. = aorta. Although both hearts shown here are similar anatomically, during life patient a had a 65-mm Hg peak systolic pressure gradient (PSG) at rest between left ventricle and systemic artery, and (b) had a zero pressure gradient at rest. With provocation, the PSG in a rose to 100 mm Hg, and in b a PSG of 75 mm Hg was produced. The heart shown in a was that of a 47-year-old woman (A68-191) who had angina, congestive cardiac failure, and systemic hypertension for 10 years. The heart shown in b was that of a 41-year-old woman (A67-72) who had angina, congestive cardiac failure, and systemic hypertension for 9 years. The heart in a weighed 750 gms, and the one in b, weighed 730 gms.

females; twelve were males. Other family members of 13 patients had similar cardiac conditions. Ten patients had systemic hypertension; 5, anemia (blood hematocrit < 35 percent); 8, atrial fibrillation; 9, bundle branch block (left in 3, indeterminate in 5, and bilateral in 1); and 1, complete heart block. The latter was preceded by left bundle branch block. Thirteen patients died naturally of the cardiac condition (8 suddenly; 5, progressive congestive cardiac failure); 7, after a cardiac operation; 3 from complications of cardiac catheterization; and 9 from noncardiac causes.

The 32 patients were divided into 3 groups (Table II) on the basis

Table II
Clinical and Necropsy Observations in Hypertrophic Cardiomyopathy: 32 Necropsy Patients

	Groups			
	I. With subaortic stenosis	*II. Without subaortic stenosis*	*III. No catheterization*	*Totals*
No. of Patients	14	11	7	32
+ FH of HD	4	9[f]	0	3
Ages (Yr) Range (Avg.)	18-70 (45)	12-55 (34)	49-78 (67)	12-78 (46)
Sex				
Female	9	6	5	20
Male	5	5	2	12
Length Symptoms (Yr) Range (Avg.)	4 mo-25 (9)	0-18 (7)	0-20[d] (3)	0-25 (7)
Hypertension[b]	4	1	5	10
LV-SA PSG (mm Hg) (Rest)	20-162 (93)	0	—	0-162
LV-SA PSG (mm Hg) (Provocation)	80-140[a] (104)	0-150[c]	—	0-150
Heart wt (Gm) Range (Avg.)	390-800 (580)	350[e]-1020 (563)	430-710 (518)	350[e]-1020 (582)
VS > LVFW	11	10	6	27
"Small" or Normal RV & LV Cavities	14	10	7	31
Endo plaque LVO	14	6	4	24
Thick Mitral Valve	14	6	4	24
Dilated Left Atrium	13	10	7	30
Normal Aortic Valve	11	11	7	29
No. patients with CA > 50% Narrowed	6[g]	0	0	6[g]

Abbreviations: CA = coronary artery; Endo = endocardial; FH = family history; HD = heart disease; LV = left ventricle; LVFW = left ventricular free wall; LVO = left ventricular outflow tract; PSG = peak systolic gradient; RV = right ventricle; SA = systemic artery; VS = ventricular septum.

[a] The PSG increased in each of the 7 patients provoked (by isoproterenol or Valsalva maneuver).

[b] Systematic blood pressure by cuff > 140 systolic or > 90 mm Hg diastolic or both.

[c] Of 10 patients provoked, PSG remained zero in 2 and increased 10 to 150 mm Hg in 8. In only 1 of 8, however, was the PSG with provocation > 32 mm Hg.

[d] Five of the 7 patients had no symptoms of cardiac dysfunction.

[e] Heart in a child, aged 12, not included in this total. His heart weighed 250 gms.

[f] No information available in 2 patients.

[g] Only 1 of the total 32 patients had left ventricular or ventricular septal scarring which extended through the entire wall (transmural).

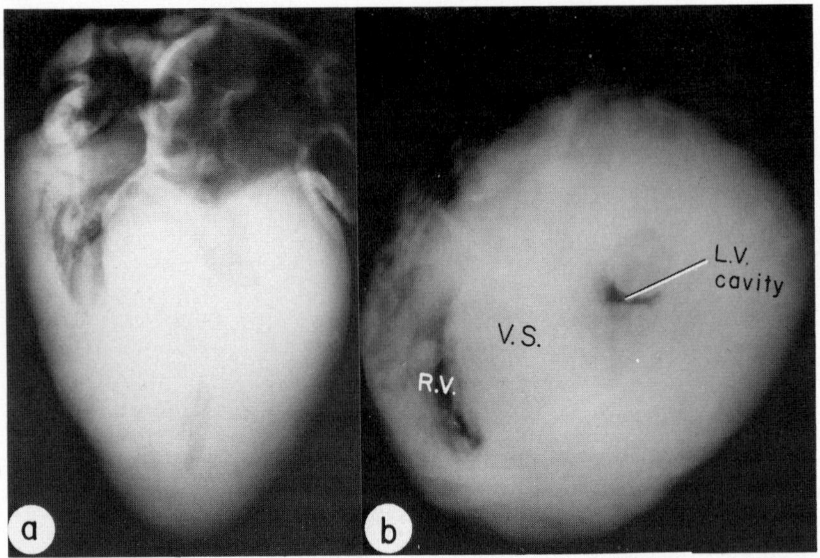

Figure 9. Hypertrophic Cardiomyopathy. Radiographs of cardiac specimens in 2 patients illustrate the extremely small left ventricular (LV) cavities which occur in this condition. A. This 36-year-old woman (A67-121) had a 75-mm Hg peak systolic pressure gradient (PSG) at rest between left ventricle and a systemic artery. B. This 41-year-old woman (A67-72) had a zero PSG at rest. Note the marked thickness of the ventricular septum (VS) and the small size of the ventricular cavity in each.

of documentation by cardiac catheterization of the presence or absence of peak systolic pressure gradient (PSG) at rest between left ventricle and a systemic artery. Fourteen patients had subaortic stenosis with PSG at rest from 20 to 162 mm Hg (average 93) (group I). Eleven patients who had zero pressure gradients at rest comprise group II; in 8 of them, however, gradients (range 10-150 mm Hg) occurred with provocation. The 7 patients in whom cardiac catheterization was not performed comprise group III. The diagnosis of IHSS was established preoperatively in 13 of 14 patients in group I, in 9 of 11 patients in group II, and in only 2 of 7 patients in group III. The fourteenth patient in group I was studied in 1956 before IHSS was recognized as a distinct entity. The other 2 patients in group II had pure mitral regurgitation believed clinically to be on a rheumatic basis. At mitral valve replacement in 1, the left ventricular wall was found to be thick and the cavity, small; IHSS, therefore, was suspected and later confirmed at postoperative catheterization. The clue to proper diagnosis of IHSS in each of the 2 patients in group III was rapidly rising systemic arterial pulses. An additional clue in 1 patient was increased

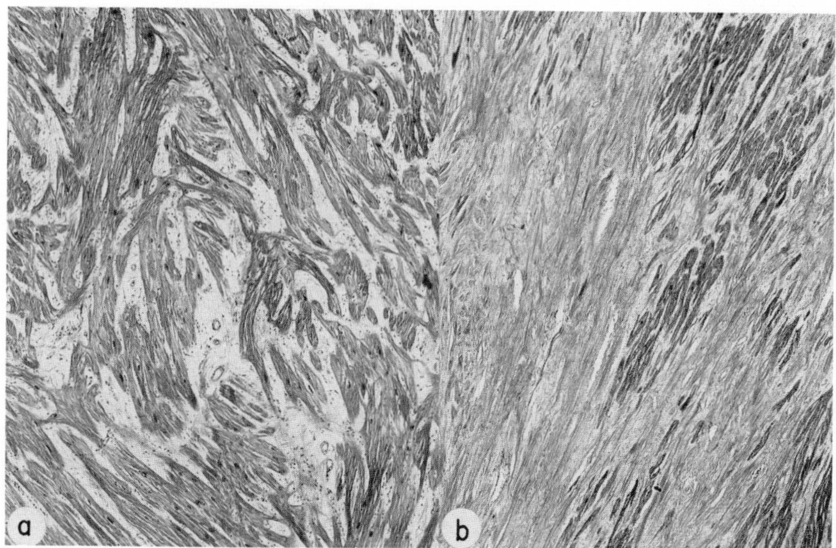

Figure 10. Hypertrophic Cardiomyopathy (A67-72). A. Photomicrographs of portions of ventricular septum showing severe derangement of orientation of myocardial fibers and increased interstitial collagen. B. Foci of replacement fibrosis also occur.

intensity of the precordial systolic murmur during the beats following premature ventricular contractions [8]. The diagnosis of IHSS in each of the 8 patients in whom this diagnosis was not established or strongly suspected clinically was made at necropsy by observing anatomic cardiac findings identical to those in patients in whom the diagnosis was established by clinical means. Six of the 8 clinically undiagnosed conditions were in group III.

The 14 patients in group I averaged 45 years of age; the 11 in group II, 34 years; and the 7 in group III, 67 years. All patients in group I had symptoms of cardiac dysfunction; 1 patient in group II and 4 in group III were asymptomatic. Whereas only 4 patients in group I had histories of similar heart disease in other family members, all 9 patients in group II in whom this information was available had positive histories. Precordial systolic murmurs ranging in intensity from grade 3/6 to 5/6 were present at some time in all 14 patients in group I. In 1 patient, however, a grade 3/6 systolic precordial murmur was audible 8 years before death when the PSG was 70 mm Hg, but when the patient was examined during the last year of life, no precordial murmur was audible. Similar murmurs occurred in 10 of 11 patients in group II, but their intensity was less (grade 3/6 in 3 patients; grade 2/6 in 4; grade 1/6 in 3). Systolic murmurs were audible

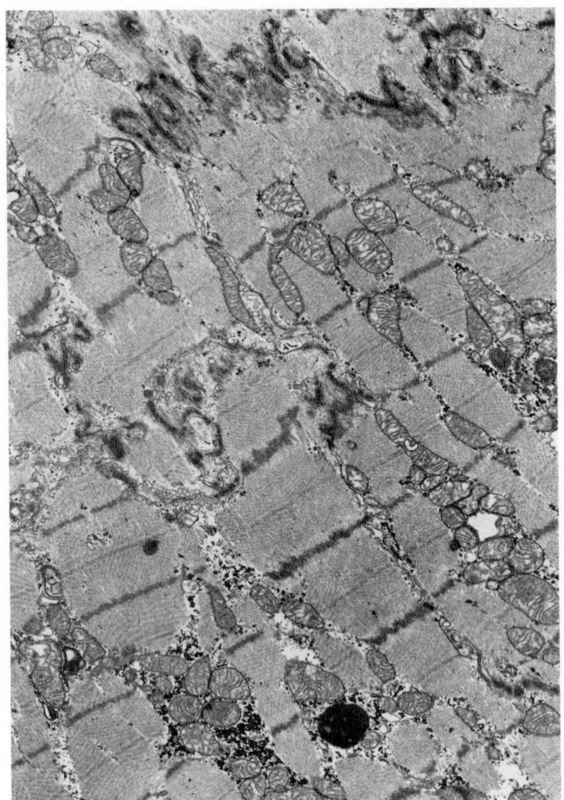

Figure 11. Hypertrophic cardiomyopathy. Part of 3 muscle cells from left ventricular outflow tract of a 30-year-old man showing normally arranged myofibrils, intercalated disc arranged end-to-end, and extensive area of side-to-side intercellular junction (×12,000).

in 6 (grade 4/6 in 1; grade 3/6 in 4) of 7 patients in group III. Three of 14 patients in group I, 4 of 11 in group II, and 1 of 7 in group III had atrial fibrillation. Of 10 patients in group I in whom left ventricular angiographic studies were performed, 4 had mitral regurgitation. Six patients in group I and 4 in group II had systolic pressure gradients between right ventricle and pulmonary artery. One of the latter patients had a 128 mm Hg PSG between right ventricular body and pulmonary artery and no PSG between left ventricle and systemic artery. His brother, however, had typical left-sided IHSS. Two patients in group I and 3 in group II had pulmonary hypertension; in only 1 patient (group I) was the pulmonary systolic pressure greater than 50 mm Hg. Three of 6 patients in group I

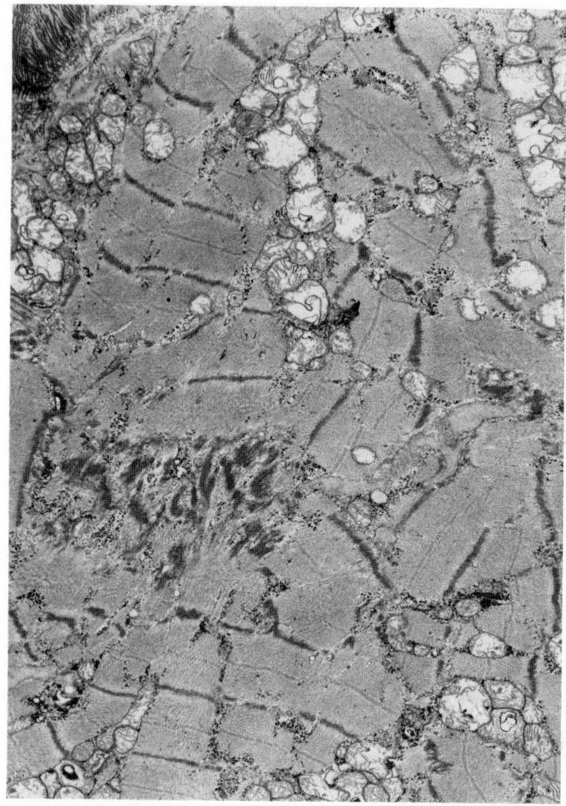

Figure 12. Hypertrophic Cardiomyopathy. Severe disorientation of myofibrils, which course in various directions, occurs in vicinity of intercalated disc from left ventricular outflow tract myocardium of 24-year-old-woman (X8,000).

and 5 of 7 patients in group II had elevated left atrial pressures; all 8 patients with elevated left atrial pressures had either mitral regurgitation or elevated left ventricular end-diastolic pressures. Nine patients in group I and 7 in group II had elevated ($\geqq$ 12 mm Hg) left ventricular end-diastolic pressures.

Necropsy cardiac observations in 32 patients are summarized in Table II. The hearts of the 31 adult patients ranged in weight from 350 to 1020 gm (avg. 582); the hearts of the 20 women averaged 511 gm, and those of the 11 adult men, 662 gm. In 27 patients, the ventricular septa were unequivocally thicker than the left ventricular free walls and in 31 patients both ventricular cavities appeared smaller than normal or normal in size. The ventricular cavities were unequivocally dilated in only

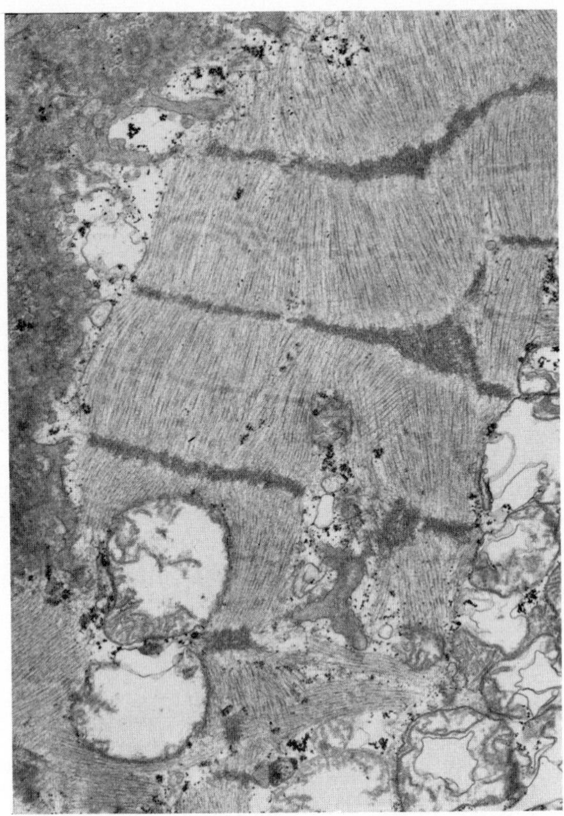

Figure 13. Hypertrophic Cardiomyopathy. Cross-weaving of myofilaments, mitochondrial damage, and asymmetric widening and splitting of Z bands are seen in left ventricular outflow tract myocardium of 39-year-old woman (X22,200).

1 patient. The mural endocardium of the left ventricular outflow tract in apposition to the anterior mitral leaflet was thickened in 24 patients. The mitral valve leaflets, particularly the anterior ones, were thickened by fibrous tissue in 24 patients. Both left and right atria were dilated in 30 patients. Except for fibromas in 2 patients and mild diffuse thickening in 1, the aortic valve cusps were normal. Foci of fibrosis were observed grossly in the left ventricular papillary muscles in 31 patients, and these structures appeared smaller than normal in all of them. Other subendocardial scars were present grossly in a number of patients. Only 1 patient had transmural fibrosis, and it was small. Except for several patients who died after cardiac operations, no foci of myocardial necrosis were present. Histologic examinations of sections of left ventricular free wall and ventricular septum

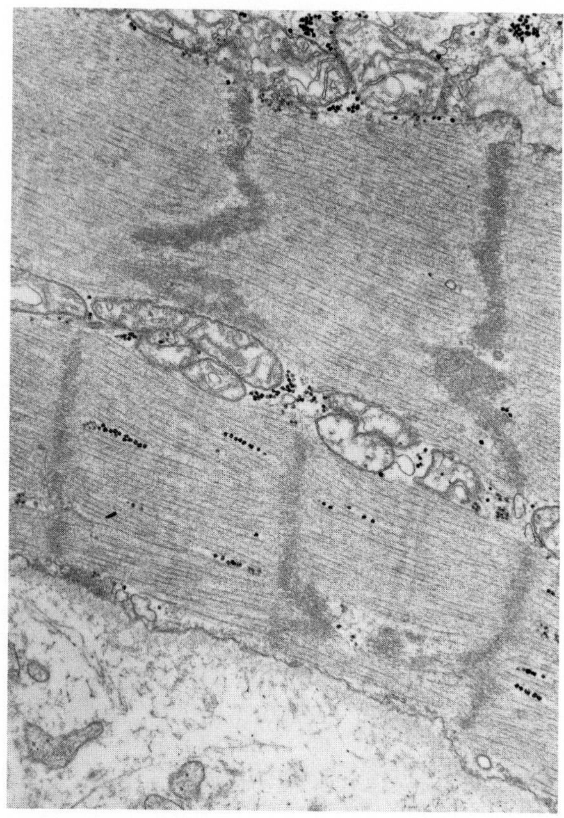

Figure 14. Hypertrophic Cardiomyopathy. Part of muscle cell from left ventricular outflow tract of 13-year-old girl shows irregular widening of Z bands and evidence of formation of new sarcomeres (i.e., incompletely separated Z band material at bottom of picture; X37,500).

disclosed interstitial and perivascular fibrosis of varying degrees in all patients and usually foci of replacement fibrosis, as well. Varying degrees of disorientation of myocardial fibers were observed in histologic sections of the ventricular septa in all 32 patients. A marked prominence of intramural coronary arteries in the ventricular septa was observed in 1 patient.

The myocardium in the left ventricular outflow tract of patients with IHSS is distinctive by light and electron microscopy. By electron microscope, Ferrans et al. [9] studied the operatively excised left ventricular outflow tract muscle in 14 patients with IHSS. Distinctive abnormalities were found in each patient. Bundles of muscle cells were severely disorganized with cells running in different directions instead of in parallel directions.

Muscle cells were wider and shorter than in cardiac hypertrophy due to other causes and showed increased cellular branching, extensive side-to-side intercellular junctions, widened Z bands, and evidence of formation of new sarcomeres. Some myofibrils were oriented obliquely or perpendicular to the longitudinal axes of the cells, and some myofilaments that originated from a single Z band inserted into Z bands of other myofibrils. Examination of left ventricular apical myocardium in 2 of the 14 patients disclosed hypertrophied but normally arranged muscle cells. The abnormal architecture of the muscle cells appears to be the basic morphologic feature of hypertrophic cardiomyopathy.

Comments on Hypertrophic (Asymmetric) Cardiomyopathy

Study of the above-described patients with hypertrophic cardiomyopathy allows delineation of characteristic anatomic features of this entity: (1) Disproportional hypertrophy of the ventricular septum; (2) Small or normal-sized left and right ventricular cavities; (3) Endocardial mural plaque, left ventricular outflow tract; (4) Thickened mitral valve; (5) Dilated left and right atria; (6) Hypertrophied free walls of all 4 cardiac chambers; (7) Normal or nearly-normal aortic valve cusps; (8) Normal-sized ascending aorta; (9) Severe abnormalities involving the organization of muscle cell bundles and the arrangement and orientation of myofibrils and myofilaments of individual muscle cells in the ventricular septum.

The major gross anatomic feature of hypertrophic cardiomyopathy is disproportional hypertrophy of the ventricular septum; that is, the ventricular septum is thicker than the left ventricular free wall. Normally, at all ages, the ventricular septum and left ventricular free wall are equal in thickness. Disproportional or asymmetric septal hypertrophy is the characteristic anatomic feature of hypertrophic cardiomyopathy. Disproportional septal hypertrophy and disorganization of the septal muscle fibers are probably the only anatomic features of hypertrophic cardiomyopathy present from birth. The other features appear secondary to these basic defects and are acquired later. Originally, it was believed that the thickest portion of the ventricular septum in this condition was that portion just below the aortic valve. Study of our 32 necropsy patients, however, clearly demonstrates that the thickest portion of the septum is about midway between the base of the aortic valve cusps and the apex of the left ventricle. The thickest portion of the septum also is usually just opposite the apex of the right ventricle. Thus, an adequate myotomy or myectomy in IHSS must include interruption or excision of myocardium located in the middle third of the septum and not just that portion close to the aortic valve.

If assymetric septal hypertrophy is considered nearly a *sine qua non* of hypertrophic cardiomyopathy, an explanation is required for the inclusion of 5 among the 32 patients in whom this feature did not occur. In all 5 patients the septum and free wall were of equal thickness. One patient, a 50-year-old woman, had undergone left ventricular outflow myotomy and myectomy 31 months earlier with total obliteration of the systolic pressure gradient. This patient clearly had disproportional septal hypertrophy before operation. Two other patients, both women, aged 33 and 46 years, respectively, had severe scarring of the ventricular septum without significant scarring of the free wall. It is probable that the scarring caused contracture of the septum. Furthermore, 1 patient had no pressure gradient at rest; the other one who, 8 years earlier, had had a 70-mm Hg peak systolic pressure gradient between left ventricle and a systemic artery and a loud precordial murmur, had no murmur when examined during her last months of life. The cause of the lack of disproportional septal hypertrophy in the fourth patient, a 65-year-old woman, is unclear. She was asymptomatic and never had evidence of cardiac dysfunction. Although she did not undergo cardiac catheterization, it is probable that she had no pressure gradient. The fifth patient, a 54-year-old woman, had no left ventricular outflow systolic pressure gradient at rest and a 25 mm Hg gradient with provocation. She was the only patient with dilated ventricular cavities, and she did not have an outflow mural plaque or a thickened mitral valve. Four of her children, however, had catheterization-documented IHSS. The heart weights in the 5 patients ranged from 370-500 gm (avg. 437), smaller average weights than those in the other 27 patients with disproportional septal hypertrophy.

The small systolic pressure gradients between right ventricular body and pulmonary trunk which occur in many patients with hypertrophic cardiomyopathy almost certainly result from severe hypertrophy of the ventricular septum, since these gradients often disappear after left ventricular myotomy with or without myectomy. The cause of the hypertrophy of the right ventricular free wall in patients with IHSS without right ventricular systolic hypertension or outflow obstruction is uncertain.

The left ventricular cavity in hypertrophic cardiomyopathy is either smaller than normal or normal in size. Most commonly, the cavity is slit-like with an S-shaped configuration. The papillary muscles actually contact one another during ventricular systole as do the anterior mitral leaflet and the mural endocardium of the left ventricular outflow tract. Fibromas, which appear to result from abnormal contact of surfaces together during ventricular contraction, were present in 2 of our patients. In one, a 19-year-old girl with a 162 mm Hg left ventricular outflow tract pressure gradient, a saccular aneurysm was present at the apex of the left ventricle.

It consisted entirely of myocardium, but its thickness was considerably less than that of the wall in other areas.

The small left ventricular cavity appears to be responsible for the thickening of the mural endocardium in the left ventricular outflow tract and also for the fibrous thickening of the mitral leaflets. It is important to recall that the mitral valve resides in the left ventricle, which being relatively small in IHSS, causes abnormal contact of the leaflets with themselves and causes the anterior leaflet to contact the mural endocardial plaque in the left ventricular outflow tract. The caudal margin of the mural endocardial plaque corresponds precisely to the distal margin of the anterior mitral leaflet. The focal fibrous thickening of the posterior mitral leaflet probably results from contact of the mitral leaflets during ventricular systole since there is not enough room in the left ventricular cavity to accommodate the leaflets and chordae easily. The ventricle and mitral leaflets in this respect may be regarded as being similar to an accordion. The mitral leaflet thickening in IHSS is somewhat analogous to that which occurs normally as a consequence of aging. With aging, the left ventricular cavity becomes smaller, presumably in response to the lowered cardiac output; the mitral leaflets, thicker; the left ventricular muscle, less compliant; and the left atrium dilates in response to increased work required to fill the small left ventricle. Similar mechanisms appear to be accelerated in IHSS.

Most patients with IHSS have some degree of mitral regurgitation. It is not related to annular dilation since the mitral annulus in this condition is smaller than normal. Furthermore, the leaflet thickening, in and of itself, is not extensive enough to cause valvular regurgitation. The most likely explanation appears to be abnormal bending of the papillary muscles, particularly the anterolateral one [10, 11] (Fig. 15). These structures may be bent abnormally by the bulging ventricular septum with resulting excessive tension on the chordae tendineae preventing closure of the mitral orifice. Although they are usually present in the papillary muscles in IHSS, focal scars cannot account for the regurgitation. Although it is usually mild in IHSS, mitral regurgitation may be the predominant clinical feature of this condition. Mitral valve replacement in IHSS is hazardous since the small left ventricular cavity is rarely capable of freely accommodating a prosthesis.

The aortic valve cusps are usually normal in patients with hypertrophic cardiomyopathy. By contrast, in discrete subaortic stenosis they are the sites of lesions produced by blood being ejected under high force and velocity through the area of narrowing, which is only about 1 cm below the base of the aortic cusps. In IHSS, the area of obstruction is farther down in the left ventricular cavity, almost certainly at the caudal margin of the left-

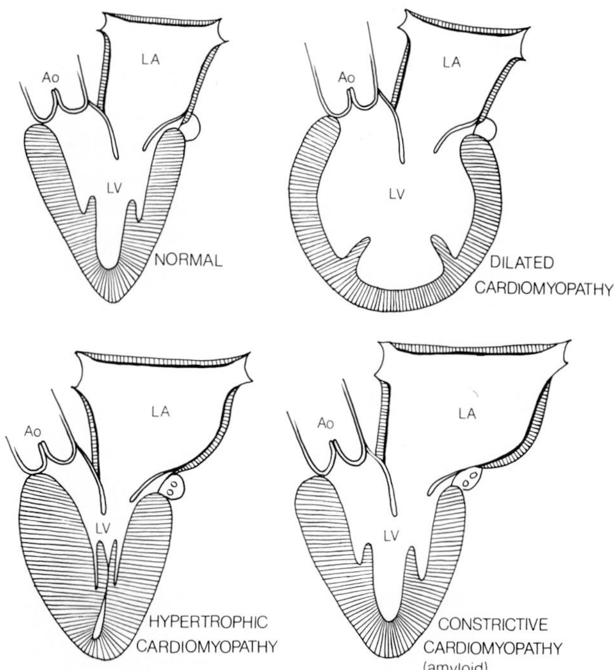

Figure 15. Cardiomyopathies. Diagram showing relative sizes of the left ventricle (LV) in the various cardiomyopathies as compared to the normal. In the dilated type, the left ventricular dilation causes the papillary muscles to be pulled laterally and caudally which may prevent the mitral orifice from closing completely in ventricular systole. In the hypertrophic type, the anterolateral and possibly the posteromedial papillary muscle is bent by the small left ventricular cavity. In amyloid heart disease, the left ventricular cavity is of normal size. LA = left atrium; Ao = aorta.

ventricular outflow endocardial plaque which corresponds to the distal margin of the anterior mitral leaflet. This site is considerably below the aortic valve cusps so that if a jet is produced, it is diffused before reaching the valve cusps.

The recent electron microscopic studies of Ferrans et al. [9] clearly demonstrate distinctive morphologic abnormalities in hypertrophic cardiomyopathy. They consist of severe disorganization of the bundles of muscle cells and of the architecture of individual muscle cells in the ventricular septum. Similar findings were not observed in the left ventricular free wall of patients with IHSS nor in the crista supraventricularis muscle of patients with tetralogy of Fallot. Abnormalities of the organization of muscle bundles and muscle cells were observed in only 10 percent of patients with idiopathic cardiomegaly of the dilated type, and in them they were minimal in degree and uncommon [2]. The biopsies in the latter patients, however, were either from the caudal portion of the right ventricle or from the left or right ventricular free walls and not from the cephalad portion of the ventricular septum as in the patients with IHSS. The disorganization of the muscle fibers in IHSS can also be detected by light microscopic examination, by which method disorganization is seldom found in subjects with idiopathic cardiomegaly of the dilated type but is observed extremely often in patients with IHSS.

ENDOMYOCARDIAL DISEASE

A cardiomyopathy of unknown etiology characterized by severe focal endocardial fibrosis of one or both ventricles, with underlying subendocardial fibrosis, and with or without associated eosinophilia, will be discussed under this heading. At necropsy, we have studied 6 patients with extensive ventricular endomyocardial fibrosis associated with severe blood eosinophilia. Two of the 6 patients were described earlier [12, 13]. Four of these patients were referred to the National Institutes of Health with a diagnosis of eosinophilic leukemia. Although one patient had a positive Philadelphia chromosome, no other features distinguished one patient from the others. We prefer to call this condition *endomyocardial disease with eosinophilia*. All 6 patients were men, aged 25 to 52 years (avg. 39). Each had had symptoms from 11 to 42 months (avg. 24). The highest leukocyte counts ranged from 79,000 to 108,000 per cu mm, and the highest percentage of eosinophils on differential smear of peripheral blood ranged from 35 to 90 percent. Although greatly increased in number, the eosinophils appeared structurally normal in each patient. Each had overt right- and left-sided congestive cardiac failure, which was the dominant clinical feature in each patient and usually the cause of death. At necropsy, the hearts weighed 420 to 530 gm (avg. 472). All 4 cardiac chambers were mildly dilated, and the walls of all 4 chambers were mildly thickened. The endocardium in the left ventricular inflow tract and apex was markedly thickened by dense fibrous tissue in each patient, and this fibrosis, devoid of elastic fibrils, was overlaid by fibrin-platelet-leukocyte-erythrocyte thrombi in every patient. Right ventricular apical endocardial scars were present in every patient, and in 2 they extended cephalad toward the tricuspid valve in the inflow portion of this chamber. Mural thrombi overlay these right ventricular fibrous plaques in 2 patients. The left ventricular myocardium immediately beneath the fibrous plaques showed some degree of replacement and interstitial fibrosis in each patient, but in all patients the myocardial scarring was limited to the inner half of the wall (subendocardium). No right ventricular myocardial scarring was observed. Eosinophilic leukocytes, usually few in number, were found in sections of heart. In 2 patients several intramural coronary arteries were plugged by fibrin-platelet thrombi with resulting foci of myocardial necrosis. Except for 1 patient with extensive coronary arterial atherosclerosis, the extramural coronary vessels were normal. No patient had had clinical evidence of acute myocardial infarction, but 1 patient had had systemic hypertension at one time. The liver (weight 1800 to 2800 gm [avg. 2200]) was enlarged in all 6 patients, but the lymph nodes were not prominent. Splenic weights were available in only 4 patients since splenectomies had been done elsewhere in 2. The splenic weights in the 4 patients were 480, 560, 560, and 1500 gm. The weights were definitely greater than those in patients with idiopathic cardiomegaly of either the dilated or hypertrophic types. Several organs, including the lungs, contained emboli with infarcts.

In addition to the 6 American patients with endomyocardial disease and eosinophilia described above, one of us (WCR) has examined the hearts of 24 patients who died in Kampala, Uganda, with endomyocardial fibrosis (EMF) without significant eosinophilia.* To our knowledge, none had peripheral blood eosinophilia greater than 15 percent. Their ages (known in 17 of the 24) ranged from 3 to 50 years (avg. 27); 3 patients were older than 40, and 6 were younger than 21. Of 16 patients in whom the sex was known, 11 were males, and 5 were females. The length of duration of symptoms of cardiac dysfunction (known in 16 patients) ranged from 2 weeks to 24 months (avg. 7 months).

At necropsy, the hearts were usually only mildly increased in weight, ranging from 370 to 500 gm. Endocardial plaquing (fibrous tissue devoid of elastic fibers) was present in the left ventricle in all 25 patients: In 14 it was severe; in 5, moderate; and in 5, mild. Right ventricular endocardial plaquing was present in 18 and absent in 6 patients; in 9 it was severe; in 2, moderate; and in 7, minimal. Thus, endocardial fibrosis involved both ventricles in 18 (75 percent) of the 24 patients. The endocardial fibrosis was located almost exclusively in the inflow tracts of the ventricles and when the plaquing was severe, it extended from the ventricular apices to beneath the posterior mitral or posterior and septal tricuspid valve leaflets. When the endocardial scars were mild, they were usually limited to the ventricular apices. The configuration of the heart, that is, the size of

* Through the courtesy of Dr. J.N.P. Davies and Dr. Monica Bishop at Albany, New York. Dr. Davies, whose name should be attached to this entity [14], brought these specimens to Albany when he moved there from Kampala, Uganda.

the various cardiac chambers and of the pulmonary trunk, depended primarily on which ventricle contained the largest deposits of endocardial scar tissue or superimposed thrombi or both. When the amount of endocardial plaquing was severe in the left ventricle and absent, mild, or moderate in the right ventricle, the heart usually had the appearance of a mitral stenotic heart; that is, the left atrium, pulmonary trunk, right ventricle, and right atrium were dilated; the left ventricular cavity was small, being constricted by the extensive endocardial scarring. The left ventricle in this situation appears to be noncompliant and acts to some extent as an impediment to flow. The mitral lesion in this circumstance, however, is not stenotic unless another disease (i.e., rheumatic) coexists, but the mitral orifice in EMF is frequently made incompetent by the mural endocardial fibrosis which adheres to the undersurface of the posterior mitral leaflet causing the latter to be immobile. When the right ventricular endocardial scarring is more severe than that in the left ventricle, the right ventricle acts as an impediment to flow. The right atrium is dilated, at times to giant proportions (1 of the 24 patients), the right ventricle is usually constricted, and the left atrium and left ventricle remain more or less normal in size. This type heart may be viewed as the tricuspid incompetent one. When the amount of endocardial plaquing is similar in both ventricles, each atrium becomes quite dilated and the ventricular cavities usually remain small or at least not dilated.

Although it is usually confined to the inflow tract, on rare occasions, the ventricular endocardial plaquing in EMF may extend into the left ventricular outflow tract as it did in 1 of the 24 patients, and it also may be present in the atria. In 1 of the 24 patients both atria contained large endocardial plaques. Infective endocarditis appears to be a frequent complication of EMF. Three of the 24 patients had superimposed bacterial endocarditis of the mitral valve, causing rupture of several chordae tendineae in each patient.

Comments on Endomyocardial Fibrosis with and without Eosinophilia

In 1936, Löffler described 2 patients with "fibroplastic parietal endocarditis with blood eosinophilia" [15]. During his lifetime Löffler saw only 2 patients with this condition which bears his name. From 1936 to 1957, 24 other patients with this condition were reported [12], and in the same year Bousser summarized clinical and pathologic findings in 13 patients with "eosinophilic leukemia" reported between 1944 and 1956 [16]. Since then "Löffler's fibroplastic parietal endocarditis with blood eosinophilia" and "eosinophilic leukemia" have been described [17] in many other patients. Each of these conditions is characterized by endocardial fibrosis of one or both ventricles and severe blood eosinophilia. Death is usually the result of congestive cardiac failure. From examination of previous reports and our 6 necropsy cases, it appears that the clinical and pathologic findings in patients with eosinophilic leukemia and Löffler's endocarditis are similar, and that these two conditions are indeed the same disease. Whether or not this entity deserves to be called leukemia remains unclear. One of our 6 patients had the Philadelphia (Ph 1) chromosome, a finding believed to be diagnostic of chronic granulocytic leukemia. Although greatly increased in number, the eosinophils in all 6 patients appeared normal morphologically: an observation quite at variance with the usual concept of leukemia. The enlargement of the liver and spleen in these patients is out of proportion to that found in most patients with congestive cardiac failure and tends to support the concept that this entity is in the leukemic category.

Certain similarities also exist between endomyocardial fibrosis of the African (EMF) and endomyocardial fibrosis with eosinophilia, described by others as Löffler's endocarditis or eosinophilic leukemia. The mural endocardial thickening in the ventricles is seen in both conditions. Recently, blood eosinophilia has been emphasized as a feature of EMF. In his initial report of 36 patients, Davies [18] mentioned that "they sometimes show an eosinophilia for which none of the causes of eosinophilia account." Of 40 necropsy patients with EMF studied by Ive and associates [19], 17 (43 percent) had eosinophilia (absolute count > 1000 per cu mm or differential count > 20 percent of the total leukocyte count). Davies speculated that the earliest lesion in EMF is infiltration of myocardium by round cells and eosinophils leading to necrosis of the endocardium and subendocardial myocardium. Thrombi form over the necrotic areas. As the mural thrombi and necrotic cardiac tissue become organized, the inflammatory cells disappear, and only dense fibrous tissue remains. In a recent study of the hearts of 16 patients who died from EMF, Connor et al. [14] found excessive amounts of acid mucopolysaccharide (AMP) in the endocardium and inner myocardium, and these authors suggested that this was "a fundamental and possible unique change" in EMF. These authors did not mention eosinophilic cell infiltration in EMF, but indeed these cells may be absent or rare in cases of Löffler's endocarditis or eosinophilic leukemia [12, 13, 15].

It appears that some patients with EMF may have eosinophilia and that others may not. In his initial report, Löffler emphasized that eosinophilia is inconstant and may disappear. It is possible that the presence or absence of eosinophilia is dependent on the length of the illness.

An attractive hypothesis is the possibility that Löffler's fibroplastic

ENDOMYOCARDIAL DISEASE AND EOSINOPHILIA
A Clinical and Pathologic Spectrum

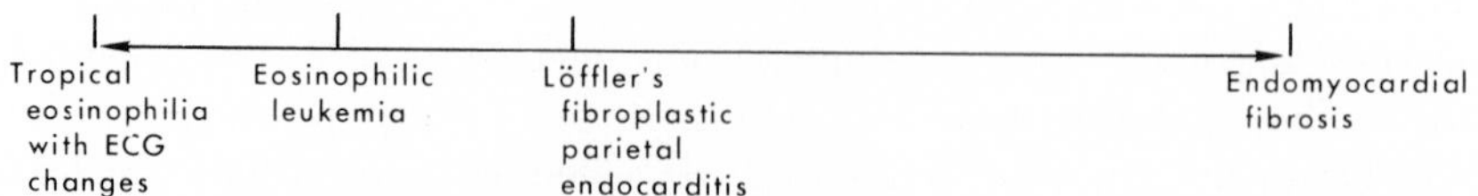

Figure 16. Endomyocardial Disease. Diagram illustrating spectrum of endomyocardial disease with and without eosinophilia. See text for explanation.

parietal endocarditis, eosinophilic leukemia (without abnormal myelopoiesis), and EMF of Davies are the same disease at different stages of development (Figs. 16-18). Patients with eosinophilia associated with a transient benign febrile illness, such as tropical eosinophilia or Löffler's pneumonia, may represent one end of the spectrum. Patients with severe EMF and no blood eosinophilia may represent the other end. Between these two extremes, there may be patients who still have eosinophilia but less extensive endocardial scarring. The latter process is still active and thus eosinophilia is still present; but as the inflammatory process dies down, cardiac scar tissue remains and eosinophilia disappears.

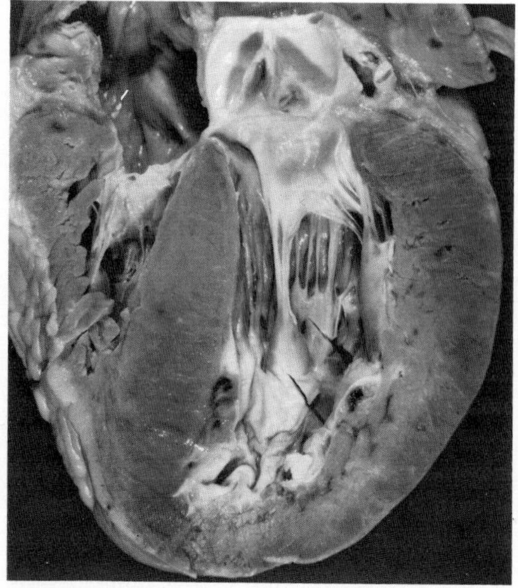

Figure 17. Endomyocardial Disease and Eosinophilia. Longitudinal section of ventricles in a 46-year-old man (A71-250) who died after a complicated illness of 42 months. He had progressive congestive cardiac failure, leukocytosis (96,000 white blood cells per cu mm) with 90 percent eosinophils on peripheral blood smear. He also had murmurs typical of aortic stenosis and regurgitation. At necropsy, the heart weighed 520 gms; large endocardial plaques were present in the apex of the left ventricle (shown here), and small ones, in the apex of the right ventricle. No intracardiac thrombi were present. (This patient was studied and cared for clinically by Dr. Sheldon Wolff, Clinical Director, National Institute of Allergy and Infectious Diseases.)

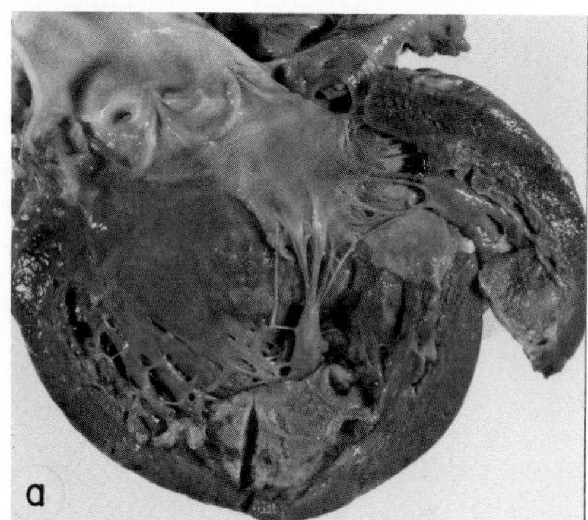

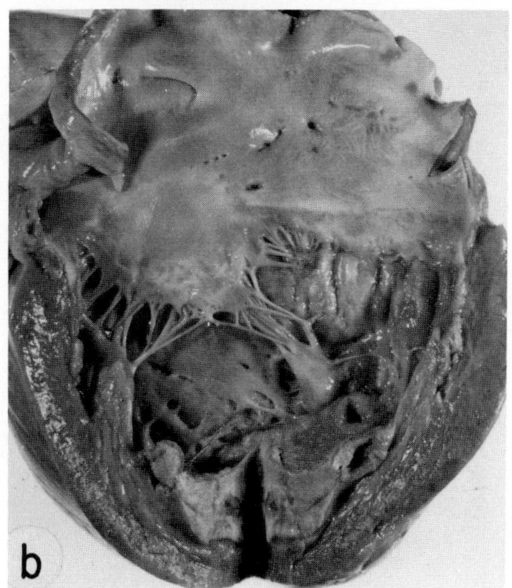

Figure 18. Davies' Endomyocardial Fibrosis of the African. a. Opened left ventricle, aortic valve, and aorta. b. Opened left atrium, mitral valve, and left ventricle. A large thrombus is present over the left ventricular apex and the posterior mitral leaflet is adherent to the underlying mural endocardium. The process involves the endocardium of the entire inflow portion of the left ventricle. The presence of the large thrombus and the absence of dense endocardial fibrous tissue probably indicates that the process in this patient was of relatively recent onset. (The photographs were given to one of us (WCR) by Dr. Gregory T. O'Connor, who spent 2 years in Kampala, Uganda.)

INFILTRATIVE CARDIOMYOPATHIES

These include various infiltrates into the walls of the cardiac chambers. The infiltrates may be localized to myocardial interstitium (amyloid, granulomas, neoplasms, acid mucopolysaccharides) or within myocardial cells (calcium, iron, glycogen and lipids). Some infiltrates, like calcium, may involve both interstitium and myocardial fibers.

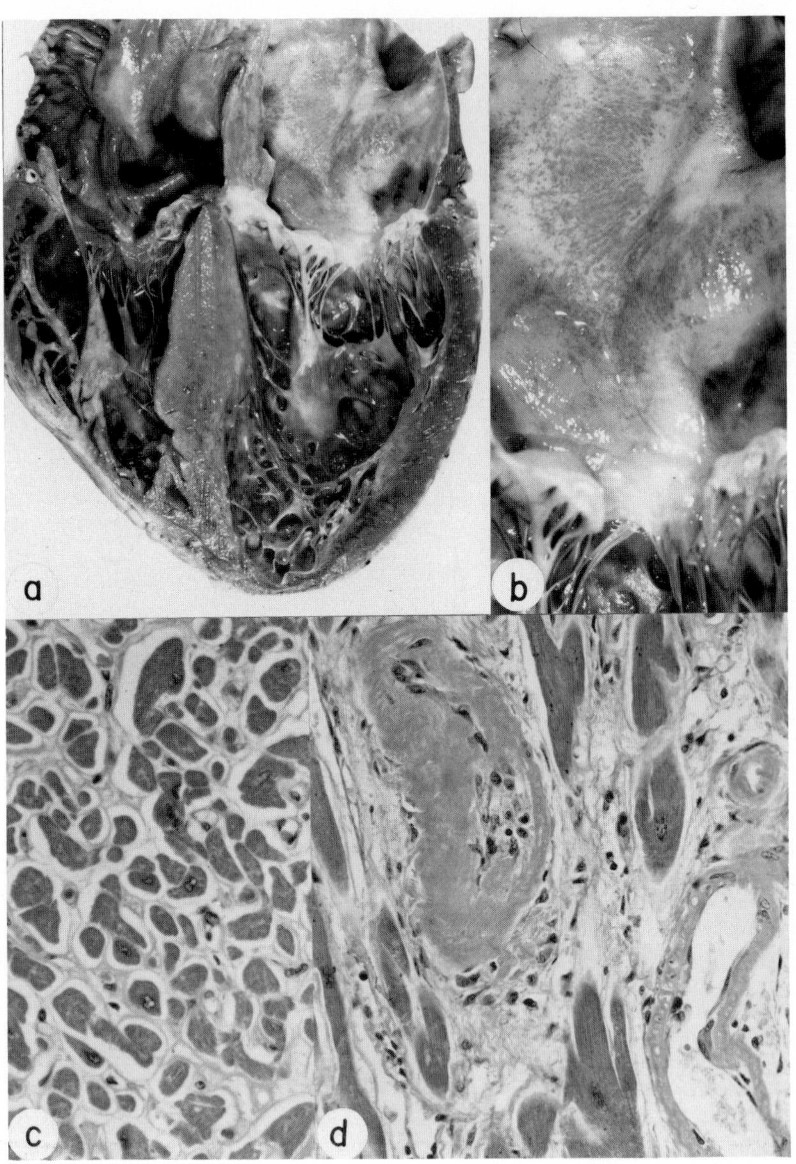

Figure 19. Cardiac Amyloidosis. a. Posterior half of the heart in an 86-year-old-man (A68-18) who had angina pectoris and congestive cardiac failure. The ventricular walls are firm and contained extensive focal fibrous scars as well as large amyloid deposits. b. Close-up of the left atrial endocardium. The wavy lesion on this endocardium represents amyloid deposits and is indicative of extensive ventricular amyloid deposits. c. Photomicrograph of interstitial deposits in the left ventricle of a 54-year-old man with severe congestive heart failure secondary to cardiac amyloidosis (X392). d. Intramural coronary artery in the same patient showing extensive amyloid deposits in its wall. Hematoxylin and eosin stains; X392 (c), X250(d).

Amyloidosis

At necropsy, we have studied 18 patients with cardiac amyloidosis (Fig. 19) extensive enough to cause cardiac dysfunction during life. Fifteen were described elsewhere [20]. The 18 patients ranged in age from 21 to 89 years (avg. 59 years): 12 were men and 6 were women. Fifteen patients had congestive cardiac failure; in none was the failure lessened by administration of digitalis. Conduction disturbances or arrhythmias developed in 11 patients, in 10 of them while they were receiving digitalis. Each of the 3 patients without congestive cardiac failure had gastrointestinal disturbances and peripheral neuropathy. Congestive cardiac failure was the cause of death in 15 of the 18 patients. Although 3 patients had histories of elevated blood pressure in the past, none had systemic hypertension during the last 3 months of life. Electrocardiograms disclosed low voltage (sum of the total R and S wave voltage in leads I, II, and III $\leqq$ 1.5 mv) in 15 patients, and patterns simulating old anterior myocardial infarction (poor R wave progression in leads V_1-V_3) or inferior myocardial infarction (Q wave in leads II, III, and aVF) in 12 patients. Chest radiographs showed cardiomegaly in 15 patients. None, however, had massive cardiac enlargement. Two patients had clinical and hemodynamic findings suggesting constrictive pericarditis, and 1 underwent thoracotomy for planned pericardiectomy.

In 14 patients amyloidosis was not associated with another systemic disease (*primary amyloidosis*), and in 4 patients another systemic disease (multiple myeloma) was present (*secondary amyloidosis*). In 16 patients amyloid was present in many body organs (*systemic amyloidosis*), and in 2 patients amyloid was present only in the heart (*isolated amyloidosis*). In 4 patients more than 1 family member had amyloidosis (*familial amyloidosis*); each had peripheral neuropathy, and 3 had vitreous opacities. The diagnosis of amyloidosis was established during life by biopsy in 13 of the 16 patients with systemic amyloidosis.

At necropsy, the hearts weighed 370 to 700 gm (avg. 498 gm). The ventricular myocardium in each patient was firm, rubbery, and noncompliant. Histologically, amyloid was present in each heart between many myocardial cells. Focal small deposits of amyloid, replacing areas of myocardium, also were found in most hearts. Both left ventricular papillary muscles of all 18 patients contained amyloid. The sinus node or atrioventricular bundle, or both, showed amyloid in 5 of 8 patients in whom these tissues were examined. Tan, waxy-appearing focal deposits of amyloid were visible grossly in the endocardium of both right and left atria of every patient and also in ventricular endocardium of 12 patients. One or more cardiac valves in each patient contained amyloid, but the deposits did not appear to impair valvular function in any patient. Amyloid occurred in the adventitia and media of intramural coronary arteries and veins of every patient, and in half of them the lumens of the intramural coronary vessels were narrowed by intimal amyloid deposits. Four patients had severe (> 75 percent) narrowing of the extramural coronary arteries by old atherosclerotic plaques, but no intimal amyloid deposits were found in these arteries. In 2 patients, however, small amyloid deposits were observed in the media of extramural coronary arteries. In Congo red preparations, the amyloid deposits stained orange and showed green birefringence. The deposits were metachromatic when stained by crystal violet. By electron microscopy, (1 patient) the cardiac amyloid deposits consisted of non-branching fibrils 80 to 130 Å (avg. 100) in diameter.

The above data and those of others indicate that amyloid in the heart must be extensive to produce cardiac dysfunction. The hearts which function improperly because of amyloid infiltration have firm rubbery non-compliant ventricular walls. Although the ventricular walls are firm, the ventricular cavities are usually not dilated.* The atria, however, usually are dilated, and the enlargement of the cardiac silhouette in this condition may well be related to the atrial dilatation rather than to the ventricular wall thickening. Most symptomatic patients with cardiac amyloidosis have congestive cardiac failure unresponsive to digitalis therapy, electrocardiographic low QRS voltage, and conduction or rhythm disturbances. The latter are particularly common after digitalis administration, which may be contraindicated in this condition. The diagnosis of clinically significant cardiac amyloidosis should be questioned in the absence of congestive cardiac failure and electrocardiographic low voltage.

Granuloma (Giant Cell Myocarditis)

Granulomas with giant cells have been observed in myocardium in a number of conditions (Table III). We have found giant cells in myocardium at necropsy in 14 patients (Table IV) excluding cases of acute rheumatic fever. The most common associated condition was infective endocarditis (4 patients), active in 2 [21, 22, 23], and healed in 2. Two patients had coronary heart disease, and another had systemic hypertension; the cause of the granulomas in these 3 patients is unknown. Two patients had rheumatoid arthritis with rheumatoid nodules in myocardium and endocardium [24, 25]. One patient had panarteritis causing pulseless disease in addition to granulomatous myocarditis [26]. Two patients had

* Cardiac amyloidosis thus joins hypertrophic cardiomyopathy (IHSS) and constrictive pericarditis as a cause of congestive cardiac failure not associated with ventricular dilatation.

Table III
Conditions Associated with Giant Cells in Myocardium

1. Infection
   a. Tuberculosis
   b. Parasites
   c. Fungi
   d. Spirochetes (syphilis)
2. Systemic noninfectious diseases
   a. Sarcoidosis
   b. Wegener's granulomatosis
   c. Panarteritis (pulseless disease)
3. Rheumatic heart disease or acute rheumatic fever
4. Rheumatoid arthritis
5. Coronary heart disease
6. Hypertensive heart disease
7. Thymoma and/or myasthenia gravis and/or myositis
8. Idiopathic

probable sarcoidosis, and in the other 2 no other associated disease was present (idiopathic). In the latter 4 patients, the number of myocardial granulomas were extensive (3-4+/4+), whereas in the other 10 patients the myocardial granulomas were sparse and small (1-2+/4+). In the 2 patients with probable sarcoidosis, granulomas also were found in other organs. In the 2 patients with idiopathic giant cell myocarditis, other organs were not available for examination. In each of the 2 patients with idiopathic giant cell myocarditis, the infiltrates focally extended through the entire thickness of the left ventricular free wall (Fig. 20). In 1 of the 2 patients with sarcoidosis, granulomas completely replaced both left ventricular papillary muscles and much of the free wall beneath them (Fig. 21). This patient came to medical attention shortly before death with pure mitral regurgitation from papillary muscle dysfunction [10].

It is evident from this and other reports that there are many causes of giant cells in the myocardium. Idiopathic giant cell myocarditis affects all ages without predilection for sex or race. Congestive cardiac failure, arrhythmias, and sudden death are common, and often the conducting as well as the working myocardium are extensively damaged. At the other end of the spectrum are patients who die from other conditions, and who are found to have giant cells in myocardium, at necropsy. The number of myocardial giant cells in the latter group of patients is usually small and of no functional significance. Patients with giant cells in the myocardium often also have giant cells in other organs or tissues.

It is difficult to distinguish idiopathic giant cell myocarditis with extracardiac involvement from sarcoidosis involving the heart and other organs. Although it rarely causes death, cardiac involvement occurs in

Table IV
Giant-Cell Myocarditis: Data in 14 Necropsy Patients

Patient	*Age (Yr)*	*Race*	*Sex*	*Associated Disease*	*CHF*	*ECG*	*Mode of death*	*Myocardial Giant Cells (1+ -4+)*	*Extracardiac Giant Cells*
1	48	W	F	Negative	+	—	CHF Arrhythmia	++++	—
2				Negative	+	CHB	CHF	+++	—
3	40	W	F	Sarcoid	+	LVH	RF CHF	+++	+ (liver)
4	26	B	F	Sarcoid	+	CHB	Arrhythmia CHF	++++	+ (liver, L,LN)
5	26	B	M	IE(active)	+	AMI	AMI 2° embolus	+[b]	0
6	17	W	F	IE(active)	+	RVH, RAD	CHF	+	0
7	42	W	M	IE(healed)	+	AF, LVH	CHF	+	0
8	10	W	F	IE(healed)[a]	+	—	CHF	++	+ (L)
9	65	W	F	RA	+	LBBB ↑P-R	CHF	++	+ (L,SC)
10	73	B	M	RA	+	LAD	Sudden	++	+ (SC)
11	15	B	M	Panarteritis	0	PVC	Operation	+[c]	+ (arteries)
12	38	B	M	CAD	+	IVCD	CHF	+	+ (liver,L)
13	50	W	M	CAD	+	OMI	Operation	+	0
14	61	W	F	HCVD Cancer, uterus	0	LVH	Shock	+	0

Abbreviations: + = positive, 0 = negative; — = information not available; ↑ = increased; AF = atrial fibrillation; AMI = acute myocardial infarction; CAD = coronary heart disease; CHB = complete heart block; CHF = congestive heart failure; ECG = electrocardiogram; HCVD = hypertensive cardiovascular disease; IE = infective endocarditis; IVCD = intraventricular conduction defect; LAD = left axis deviation; LBBB = left bundle branch block; L = lung; LN = lymph nodes; OMI = old myocardial infarction; P-R = P-R interval; PVC = premature ventricular contractions; RA = rheumatoid arthritis; RAD = right axis deviation; RF = renal failure; RVH = right ventricular hypertrophy; SC = subcutaneous tissue.

[a] Complex congenital malformation of heart and great vessels also.

[b] Septic coronary embolus occluding left anterior descending artery.

[c] Giant cell arteritis also involved the coronary arteries but produced no significant obstruction.

about 20 percent of patients with sarcoidosis [27]. The non-caseating granulomas are usually located in the ventricular septum and free wall and occasionally in the pericardium. The myocardial granulomas apparently may progress to fibrous scars without residual granulomatous inflammation as exemplified in a patient studied by us. Degeneration of myocardial cells may occur also [28]. Arrhythmias, conduction disturbances, and sudden

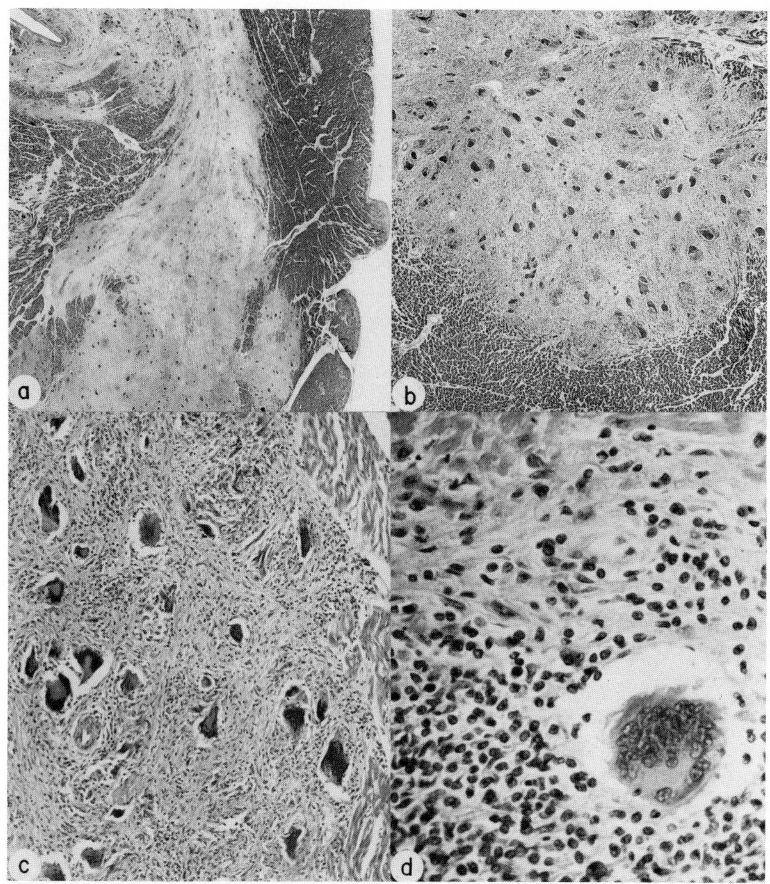

Figure 20. Giant-Cell Myocarditis, Idiopathic Type. This 49-year-old, obese, Indian woman had been well until 2 months before death when syncope appeared. When she was hospitalized, her electrocardiogram disclosed complete heart block with a ventricular rate of 32 beats per minute. The blood pressure was 140/70 mm Hg. No murmurs were audible. Chest radiograph showed moderate cardiomegaly. A month after the episode of syncope, acute pneumonia developed, shortly followed by evidence of congestive cardiac failure. Three days before death, substernal chest pain occurred and the electrocardiogram then showed changes consistent with acute myocardial infarction. Congestive heart failure persisted. Cardiac arrest followed a seizure. At necropsy, the heart weighed 430 gms. Large, white firm infiltrates were present in the cephalad portion of the muscular ventricular septum and in the anterolateral papillary muscle of the left ventricle. a, b, c, d. Histologic examination of the infiltrates disclosed them to be composed of fibrous tissue containing numerous giant cells and some mononuclear cells. Special stains for acid-fast organisms, other bacteria, and fungi were normal. The heart was the only organ containing granulomas. a. Includes full thickness of ventricular septum to show the extensiveness of the infiltrates. b, c, and d. Progressive higher power photomicrographs of the giant-cell infiltrates. Some of the giant cells contained over 50 nuclei. Hematoxylin and eosin stains: ×11, a; ×85, c; ×130, d.

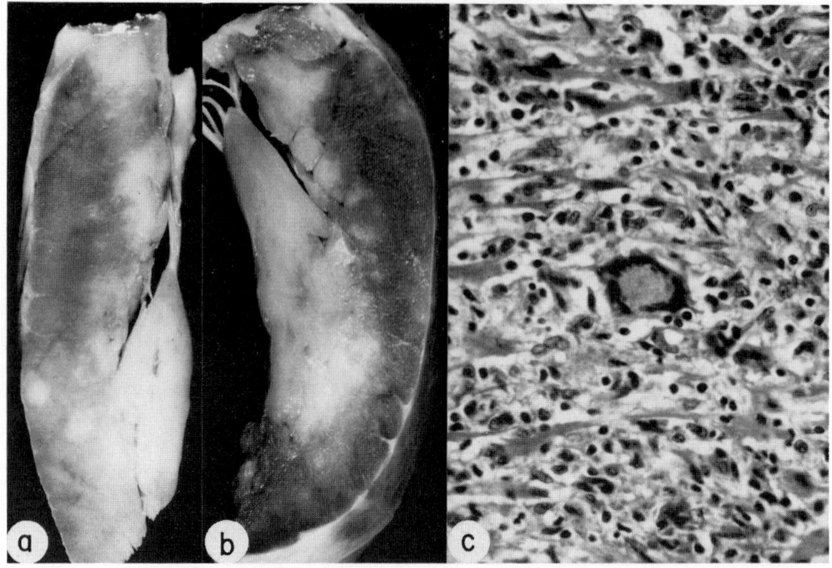

Figure 21. Giant-Cell Myocarditis Secondary to Sarcoidosis. a. Longitudinal section through the anterolateral papillary muscles. b. Posteromedial papillary muscles in a 26-year-old woman (PGGH ※ A-70-541) who had been asymptomatic until 10 days before death when dyspnea appeared. The dyspnea rapidly worsened and when hospitalized on the day of death, she was in acute pulmonary edema. The blood pressure was 80/70 mm Hg, heart rate 160 beats per minute, and a grade III-IV/VI pansystolic blowing murmur, which radiated to the axilla, was audible. Chest radiograph showed congested lungs, cardiomegaly, and prominent hilar adenopathy. Electrocardiogram showed nonspecific ST-T wave changes and atrial hypertrophy. She developed complete heart block and died shortly thereafter. a and b. At necropsy, large, firm white deposits were present in the walls of all 4 cardiac chambers and completely replaced both left ventricular papillary muscles. On histologic section, the firm white areas represented hard granulomas typical of sarcoidosis. c. Hematoxylin and eosin stain (X400). Similar hard granulomas were present in lymph nodes, liver, spleen, and lung. Stains for acid-fast organisms, other bacteria, and fungi were negative. [Kindly submitted to one of us (W.C.R.) by Dr. James Hutchinson.]

death may occur. Probably some patients previously reported as having idiopathic giant cell myocarditis actually had sarcoidosis.

Giant cell myocarditis has a varied etiology and probably represents an unusual reaction of the myocardium to antigens or stimuli of varying types. Clinically, the diagnosis of giant cell myocarditis cannot be established without myocardial biopsy; negative biopsy does not rule out this entity.

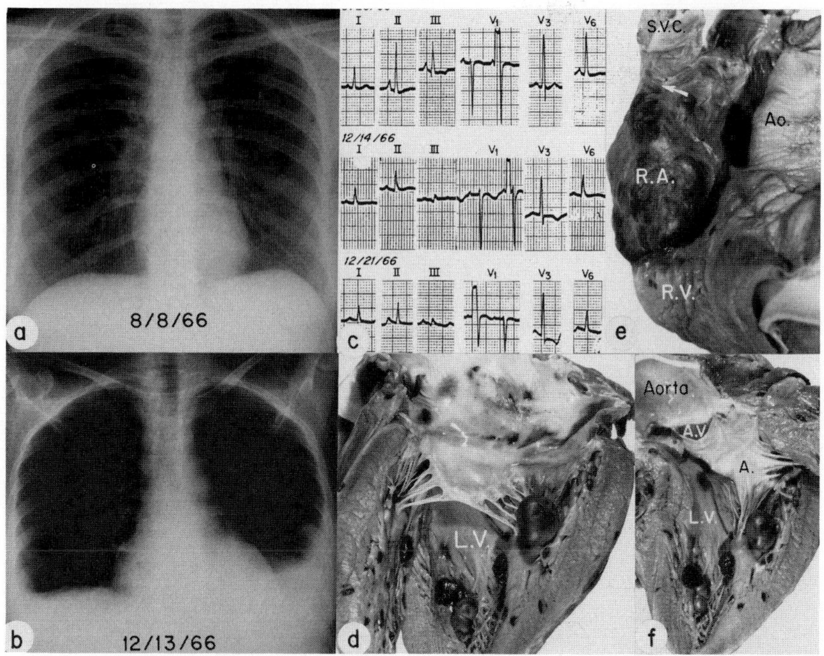

Figure 22. Secondary Tumor (Melanoma) to the *Heart*. a and b. Chest radiographs. c. Electrocardiogram. d, e, f. Heart specimen. This 25-year-old woman (A66-243) died 3 years after removal of a melanoma from the back. An intermittent atrial gallop and a systolic precordial murmur were present during the last 6 weeks of life. The electrocardiograms show sinus tachycardia, progressive decrease in QRS voltage in the limb leads, and the development of nonspecific ST-T wave changes. The chest x-ray in a is normal, whereas the one in b shows pleural and possibly pericardial effusions. These effusions were probably the result of a reaction to bis-beta-chloroethyl nitrosourea (BCNU) given 5 days earlier (17 days before death) since at necropsy no pericardial or pleural effusion were present, and the heart weighed only 240 gms. Thus, it would appear that treatment itself was the cause of failure in the patient although the intracardiac tumor nodules may have played a role. d. Opened left trium, mitral valve and left ventricle (LV). e. Opened left ventricle, aortic valve (AV), and aorta. A = anterior mitral leaflet. Several black tumor deposits are present in the left ventricle. f. Exterior of heart showing extensive tumor deposits in right atrium (RA). The arrow indicates the region of the sinus node. SVC = superior vena cava; RV = right ventricle; Ao = aorta.

Neoplasm

Through publications, many of which are case reports, neoplastic disease of the heart (Figs. 22, 23) has received far more attention than it deserves. Most tumors in the heart represent metastases from primary tumors elsewhere, the most common being in lung and breast. The majority

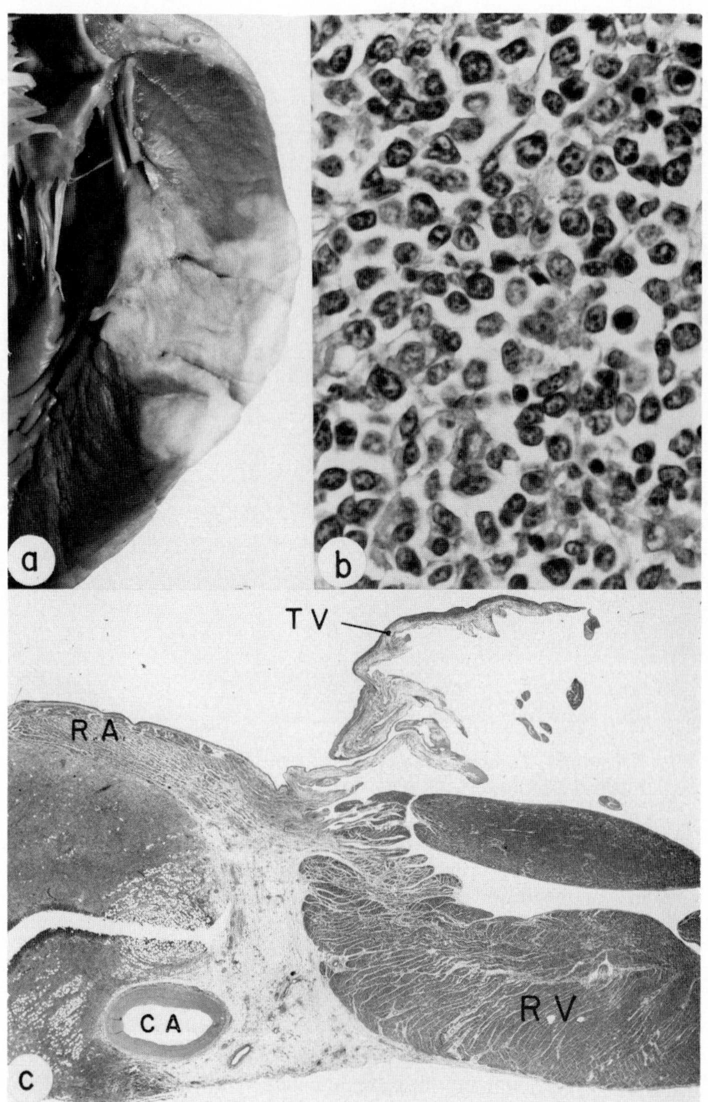

Figure 23. Secondary Tumor (Undifferentiated Lymphoma) to heart. This 59-year-old woman (A63-119) had extensive deposits of tumor in the right atrium, left ventricle, and pericardium but no signs or symptoms of cardiac dysfunction. Tumor was present at necropsy in 16 organs and tissues. A. Longitudinal section of portions of left ventricular wall showing a through-and-through tumor deposit. B. Photomicrograph of an area of tumor nodule (X628). C. Photomicrograph of a section of right atrium (RA), tricuspid valve (TV) leaflet, and right ventricle (RV) showing extensive infiltration by tumor in the adipose tissue in the right atrioventricular sulcus. CA = coronary artery. Hematoxylin and eosin stains X5 (C), X628(B).

of secondary tumors invade only epicardium (tumor limited to parietal pericardium should not be considered as involving the heart) and relatively few of them penetrate into myocardium. Secondary tumors attaching to the endocardium initially with invasion of myocardium thereafter are far less frequent, although this pathway is the usual one for tumors originating in the kidneys or adrenal glands. Primary tumors of the heart more often originate from the endocardium, the most common one being myxoma which is nearly always benign. Primary malignant tumors of the heart are rare, indeed, and usually are sarcomas.

At necropsy, one of us (WCR) has examined the hearts of 686 patients who died of acute leukemia (420 patients) [29], or lymphoma (196 patients) [30], or malignant melanoma (70 patients) [31]. Several observations which resulted from these studies may be summarized as follows. Although metastases to the heart in these 3 malignancies occurred relatively frequently (64 percent in melanoma; 37 percent in acute leukemia; 24 percent in lymphoma), symptoms of cardiac dysfunction occurred infrequently. Indeed, the frequency of dyspnea, chest pain, effusions into body cavities, precordial murmurs, ventricular gallops, edema, and electrocardiographic disturbances was similar in the patients *with* and in those *without* cardiac leukemia or lymphoma. Moreover, these clinical findings were most often the result of mediastinal, pleural, or pulmonary leukemia or lymphoma, anemia, hypoalbuminemia, or an underlying cardiac condition. Electrocardiograms were abnormal in 61 percent of 33 patients with cardiac lymphoma and in 62 percent of 104 patients with lymphoma but without tumor nodules in the heart. Controls of this type for patients with secondary cardiac neoplasms were not found in previous reports of cardiac metastases. Signs or symptoms of cardiac dysfunction could be attributed to lymphomatous involvement of the heart in only 5 of the 48 patients with cardiac lymphoma and to fewer than 20 of the 156 patients with cardiac infiltration by leukemia cells. Most patients with cardiac symptoms had extensive neoplastic involvement with hemorrhage into the pericardial sac or huge tumor deposits within a chamber or a cardiac wall. Most often, however, even huge tumor nodules in a cardiac chamber or wall were clinically silent. It is possible, however, that cardiac symptoms were masked or overshadowed by clinical manifestations resulting from tumor deposits in other body organs or tissues.

The three reports above were discussed because, to our knowledge, they were the first reports in which (1) necropsy data were obtained by reexamination of the hearts, both grossly and histologically by only one or two observers rather than accepting the information listed in the autopsy protocols; and (2) the clinical data were obtained in patients with the same neoplasm but no cardiac metastases as well as in the patients with cardiac metastases. These studies also demonstrated that many previously proposed criteria for clinically determining the presence of cardiac metastases were unreliable. In a patient with a malignant neoplasm and without previous cardiac disease, the following clinical findings strongly suggest the presence of cardiac metastases: (1) acute pericarditis, (2) cardiac tamponade or constriction, (3) rapid increase in the size of the cardiac silhouette by radiography, (4) onset of an ectopic tachycardia, (5) development of second- or third-degree atrioventricular block, and (6) onset of unequivocal cardiac failure. Cytologic examination of pericardial fluid and angiography obviously increase the accuracy in establishing a diagnosis of cardiac metastases.

Calcium

Calcium is most commonly observed in the heart in the coronary arteries, mitral annulus, aortic and scarred mitral valve cusps, in large myocardial scars, and in pericardium. In these circumstances, the calcific deposits are extracellular. This discussion, however, concerns calcific deposits within individual myocardial fibers (Fig. 24), also a frequent occurrence. Focal calcific deposits in myocardial cells are frequently observed in patients dying after periods of prolonged shock or of renal failure [32]. We have observed this lesion most frequently in patients dying after cardiac operations [33]. Its cause is uncertain although severe hypoxia is the most likely explanation, and the lesion may be produced experimentally by this means [34]. High serum levels of calcium also may be a factor. The fibers infiltrated by calcium are always necrotic. Probably, normal myocardial cells will not calcify. Thus, so-called metastatic calcification of the heart does not occur. Deposition of calcium salts into individual myocardial cells represents dystrophic calcification. When the lesions are extensive, it is probable that cardiac dysfunction may result. We have observed two hearts of patients dying with severe uremia in whom nearly every myocardial fiber was calcified. The myocardium in each felt like shark's skin. We also have observed huge deposits of calcium throughout the left ventricular wall in a 19-year-old man from Uganda. The cause was unknown. Massive myocardial calcification has been reported by others [35].

Iron

It is now clear that extensive iron deposits in myocardial cells cause cardiac dysfunction (Fig. 25). Buja and Roberts [36] studied 19 patients with cardiac iron deposits: The ventricular iron deposits were grossly visible in 9 patients, and by light microscopy only, in the other 10. Each of

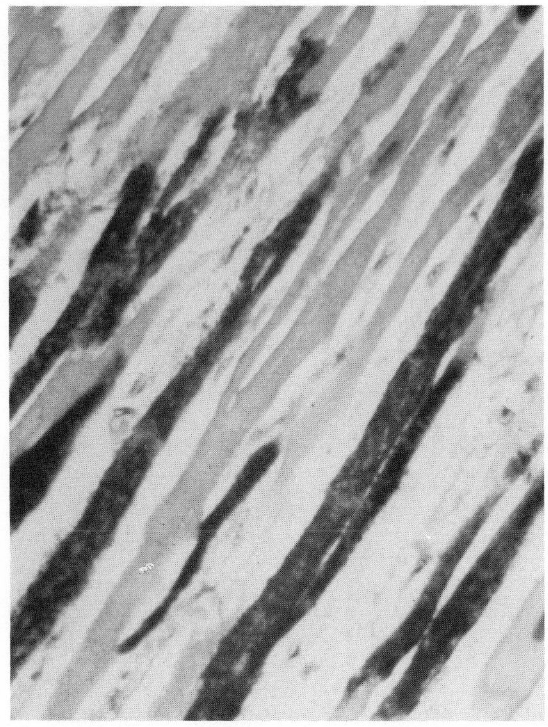

Figure 24. Myocardial Fiber Calcification. This 46-year-old woman (A66-146) died 20 days after replacement of the mitral and tricuspid valves with prosthetic valves. Preoperatively, she had a stenotic mitral valve and a purely incompetent tricuspid valve. During the entire postoperative period she had evidence of severely low cardiac output. Calcification of individual myocardial fibers was widespread at necropsy. The cause of this lesion is uncertain, but hypoxia probably plays a role in its formation. Hematoxylin and eosin stain (X187).

the 9 patients with grossly visible iron had clinical evidence of cardiac dysfunction (congestive cardiac failure in 7), whereas none of the 10 with microscopically visible iron had cardiac dysfunction. All 9 patients with grossly visible iron had abnormal electrocardiograms, mainly arrhythmias and conduction disturbances. Cardiac iron deposits were not distributed uniformly. The deposits were always most extensive in ventricular myocardium, less in atrial myocardium, and least in conducting as contrasted to working myocardium. The patients with supraventricular arrhythmias, however, had the largest atrial deposits of iron. Extensive cardiac iron deposits not only occurred in patients with idiopathic hemachromatosis but also in patients who received more than 100 units of whole blood (500 ml per unit) unless bleeding diatheses coexisted. Extensive cardiac iron

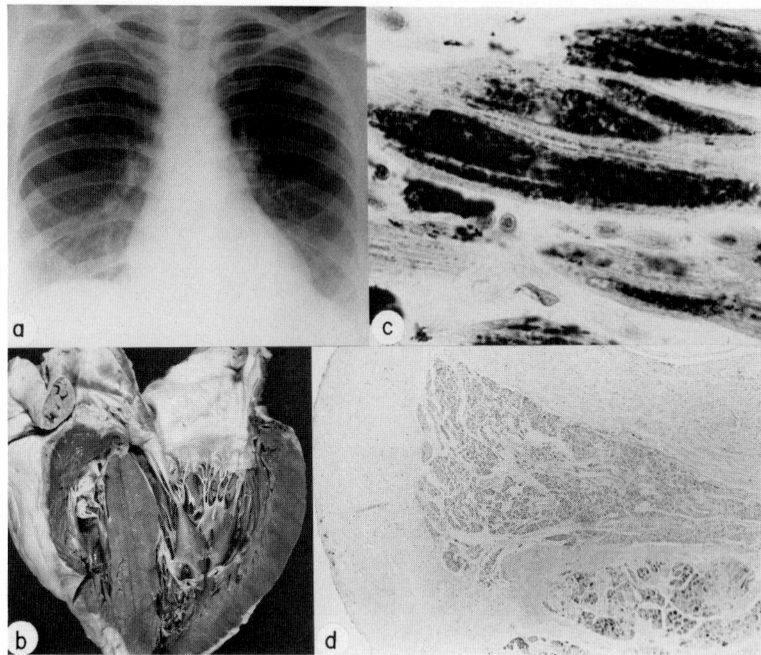

Figure 25. Cardiac hemosiderosis. This is a 42-year-old woman (A68-327) with sickle-cell anemia. She had received 260 units of blood when congestive cardiac failure developed 6 years before death. a. Chest radiograph showed cardiomegaly. By the time of death she had received 359 units of blood (90 gm iron). b. At necropsy, the walls of the right and left ventricles and left atrium were rusty brown due to extensive iron deposits. The right atrial wall in contrast was tan (b), and only minute particles of iron were present in it by histologic examination. c. Photomicrograph of several myocardial cells showing huge deposits of iron in them (Prussian blue stain, X1000). Despite large deposits of iron in working myocardium, no iron deposits were observed in conducting myocardium. d. Section of the bundle of His with no iron deposits are present in it (Prussian blue stain, X40).

deposits also occurred in patients with chronic anemia and hepatic cirrhosis who received less than 100 units of blood. The iron heart is not a strong heart but a weak one.

Glycogen

A deficiency of one or more of the enzymes involved in the biosynthesis and degradation of glycogen produces glycogen-storage disease, of which at least 8 types have been described [37]. Cardiac involvement occurs in types II, III, and IV. Most cases of glycogen storage causing cardiomegaly belong to type II (Pompe's disease), caused by a deficiency of α-1,

4-glucosidase, a lysosomal enzyme that hydrolyzes glycogen to glucose. The glycogen within cardiac muscle cells is biochemically and morphologically normal (β particles, 250 to 400 Å in diameter), but is present in excessive amounts both within lysosomes and free in the cytoplasm [38, 39]. As a result the heart enlarges, sometimes to a marked degree, and congestive cardiac failure supervenes. Survival rarely extends beyond infancy or early childhood. Microscopically, the muscle cells show a characteristic lacework pattern, with large, clear central spaces (which represent the sites of glycogen deposition) and a peripheral rim of compressed cytoplasm. Endocardial fibroelastosis involving at least the left ventricle usually is present also [40]. Although the deposits of glycogen usually involve all myocardial cells relatively uniformly, on occasion the fibers in the ventricular septum may contain disproportionately excessive quantities of glycogen which may lead to subaortic stenosis [41].

Myocardial involvement occurs to a variable extent in type III glycogenosis (glycogen-debranching-enzyme deficiency) [37]. In type IV glycogenosis (branching-enzyme deficiency), deposits of abnormal glycogen are found free in the cytoplasm of cardiac muscle cells, hepatocytes, and a variety of other cell types [42]. These glycogen deposits are basophilic (in contrast to those in other glycogenoses, which are unstained in hematoxylin-eosin preparations) and are composed of nonbranching fibrils that measure from 40 to 80 Å in diameter. These fibrils resemble those of the basophilic carbohydrate deposits in basophilic degeneration of the heart [43, 44]. It has been suggested that congenital rhabdomyoma of the heart, in which the tumor cells contain large amounts of glycogen, may be a localized form of glycogen-storage disease [45]. Small foci of basophilic degeneration of the heart are common findings at necropsy, particularly in the older age group. Extensive basophilic degeneration is found frequently in myxedema and occasionally in congestive and hypertrophic cardiomyopathy. Its functional significance is unknown.

In addition to the observations mentioned above, glycogen deposits have been reported in cardiac muscle cells in idiopathic cardiomyopathy of infants [46] and in adults with beer-drinker's cardiomyopathy [47] or familial cardiomyopathy [48]. Except in the latter patients, the glycogen deposits were localized within myocardial cell mitochondria. Recently, Buja et al. [49] showed that intramitochondrial glycogen deposits develop in canine myocardium as a delayed response to prolonged periods (30 to 45 minutes) of anoxic cardiac arrest. Furthermore, we have observed intramitochondrial glycogen in myocardium of patients with Fallot's tetralogy. It would appear, therefore, that such deposits in cardiac muscle cells represent a type of response to injury rather than to a specific type of cardiomyopathy.

Lipids and Mucopolysaccharides

Infiltration of the cytoplasm of cardiac muscle cells by lipid droplets (fatty degeneration) occurs as a nonspecific abnormality in a great variety of disorders, including hypoxia.

Fabry's disease (angiokeratoma corporis diffusum universale) may be singled out among the lipid-storage diseases as the one in which extensive and clinically significant (cardiomegaly and congestive cardiac failure) accumulation of glycolipid occurs in cardiac muscle cells [50]. In this condition, glycolipid deposits also are present in endothelium and vascular smooth muscle as well as in most other tissues of the body. The disease results from a deficiency of ceramide trihexosidase, an enzyme which hydrolyzes ceramide trihexoside. This glycolipid accumulates in the form of birefringent granules composed of concentric or parallel lamellae spaced 40 to 65 Å apart. In ordinary histologic preparations, the deposits are dissolved and the cardiac muscle cells resemble those in type II glycogenosis. In cardiac muscle cells of a patient with Hurler's disease, we also observed small lipid deposits composed of parallel or concentric lamellae. The deposits, the composition of which is unknown, were extensive in smooth muscle cells of coronary arteries also.

SECONDARY CARDIOMYOPATHIES (ASSOCIATED WITH A KNOWN CONDITION)

Generalized Infections

Virtually all organisms may attack myocardium, and inflammation of myocardium is common in patients with generalized infections of all types [51]. Many viruses, including those causing measles, mumps, chicken pox, and so forth, may alter myocardial function and structure. Fatal myocardial disease due to mumps has been reported [52] (Fig. 26). Coxsackie B viruses are generally known to cause myocarditis and pericarditis in man [53]. The possibility that at least some cases of "idiopathic" dilated type of cardiomyopathy are of viral etiology has been the subject of considerable speculation [53]. Although they have been observed in acute viral myocarditis in humans and experimental animals [53, 54], virus-like particles in cardiac muscle cells have been reported, to our knowledge, in only one patient [55] with long-standing congestive cardiomyopathy. This patient, however, died soon after developing a flulike illness. Preexisting myocardial damage may increase the susceptibility of the heart to viral infections [54]. Ferrans et al. [2] did not find viral particles in any of 31 myocardial biopsies

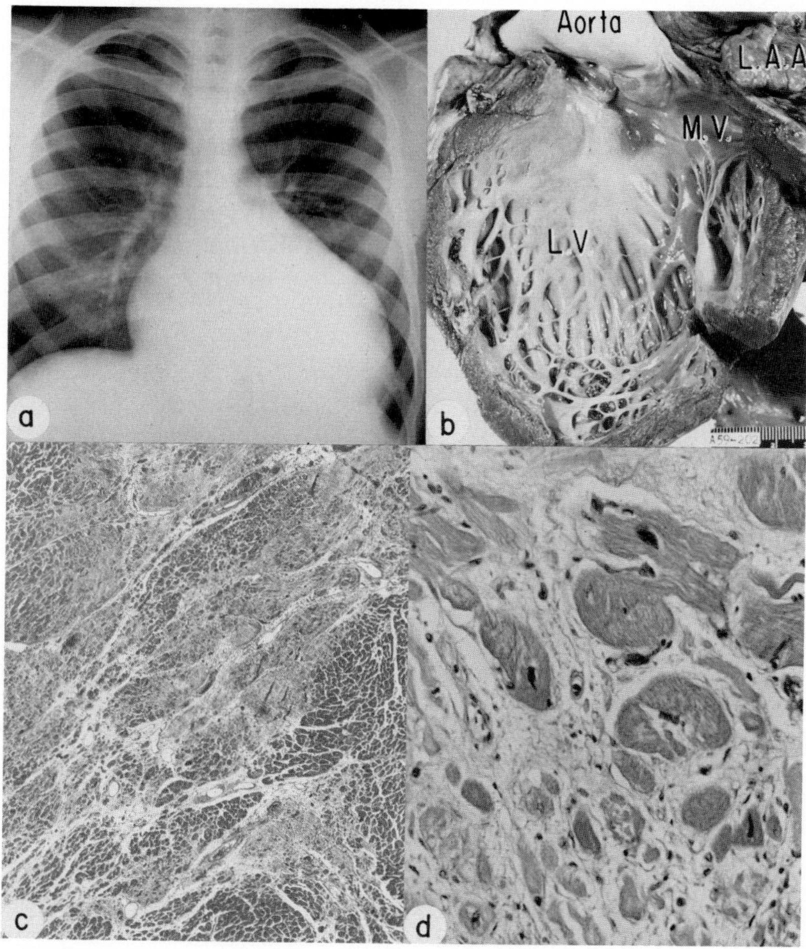

Figure 26. Mumps of the Heart. This 17-year-old boy (A59-202) died 8 months after the onset of well-documented mumps. At the time of the acute illness tachycardia was noted; it persisted, the heart progressively enlarged, and congestive heart failure appeared. He died of the latter. a. Chest radiograph showing cardiomegaly. b. Opened left ventricle (LV), aortic valve, and aorta. The chamber is dilated and the endocardium is mildly but diffusely thickened. MV = anterior mitral leaflet; LAA = left atrial appendage. The heart weighed 550 gms. Thrombi are present in the apex. c. Photomicrograph of portion of left ventricular wall showing replacement fibrosis (Masson stain, X35). d. Close-up view of another area showing degeneration of myocardial fibers and loose interstitial fibrosis (Hematoxylin and eosin stain, X235).

from patients with congestive cardiomyopathy. If viruses play a role in the pathogenesis of congestive cardiomyopathy, it must be assumed either that they are present in cardiac muscle only during the initial, acute phase of damage, which would be followed by a chronic phase of progressive cardiac damage in the absence of viral particles or that they remain, morphologically undetected, during the phase of progressive deterioration. In the latter circumstances, unusual mechanisms (such as those operative in the slow-virus types of infections of the nervous system) must be postulated to account for the chronicity of such cardiac viral infections.

Numerous species of rickettsiae, fungi, bacteria, and parasites have been reported to invade the myocardium. With the notable exceptions of *Toxoplasma gondii* and *Trypanosoma cruzi*, these agents mostly cause acute lesions that do not present clinical or pathologic syndromes such as those in the cardiomyopathies. In some patients, the picture of congestive cardiomyopathy has been shown to result from Toxoplasma infection. Probably the most common myocardial infection throughout the world is Chagas' disease, an acute, subacute, or chronic illness resulting from infection by *Trypanosoma cruzi*. This infection is endemic in large areas of South America. Characteristically, the hearts of patients with chronic Chagas' disease are very dilated, the apical ventricular walls are thinned, usually resulting in either functional or anatomic aneurysms at these sites, and mural thrombi are common (Fig. 27). Histologically, a diffuse inflammatory reaction may be present in addition to the apical scarring.

Collagen Disease

All collagen diseases may affect myocardium. Rheumatic fever, rheumatoid arthritis, systemic lupus erythematosus, however, usually have a greater effect on the cardiac valves than on the myocardium. Most patients dying today with these conditions had received steroid medication, which significantly alters the response of the tissues to these diseases. Involvement of myocardium in polyarteritis nodosa usually results from its involvement of the coronary arteries rather than a primary affect on myocardium. Scleroderma (progressive systemic sclerosis), however, may cause myocardial fibrosis without involvement of the coronary arteries. Cardiac disease in most patients with scleroderma, however, is secondary to systemic hypertension from renal involvement or to cor pulmonale from the vascular and parenchymal involvement of the lung. Congestive heart failure in scleroderma in the absence of systemic hypertension or extensive sclerodermatous pulmonary disease is rare. Myocardial involvement in dermatomyositis is also rare.

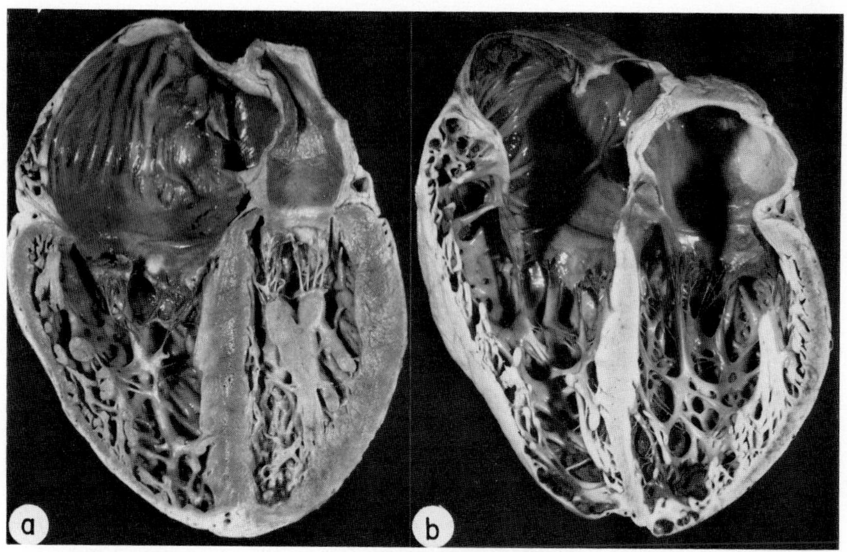

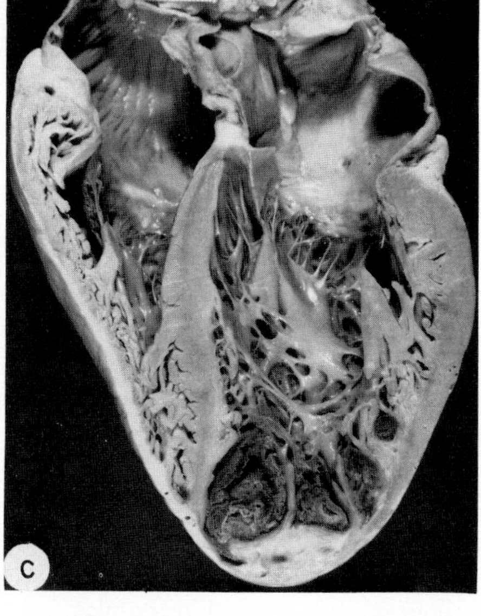

Figure 27. Chagas' disease. Hearts of 3 patients who died of this disorder. The anterior half of each specimen has been removed showing the 4 walls and cavities. a. The right side of the heart is more dilated than the left side. Although there is scarring of the apical portions of each ventricle, no intracavitary thrombi or ventricular aneurysms are present. Weight is 350 gms. b. In this specimen both ventricles are dilated to about equal proportions. The apical walls of both ventricles are extremely thinned and thrombi are present above the thinned portions of each ventricle. Weight is 560 gms. c. The left ventricle is more dilated than is the right one. The apical wall of the left ventricle is scarred and a large thrombus is present in it. During life, a ventricular aneurysm was probably present in this area. The wall is hypertrophied. Weight is 390 gms. (These hearts were submitted to one of us (WCR) by Dr. João B. M. Janini, Chief of Pathology, University of Brasilia, Brasilia, Brazil. We are indebted to him for allowing us to study these cases.)

Endocrine Disorders

Large doses of thyroxine produce nonspecific changes in the sarcoplasmic reticulum and mitochondria of cardiac muscle of experimental animals. The relevance of these changes to those (cardiac hypertrophy and dilatation) in thyrotoxic heart disease in humans remains undetermined. When uncomplicated, thyrotoxicosis is seldom fatal; the light microscopic findings of heart wall have been nonspecific [56], and no ultrastructural studies of myocardium have been reported.

Congestive cardiac failure and cardiomegaly are common in patients with acromegaly [57], but systemic hypertension is usually also present, and thus the influence of growth hormone on myocardium is difficult to evaluate. At necropsy, one of us (WCR) has studied 7 patients with acromegaly. Their ages ranged from 28 to 76 years (avg. 51) and symptoms of this disorder were present in them from 2 to 23 years. All but 1 had symptoms for 12 years or more. Three patients died suddenly and unexpectedly, presumably from an arrhythmia. Five of the 7 were known to have systemic hypertension, and their hearts weighed 390 to 700 gm (avg. 534). The sixth patient never had evidence of cardiac dysfunction, and his heart weighed 330 gm and appeared normal. The seventh patient who, although also normotensive, presented initially with congestive cardiac failure at age 31 was killed in an auto accident 2 years later. His electrocardiogram showed low voltage and poor R-wave progression across the precordium. Cardiac catheterization disclosed a left ventricular end-diastolic pressure of 28 mm Hg with a normal cardiac index (3.0 liter/minute/m^2). At necropsy, his heart weighed 650 gm. The left ventricle contained mural thrombi, and histologically, a few mononuclear cell infiltrates were found in the left ventricular wall. The myocardial fibers were hypertrophied, and the left ventricular endocardium was focally thickened. Thus, this patient's heart was typical of idiopathic cardiomegaly, and yet he proved to have acromegaly with an acidophilic adenoma of the pituitary gland although he never had systemic hypertension.

Structural changes produced by adrenal cortical hormones appear responsible for the skeletal muscle weakness which develops in patients with Cushing's syndrome [58]. Although cortisone and aldosterone also induce changes in myocardial ultrastructure, patients with Cushing's syndrome or with hyperaldosteronism usually also have systemic hypertension and electrolyte imbalance, factors which prevent clear evaluation of the direct effects of these agents on myocardium. Excessive deposits of adipose tissue in the epicardium and between myocardial fibers are found in patients with hyperadrenocorticism and in those receiving steroid medication for prolonged periods of time. Focal myocarditis has been observed in patients with pheochromocytoma [59]. Although systemic hypertension, either paroxysmal or persistent, is virtually always present in patients with pheochromocytoma, the myocardial histopathology in these patients is different from that in patients with systemic hypertension and resembles that in experimental animals given large doses of epinephrine or norepinephrine [60].

Metabolic Disorders

Kwashiorkor, which affects infants and children, has been considered the classic example of protein deficiency, although vitamins, minerals, and calories also are deficient. The myocardium in this condition, like voluntary muscle, atrophies, and although the ventricular chambers may be dilated, they are usually small [61]. Histologically, the intramyocardial capillaries are dilated, the interstitium is edematous, the myocardial cells are small, and sometimes vacuolated. Usually the myocardium is pale and the subepicardial adipose tissue is severely atrophied. It is probable that the atrophied heart is a poor pump. Experimental protein malnutrition in monkeys causes myocardial fiber coagulation, fragmentation, and hydropic degeneration and interstitial inflammation early, and myocardial cell atrophy and interstitial fibrosis late but no endocardial lesions [62].

Cardiac lesions, which involve the mitochondria, in particular, have been described in animals with pure, experimentally induced thiamine deficiency (beriberi). Although this disease has been listed as the classic, primary vitamin deficiency affecting the heart, beriberi seldom occurs in humans in the absence of other nutritional deficiencies. The heart in this condition is stated to be enlarged; the myocardial interstitium, edematous, and occasionally focally fibrotic; and the endocardium, focally thickened.

Severe and chronic anemia may cause ventricular hypertrophy and dilatation which are reversible on correction of the anemia. In addition to the indirect effects that result from anemia, iron deficiency appears to exert a direct effect on the myocardium, at least in experimental animals. This effect, which presumably is mediated through deficiency of iron for synthesis of myoglobin and cytochromes, is manifested by marked enlargement and increase in numbers of mitochondria in cardiac muscle.

In both humans and experimental animals, hypokalemia can cause focal necrosis of myocardial cells with interstitial inflammation and subsequent fibrosis [63]. Myocardial necrosis and calcification occur in magnesium deficiency [64].

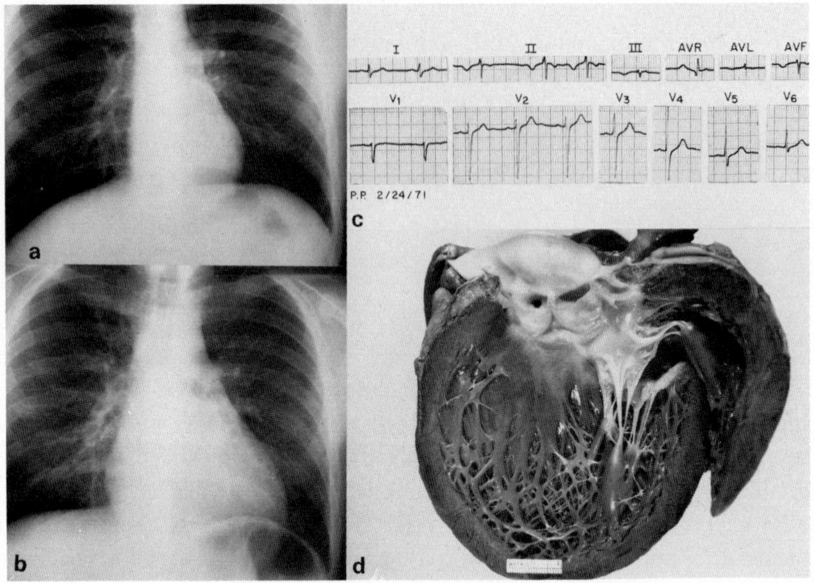

Figure 28. Drug-induced cardiomyopathy. This 19-year-old boy (A71-48) died in "massive" congestive cardiac failure following treatment of his acute myelogenous leukemia with daunorubicin. A. and B. Chest radiographs show progressive cardiomegaly. C. The electrocardiogram was recorded several days before death. D. Opened left ventricle, aortic valve, and aorta. The chamber is considerably dilated. Although no foci of myocardial fibrosis or necrosis were observed grossly, considerable interstitial fibrosis and myocardial cell degeneration were observed on histologic examination. Several other patients have been observed by us in whom cardiomegaly and congestive cardiac failure followed daunorubicin therapy.

Physical Forces, Drugs, and Metals

Trauma (contusions) and *radiation* are well-recognized causes of myocardial cell damage or interstitial myocardial fibrosis or both. Probably far more drugs than we realize cause alteration in myocardial structure. Digitalis, isoproterenol, ephedrine, and a variety of other sympathomimetric agents, diuretics (through electrolyte disturbances), antibiotics, emetine, and so forth have all been shown to damage myocardial cells. Daunorubicin therapy in leukemic patients has caused generalized cardiomegaly and a clinical picture similar to that of idiopathic cardiomegaly (Fig. 28). Histologically, the myocardial fibers have had altered staining characteristics and abnormal nuclei. Cobalt, arsenic, antimony, fluoride, mercury, and lead have all been shown to alter myocardial structure and function. A beer-

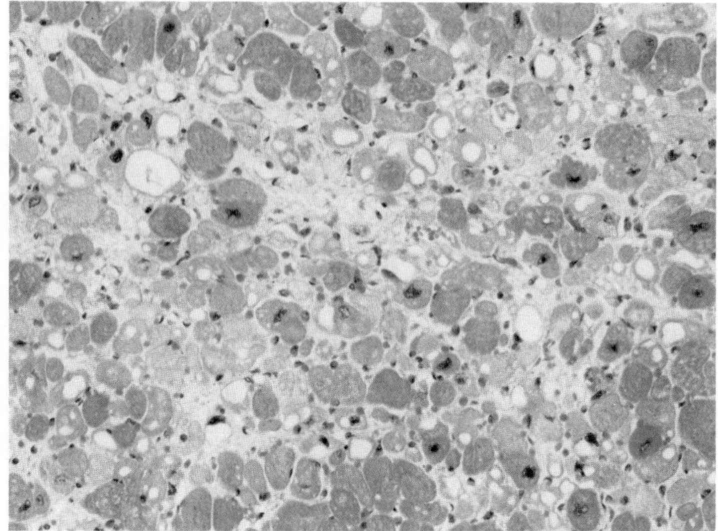

Figure 29. Cobalt (Beer-Drinkers') Cardiomyopathy. This 30-year-old man had been ill for only 4 weeks. Photomicrograph showing severe degeneration and loss of myocardial fibers, vacuolization of same fibers, and interstitial fibrosis. (The section from which this photomicrograph was prepared was submitted by Dr. Jean-Louis Bonenfant of Quebec.)

drinker's cardiomyopathy (Fig. 29) appears to be the result of combined protein deficiency and cobalt toxicity [65, 66]. Snake and scorpion venom also appear to have a direct toxic affect on myocardial cells.

Neurologic Disorders

Friedreich's ataxia, progressive muscular dystrophy, and myotonic muscular dystrophy (all discussed elsewhere: see Chapter 13 by Perloff) are each associated with myocardial dysfunction. It is not clear how much is the result of narrowing of the intramural coronary arteries and how much is the result of myocardial fibrosis unassociated with intramural coronary disease.

REFERENCES

1. Ali, N., Ferrans, V.J., Roberts, W.C., and Massumi, R.A.: Clinical evaluation of transvenous catheter technique for endomyocardial biopsy. Chest (in press).
2. Ferrans, V.J., Massumi, R.A., Shugoll, G.I., Ali, N., and Roberts, W.C.:

Ultrastructural studies of myocardial biopsies in 45 patients with obstructive or congestive cardiomyopathy. In, Brink, A.J. and Bajusz, E. (Eds.): Recent Advances in Studies on Cardiac Sıructure and Metabolism, Vol. 2, The Cardiomyopathies (University Park Press, Baltimore, in press).

3. Falcone, M.W. and Roberts, W.C.: Atresia of right atrial ostium of coronary sinus unassociated with persistence of left superior vena cava: A clinico-pathologic study of 4 adult patients. Am Heart J 83:604-611, 1972.
4. Walsh, J.J., Burch, G.E., Black, W.C., Ferrans, V.J., and Hibbs, R.G.: Idiopathic myocardiopathy of the puerperium (post-partal heart disease). Circulation 32:19, 1965.
5. Demakis, J.G. and Rahimtoola, S.H.: Peripartum cardiomyopathy. Circulation 44:964, 1971.
6. Hibbs, R.G., Ferrans, V.J., Black, W.C. Weilbaecher, D.G., Walsh, J.J., and Burch, G.E.: Alcoholic cardiomyopathy: An electron microscopic study. Am Heart J 69:766-779, 1965.
7. Bulloch, R.T., Pearce, M.B., Murphy, M.L., Jenkins, B.J., and Davis, J.L.: Myocardial lesions in idiopathic and alcoholic cardiomyopathy: Study by ventricular septal biopsy. Am J Cardiol 29:15, 1972.
8. Ewy, G.A., Marcus, F.I., Bohajalian, O., Burke, H.L., and Roberts, W.C.: Muscular subaortic stenosis. Clinical and pathologic observations in an elderly patient. Am J Cardiol 22:126, 1968.
9. Ferrans, V.J., Morrow, A.G., and Roberts, W.C.: Myocardial ultrastructure in idiopathic hypertrophic subaortic stenosis. A study of operatively excised left ventricular outflow tract muscle in 14 patients. Circulation 45:769-792, 1972.
10. Roberts, W.C. and Cohen, L.S.: Left ventricular papillary muscles. Description of the normal and a survey of conditions causing them to be abnormal. Circulation 46:138-154, 1972.
11. Perloff, J.K. and Roberts, W.C.: The mitral apparatus—Functional anatomy of mitral regurgitation. Circulation 46:227-239, 1972.
12. Roberts, W.C., Liegler, D.G., and Carbone, P.P.: Endomyocardial disease and eosinophilia. A clinical and pathologic spectrum. Am J Med 46:28, 1969.
13. Roberts, W.C., Buja, L.M., and Ferrans, V.J.: Löffler's fibroplastic parietal endocarditis, eosinophilic leukemia, and Davies' endomyocardial fibrosis: The same disease at different stages? Pathol Microbiol 35:90, 1970.
14. Connor, D.H., Somers, K., Hutt, M.S.R., Manion, W.C., and D'Arbela, P.G.: Endomyocardial fibrosis in Uganda (Davies' disease). Am Heart J 74:687, 1967, and Ibid 75:107, 1968.
15. Löffler, W.: Endocarditis parietalis fibroplastica mit bluteosinophile. Schweiz Med Wochschr 66:817, 1936.
16. Bousser, J.: Eosinophilie et leucemie. Sang 28:553, 1957.
17. Odeberg, B.: Eosinophilic leukemia and disseminated eosinophilic collagen disease—a disease entity? Acta Med Scand 177:129, 1965.
18. Davies, J.N.P.: Endocardial fibrosis in Africans. E African Med J 25:10, 1948.
19. Ive, F.A., Willis, A.J.P., Ikeme, A.C., and Brockington, I.F.: Endomyocardial fibrosis and filariasis. Quart J Med 36:495, 1967.
20. Buja, L.M., Khoi, N.B., and Roberts, W.C.: Clinically significant cardiac amyloidosis. Clinicopathologic findings in 15 patients. Am J Cardiol 26:394, 1970.
21. Buchbinder, N.A. and Roberts, W.C.: Left-sided valvular active infective endocarditis. A study of 45 necropsy patients. Am J Med 53:20, 1972.

22. Roberts, W.C. and Buchbinder, N.A.: Right-sided valvular infective endocarditis. A clinico-pathologic study of 12 necropsy patients. Am J Med 53:7, 1972.
23. Buchbinder, N.A. and Roberts, W.C.: Active infective endocarditis confined to mural endocardium. A study of 6 necropsy patients. Arch Pathol 93:435, 1972.
24. Carpenter, D.F., Golden, A., and Roberts, W.C.: Quadrivalvular rheumatoid heart disease associated with left bundle branch block. Am J Med 43:922, 1967.
25. Roberts, W.C., Kehoe, J.A., Carpenter, D.F., and Golden, A.: Cardiac valvular lesions in rheumatoid arthritis. Arch Intern Med 122:141, 1968.
26. Roberts, W.C. and Wibin, E.A.: Idiopathic panaortitis, supra-aorta arteritis, granulomatous myocarditis and pericarditis. A cause of pulseless disease and possibly left ventricular aneurysm in the African. Am J Med 41:453, 1966.
27. Porter, G.H.: Sarcoid heart disease. New Engl J Med 263:1350, 1960.
28. Ferrans, V.J., Hibbs, R.G., Black, W.C., Walsh, J.J., and Burch, G.E.: Myocardial degeneration in cardiac sarcoidosis: Histochemical and electron microscopic studies. Am Heart J 69:159, 1965.
29. Roberts, W.C., Bodey, G.P., and Westlake, P.T.: The heart in acute leukemia. A study of 420 autopsy cases. Am J Cardiol 21:388, 1968.
30. Roberts. W.C., Glancy, D.L., and DeVita, V.T., Jr.,: Heart in malignant lymphoma (Hodgkin's disease, lymphosarcoma, reticulum cell sarcoma and mycosis fungoides). A study of 196 autopsy cases. Am J Cardiol 22:85, 1968.
31. Glancy, D.L. and Roberts, W.C.: The heart in malignant melanoma. A study of 70 autopsy cases. Am J. Cardiol 21:555, 1968.
32. Terman, D.S., Alfrey A.C., Hammond, W.S., Donndelinger, T., Ogden, D.A. and Holmes, J.H.: Cardiac calcification in uremia. A clinical, biochemical and pathologic study. Am J Med 50:744, 1971.
33. Roberts, W.C. and Morrow, A.G.: Causes of early postoperative death following cardiac valve replacement. Clinico-pathologic correlations in 64 patients studied at necropsy. J Thorac Cardiovasc Surg 54:422, 1967.
34. Buja, L.M., Levitsky, S., Ferrans, V.J., Souther, S.G., Roberts, W.C., and Morrow, A.G.: Acute and chronic effects of normothermic anoxia on canine hearts. Light and electron microscopic evaluation. Circulation (Suppl) 43 and 44:1-44, 1971.
35. Testelli, M.R. and Pilz, C.G.: Massive calcification of the myocardium. A report of two cases, one associated with nephrocalcinosis. Am J Cardiol 14:407, 1964.
36. Buja, L.M. and Roberts, W.C.: Iron in the heart. Etiology and clinical significance. Am J Med 51:209, 1971.
37. Howell, R.R.: The glycogen-storage diseases. In, Stanbury, J.B., Wyngaarden, J.B., and Fredrickson, D.S. (Eds.): The Metabolic Basis of Inherited Disease, 3rd ed. McGraw-Hill, New York, 1972, pp. 149-173.
38. Garancis, J.C.: Type II Glycogenosis. Biochemical and electron microscopic study. Am J Med 44:289, 1968.
39. Bordiuk, J.M., Legato, M.J., Lovelace, R.E., and Blumenthal, S.: Pompe's disease. Electromyographic, electron microscopic, and cardiovascular aspects. Arch Neurol 23:113, 1970.
40. Ruttenberg, H.D., Steidl, R.M., Carey, L.S., and Edwards, J.E.: Glycogen-storage disease of the heart. Hemodynamic and angiocardiographic features in 2 cases. Am Heart J 67:469, 1964.
41. Ehlers, K.H., Hagstrom, J.W.C., Lukas, D.S. Redo, S.F., and Engle, M.A.:

Glycogen-storage disease of the myocardium with obstruction to left ventricular outflow. Circulation 25:96, 1962.

42. Reed, G.B., Dixon, J.F.P., Neustein, H.B., Donnell, G.N., and Landing, B.H.: Type IV Glycogenosis. Patient with absence of a branching enzyme -1, 4-Glucan: -1, 4-Glucan 6-Glycosyl transferase. Lab Invest 19:546, 1968.
43. Rosai, J. and Lascano, E.F.: Basophilic (mucoid) degeneration of myocardium. A disorder of glycogen metabolism. Am J Pathol 61:99, 1970.
44. Kosek, J.C. and Angell, W.: Fine structure of basophilic myocardial degeneration (BMD). Arch Pathol 89:491, 1970.
45. Hudson, R.E.B.: Cardiovascular Pathology. Baltimore, Williams & Wilkins, pp. 1581-1586, 1965.
46. Auger, C. and Chenard, J.: Quebec beer-drinkers' cardiomyopathy: Ultrastructural changes in one case. Can Med Assoc J 97:916, 1967.
47. Bulloch, R.T., Murphy, M.L., and Pearce, M.B.: Fine structural lesions in the myocardium of a beer drinker with reversible heart failure. Am Heart J 80:629, 1970.
48. Battersby, E.J. and Glenner, G.G.: Familial cardiomyopathy. Am J Med 30:382, 1961.
49. Buja, L.M., Ferrans, V.J., and Levitsky, S.: Occurrence of intramitochondrial glycogen in canine myocardium after prolonged anoxic cardiac arrest. J Molec Cell Cardiol 4:237, 1972.
50. Ferrans, V.J., Hibbs, R.G., and Burda, C.D.: A histochemical and electron microscopic study of the heart in Fabry's disease. Am J Cardiol 24:95, 1969.
51. Gore, I. and Saphir, O.: Myocarditis. A classification of 1402 cases. Am Heart J 34:827, 1947.
52. Roberts, W.C. and Fox, S.M., III: Mumps of the heart. Clinical and pathologic features. Circulation 32:342, 1965.
53. Burch, G.E. and Giles, T.D.: The role of viruses in the production of heart disease. Am J Cardiol 29:231, 1972.
54. Ablemann, W.H.: Virus and the heart. Circulation 44:950, 1971.
55. Hibbs, R.G., Ferrans, V.J., Black, W.C., Walsh, J.J., and Burch, G.E.: Virus-like particles in the heart of a patient with cardiomyopathy: An electron microscopic and histochemical study. Am Heart J 69:327, 1965.
56. McEarchern, D. and Rake, G.: Study of the morbid anatomy of hearts from patients dying with hyperthyroidism. Bull Johns Hopkins Hosp 48:273, 1931.
57. Hejtmancik, M.R., Bradfield, J.Y., Jr., and Herrmann, G.R.: Acromegaly and the heart. A clinical and pathologic study. Ann Intern Med 34:1445, 1951.
58. Afifi, A.K., Bergman, R.A., and Harvey, J.C.: Steroid myopathy; clinical histologic and cytologic observations. Johns Hopkins Med J 123:158, 1968.
59. Van Vliet, P.D., Burchell, H.B., and Titus, J.C.: Focal myocarditis associated with pheochromocytoma. New Engl J. Med 274:1102, 1966.
60. Ferrans, V.J., Hibbs, R.G., Walsh, J.J. and Burch, G.E.: Histochemical and electron microscopical studies on the cardiac necroses produced by sympathomimetic agents. Ann N Y Acad Sci 156:309, 1969.
61. Smythe, P.M., Swanepoel, A., and Campbell, J.A.H.: The heart in Kwashiorkor. Br Med J 1:67, 1962.
62. Chauhan, S., Nayak, N.C., and Ramalingaswami, V.: The heart and skeletal muscle in experimental protein malnutrition in rhesus monkeys. J Pathol Bacteriol 90:301, 1965.

63. Emberson, J.W. and Muir, A.R.: Changes in the ultrastructure of rat myocardium induced by hypokalemia. Quart J Exp Physiol 54:36, 1969.
64. Heggtveit, H.A., Herman, L., and Mishra, R.K.: Cardiac necrosis and calcification in experimental magnesium deficiency. Am J Pathol 45:757, 1964.
65. Bonenfant, J. L., Auger, C., Miller, G., Chenard, J., and Roy, P.E.: Quebec beer-drinkers' myocardosis: Pathological aspects. Ann N Y Acad Sci 156:577, 1969.
66. Grinvalsky, H.T. and Fitch, D.M.: A distinctive myocardiopathy occurring in Omaha, Nebraska: Pathological aspects. Ann N Y Acad Sci 156:544, 1969.

JOHN W. VESTER, M.D.

Hemodynamics and Myocardial Metabolism Studies and their Application to Myocardial Diseases

INTRODUCTION

This book is being written for all those physicians and students of medicine who are interested in cardiology. A treatise of this subject that is adequate to the needs of the laboratory investigator would be of a length and degree of detail far beyond the interest of the busy practicing internist. Accordingly, the aim of this chapter will be to present a distillate of the current literature in a clear, simple, and straightforward fashion. Detail will be kept to a minimum, and references will be given to appropriate review and original articles for those who wish to expand their familiarity with any given point.

The function of the heart is that of a pump that uses energy to transfer fluids from one compartment to another. The heart is a somewhat more complex pump than most mechanical ones because it contains the machinery for deriving the energy necessary from chemical fuels as an integral part of the pumping mechanism itself. Therefore, one must consider the supply and extraction of substrates as a starting place. Here, substrate includes not only the fuels (primarily carbohydrate and fat) but oxygen, as well. Next, there must be a consideration of the sequence of chemical changes of these substrates which result in the transfer of the energy inherent in the fuels to a chemical coin of exchange that can be used to drive the contractile process. This will lead, then, to a review of present understanding of the mechanism whereby chemical energy can be used to cause the shortening of the individual muscle fibers that are the central event in the contractile process. At this point, we shall begin a more physiologic consideration of the mechanism of cardiac action. The amount of muscular work that can be derived from the breakdown of a given amount of an energy-rich compound is affected by a number of factors, such as myocardial fiber length, tension, and so forth. This field embodies muscle mechanics and hemodynamics.

With this basis of understanding of normal biochemistry and physiology established, in the remainder of the chapter an attempt will be made to relate what information has been obtained concerning the site or sites of breakdown in the orderly transition from substrate-contained energy to pumping efficiency in the various disease states of the myocardium.

BIOCHEMISTRY

In the introduction to this chapter, it was stated that the review of the metabolism of the heart would begin with the consideration of the substrate extraction by the heart muscle. This requires that we focus our attention on the coronary circulation from which the substrates are extracted. The amount of blood delivered to the heart muscle is generally expressed in terms of the amount supplied to 100 gm of muscle per minute. The reason for this is that the vast majority of the methods used for measuring coronary blood flow are variations on the nitrous oxide method originally developed by Kety and his coworkers. [1]. The calculations for this method require expression of results on the basis of tissue weight. Many studies of coronary blood flow have been published, and the data contained in Best and Taylor's *Textbook of Physiology* are taken as representative [2]. At rest, the data obtained for both man and the dog are in agreement. With the left ventricular cardiac work index set at approximately 3.5 to 4.5 kg-m per minute per square meter of body surface, the left coronary blood flow has been measured to range between 72 and 85 ml/100 gm of left ventricle per minute.

Bove and colleagues [3] measured the muscle weights of the various chambers and septa of the hearts from both normal and abnormal patients. When one adds together the mean weight that they cite for left ventricle plus septum, the right ventricle, the left atrium, and the right atrium, one arrives at the figure of 247.4 gm of muscle as a mean figure in the average normal heart. If one is safe in extrapolating from data derived for left ventricular muscle to all the rest of the muscle in the heart (and such an extrapolation may not be safe when one considers that the work load of the left ventricle is much greater than that of the other chambers), one can apply a correction figure of 2.47 to data expressed for 100 gm of left ventricle muscle to obtain a figure that would apply to all the muscle of the heart. Such a correction applied to the above-quoted left ventricle muscle flow data would produce a figure of 178 to 211 ml of blood per minute for the muscle of the heart of an average person, at rest. Since such a correction is potentially likely to be inaccurate, the authors will not use it further here, but it was quoted for those who do. The potential of these quoted amounts of blood flow to vary widely is apparent from recorded observations of dogs under stress conditions showing left ventricular coronary blood flows as high as 600 ml per 100 gm of left ventricle per minute.

The muscle of the heart extracts far more oxygen from the blood passing through it than the rest of the body does. Arterial blood of a normal person is said to contain, as an average, 19.8 ml of oxygen per 100 ml of blood [4]. Mixed venous blood contains about 15 ml of oxygen per 100 ml of blood. Coronary sinus venous blood, however, contains only 4 to 5 ml of oxygen per 100 ml of blood [2]. Hence, the myocardium generally extracts oxygen so that the AV difference is approximately 12 to 14 ml per 100 ml of blood. Since this extraction generally changes very little, increased oxygen uptake by the muscle of the heart is generally accomplished by variations in coronary blood flow.

The factors that affect the demand of the myocardium for oxygen have been studied in great detail by many investigators, and a complete recapitulation of this research is beyond the scope of this chapter. The recent review of the subject by Braunwald is quite inclusive and is recommended to the reader both for its content and its extensive bibliography [5].

First, the bulk of the oxygen used by the heart is related to contraction. The oxygen uptake of the arrested heart is around 2 ml per minute per 100 gm of left ventricular muscle, whereas the contracting heart uses in the neighborhood of 8 ml per 100 gm left ventricular muscle. Isolated animal heart preparations have been put to very good use in attempts to measure those factors which affect the demand of the myocardium for oxygen. These factors are listed in Table I, taken from Braunwald [5].

The use of an isolated dog-heart preparation in which cardiac output and the arterial pressure against which the heart contracts could be controlled and regulated has yielded some very interesting observations. If one knows the stroke volume of the beating heart and the resistance against which it must move the ejected blood, it is possible to calculate the work done by the heart, and express it in kilogram meters per minute. As one would expect, increasing the amount of work done by the heart by increasing one or the other of these variables (output or resistance) increases the amount of oxygen taken up. However, the relationship between oxygen consumption and work done by the heart is not a simple linear

Table I
Determinants of Myocardial Oxygen Consumption

1. Tension development
2. Contractile state
3. Heart rate
4. Basal cost
5. Depolarization
6. Direct metabolic effect of catecholamines
7. Activation
8. Maintenance of active state
9. Shortening against a load-Fenn effect

Reprinted from [5] with the permission of the author and publisher.

one. Though, in general, increases in work done do indeed require increasing oxygen uptake, it is not possible to estimate accurately the energy needs of the heart from the work produced by it when work is calculated in the classic manner as the product of developed pressure and stroke volume.

A more useful device for predicting oxygen need is the tension-time index. If one graphs the ventricular pressure pulse curve and integrates the area under the curve, one can come up with a number that expresses the total amount of tension exerted inside the ventricle during the time of ventricular contraction. Since it involves tension and time, it is expressed as millimeters of mercury seconds. If, for example, the duration of systole is kept constant, an increase in the peak pressure exerted will perforce increase the area under the curve and the tension-time index. The results of this type of study were more satisfying in that a very close relationship could be demonstrated between developed intraventricular pressure and myocardial oxygen consumption.

The likelihood of the existence of other determinants of myocardial oxygen consumption, however, was pointed out in that exercise and catecholamines, for example, could produce discrepancies in the relationship between the tension-time index and myocardial oxygen consumption. The experimental technique was then modified in order to study the effect of changes in velocity of contraction on myocardial oxygen consumption. Aortic pressure and cardiac rate were controlled and kept constant as was left ventricular output. As a result, then, cardiac work remained constant under all conditions, but velocity of contraction could be varied. Calcium infusions, norepinephrine infusions, and paired electrical stimulation are all known to increase the velocity of cardiac contraction. (Since all readers of this book may not be familiar with the significance of "paired stimulation," it will be explained further. The work on "paired stimulation," published by Ross and his coworkers [6], is based on evidence that the contraction after an extrasystole is of greater contractile force than regularly occurring contractions of the heart. The contraction timing of an isolated heart preparation is taken over by an electrical stimulator, at a standard rate. When a regular rhythm is established, impulses are then delivered at a very short time after the regularly occurring impulse that results in contraction. When this second impulse is delivered from 180 to 230 msec after the regular stimulus, a second ventricular depolarization can be observed electrocardiographically, but there is little or no detectable mechanical extrasystolic contraction. The next contraction after this electrical extrasystole shows an augmentation in rate of development contractile force of the left ventricle. If this pairing of stimuli continues, the augmentation of ventricular performance continues to increase progressively over the next 4 or 5 beats and then remains constant for several hours). When these three maneuvers (calcium infusion, norepinephrine infusion, and paired electrical stimulation) were evaluated, it was found that each of them was capable of increasing the velocity of left ventricular contraction by approximately 50 percent (Fig. 1) [7]. Whenever norepinephrine or calcium was infused into the heart to which paired electrical stimuli were being applied, a further augmentation of left ventricular contraction velocity occurred so that the total increase in left ventricular ejection velocity was 100 percent greater than the control velocity. All maneuvers increased myocardial oxygen consumption. Norepinephrine, calcium, or paired electrical stimulation alone resulted in approximately 40 percent increase in myocardial consumption uptake. When calcium or norepinephrine infusions were added to the heart receiving paired electrical stimuli, the increase in myocardial oxygen uptake was approximately 100 per cent greater than control. By definition, however, left ventricular work was not altered. Since all the maneuvers that increased the peak ejection velocity shortened the duration of ejection, the tension time index was actually decreased. These studies, then, indicate clearly that increasing the velocity of contraction increases myocardial oxygen uptake with no change in work done and with an actual decrease in tension-time index.

Another important determinant of myocardial oxygen uptake is the basal tension state of the myocardium. Covell et al. [8], delineated this factor in their studies of the effect of digitalis glycosides on the failing and non-failing isolated animal heart (Fig. 2). Since cardiac rate, stroke volume, and mean aortic pressure were held constant as in the previous studies, work done was constant at all times. The peak aortic flow rate is an indicator of the rate of ventricular wall contraction. Another indicator of the rate of ventricular wall contraction is the rate of change of the pressure inside the ventricular cavity as a function of time during the contractile

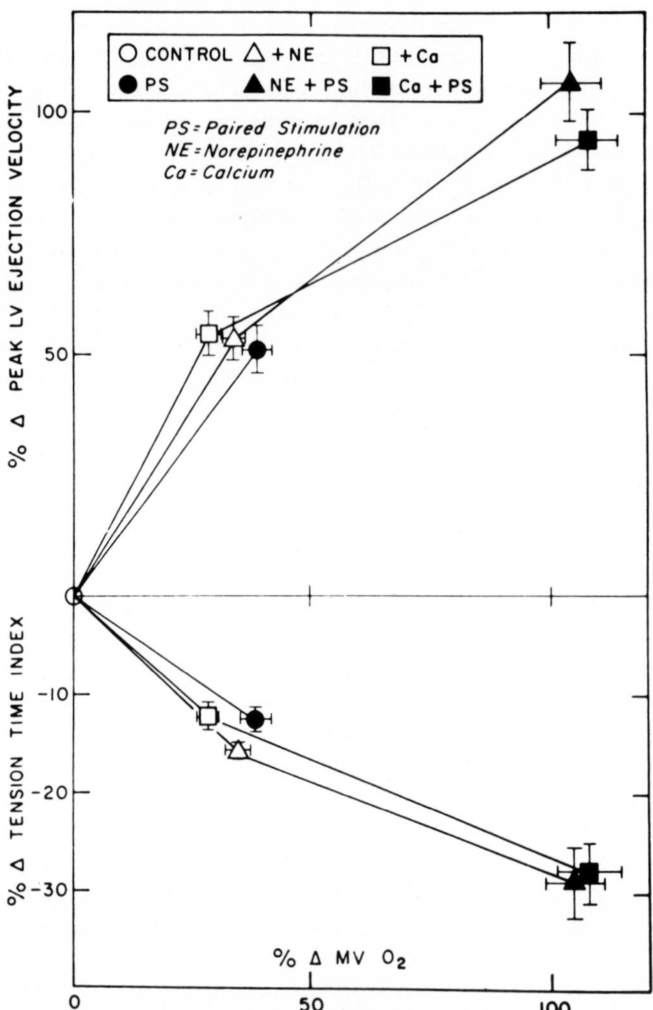

Figure 1. Relation of percent change in peak velocity of left ventricular ejection and of left ventricular TTI with the percent increase in MVO_2 for all the inotropic interventions used in paired experiments in 8 dogs. Inotropic interventions as shown on graph. Cross bars = 1 se of mean. (From Sonnenblick, E.H., Ross, J. Jr., Covell, J.W., Kaiser, G.A., and Braunwald, E.: Velocity of contraction as a determinant of myocardial oxygen consumption. Am J Physiol 209:919, 1965, by permission.)

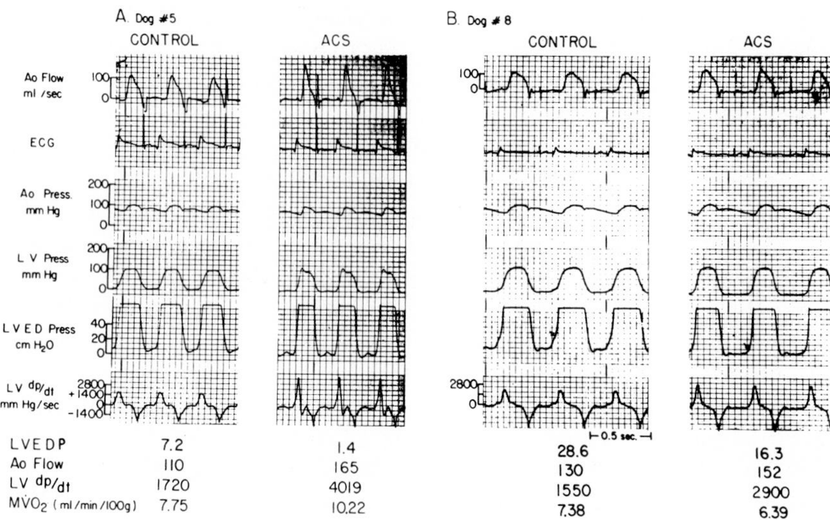

Figure 2. A and B. Representative tracings obtained from two experiments. (From Covell, J.W., Braunwald, E., Ross, J. Jr., and Sonnenblick, E.H.: Studies on digitalis. XVI. Effects on myocardial oxygen consumption. J Clin Invest 45:1535, 1966, by permission.)

event. This is alluded to in figure 2 in calculus shorthand as *dp/dt.* It will be seen that the nonfailing heart increased its contraction rate very markedly as a consequence of treatment with acetyl strophanthidin and that this increase in contractile rate was accompanied by a marked increase of oxygen uptake of the myocardium, denoted MVO (milliliters per minute per 100 gm). Though the rate of tension generation has increased, the amount of work done is unchanged though the oxygen cost is increased. Therefore, in this instance, the administration of acetyl strophanthidin to the non-failing heart produced a genuine decline in efficiency. In another dog, in which acute heart failure was induced by elevating the left ventricular end diastolic pressure, acetyl strophanthidin likewise produced a marked increase in contraction rate. In this case, however, the oxygen uptake actually showed a slight decrease. The explanation for this apparent paradox lies in the change produced in the basal tension state of the ventricular wall. In the nonfailing heart, the left ventricular end-diastolic pressure was low to begin with, and therefore it could not be decreased to any significant degree by the acetyl strophanthidin treatment so that there was no significant change in the basal tension state of the myocardium. Accordingly, the net change in oxygen uptake represented only the increase in contractility, and therefore, an increase in the total amount of oxygen taken up. In the failing heart, however, the left ventricular volume declined to a value almost half of the control state when acetyl strophanthidin was administered. As a consequence, there was a very marked lowering of the basal tension on the myocardium as cardiac volume was decreased. In the failing heart, then, one had a decrease in oxygen requirement resulting from the decrease in the basal tension state of the myocardium balancing off the increase in oxygen uptake resulting from the increase in contractility. The net result here, then, was a slight decline in oxygen uptake.

Covell, Braunwald, and associates suggest that these observations may help to explain some clinical results of digitalis treatment. If a patient with coronary artery disease and without heart failure were given digitalis, the increase in oxygen consumption could very likely lead to the appearance or augmentation of angina. On the other hand, the patient with coronary artery disease and heart failure would be benefited by the administration of digitalis in that an increase of myocardial contractility could be achieved with no net increase in myocardial oxygen consumption [8].

When one considers the ability of increased myocardial contractility to cause increased myocardial oxygen consumption, it is no surprise that cardiac suppressant drugs such as propranolol and procainamide are able to reduce myocardial oxygen consumption when myocardial wall tension is held constant. Graham et al. [9] has demonstrated this reciprocal relationship between contraction rate (V Max) and wall tension. Hence, a given level of myocardial oxygen consumption can be achieved either with a relatively high level of V Max and low-peak developed tension or with a relatively low level of V Max and high-peak developed tension.

An increasing heart rate also increases myocardial oxygen consumption. This has been amply studied and most recently reviewed by Boerth and coworkers [10]. Because an increasing heart rate causes the heart to increase its wall tension more often per unit time, it would be expected to increase myocardial oxygen consumption, and it does. In addition, however, an increasing rate not only increases the force of the contraction (the Bowditch effect) but it increases contraction rate as well. Thus with an increasing heart rate, myocardial oxygen consumption is increased both because of the increasing frequency of development of tension and the increase in rate of contraction. Tension development, contractile state, and heart rate are among the major factors governing the amount of oxygen used by the myocardium, as listed in Table I.

The basal oxygen uptake of the nonbeating heart declines from the value of 8 to 15 ml per minute per 100 gm of the contracting heart to approximately 2 ml per minute per 100 gm as stated above. If one produces electromechanical dissociation by perfusing the coronary bed with blood from which calcium has been extracted by treatment with an ion-exchange resin, one has a preparation in which a study of the cost of depolarization can be made. If propagated depolarizations are induced in this preparation by stimulating the heart electrically, one finds that the oxygen cost, at a rate of 100 cycles per minute, is about 0.04 ml of oxygen per minute per 100 gm as a direct consequence of the depolarization process.

Since catecholamines are known to have a number of other effects on living cells besides increasing the contractility of the myocardium, the possibility of a direct metabolic effect of catecholamines on cellular metabolism must be considered. If one perfuses a heart preparation with excess potassium so that the heart is arrested, the direct metabolic effect of catecholamines can be quantitated. This has been done [11], and it has been found that the increase in oxygen consumption produced by catecholamine treatment is only 5 to 10 percent as great in the noncontracting heart as when the same doses were given to hearts that were capable of contraction.

Depolarization of the myocardium results in activation of the contractile apparatus of the muscle by ionic calcium released from the sarcoplasmic reticulum. The energy cost of this process appears to be very small. Another possible cost of oxygen would be that of maintaining whatever level of active state has been developed at any given time. An attempt has been made to look at this by abruptly decreasing all pressure in an isovolumetrically contracting ventricle midway through one contraction. This has been found to decrease the oxygen consumption by only 10 percent, suggesting that the energy cost of maintenance of a given activation state is likewise small.

In an earlier part of this discussion, the relationship between tension state of the myocardium and oxygen consumption was discussed. The heart with increased end-diastolic pressure has a greater tension in its wall and a greater oxygen consumption as a result thereof. This increase in tension in the wall, leading as it does, to diastolic stretching of the fibers is considered a "preload." This stretching of the muscle by preloading enables the heart to increase the amount of tension developed without paying the price of a decrease in the velocity of contraction. This is one of the factors that contributes to the Starling law. The increased "payoff" of tension developed without decrease in velocity of contraction obtains up to a stretching of about 45 percent from initial length. The load imposed on a muscle by a preload exerts its effect in both the resting and contracting state. Another kind of load that also has an effect on tension development is called "afterload." As is apparent from the name, this is a load that imposes an effect on a muscle only after the initiation of contraction. In the intact human, preload can be imposed by elevations in end-diastolic pressure in the ventricle. An afterload is imposed by impedance to ejection

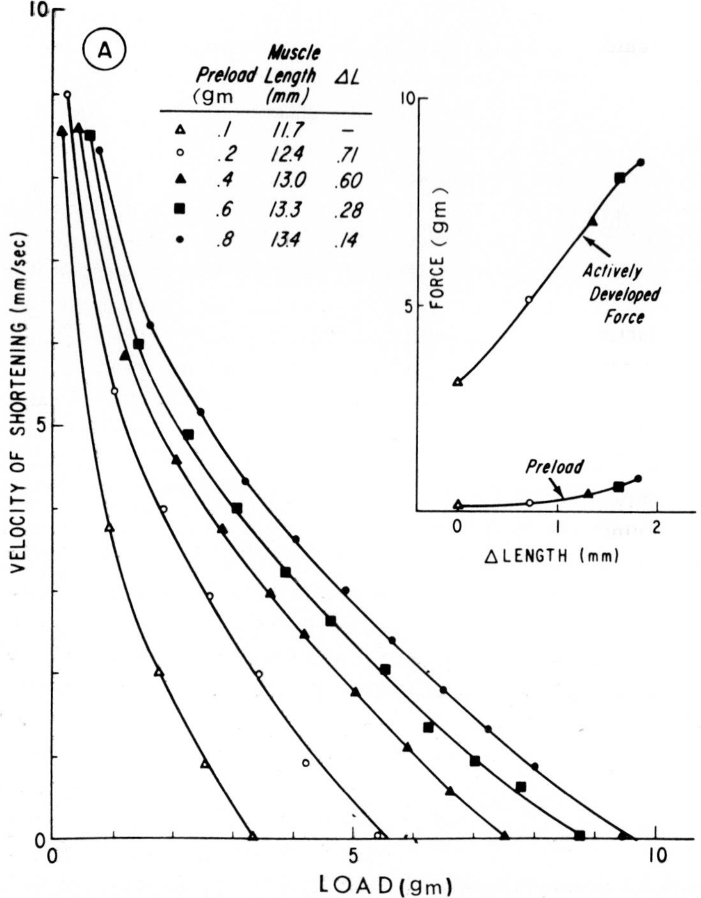

Figure 3. Force velocity curves of cat papillary muscle with increasing muscle length. Ordinate: initial velocity of isotonic shortening; abscissa: load. As the resting muscle is stretched by the application of increasing amounts of preload, the muscle is made capable of tolerating greater loads applied as afterload. Thus increasing preload increases the amount of contractile force that can be developed by the muscle. If one extrapolates back to the zero position and looks at the initial velocity of shortening, one can see that applying preload does not change the initial velocity of shortening. (From Sonnenblick, E.H.: Series elastic and contractile elements in heart muscle: Changes in muscle length. Am J Physiol 207: 1330, 1964, by permission.)

of blood from the ventricular cavity. Semilunar valvular stenosis and pulmonary or systemic hypertension are clinical examples of impedance to ejection. Figure 3 graphically shows the effect of preload on muscle contraction [12]. Figure 4, on the other hand, demonstrates the effect of

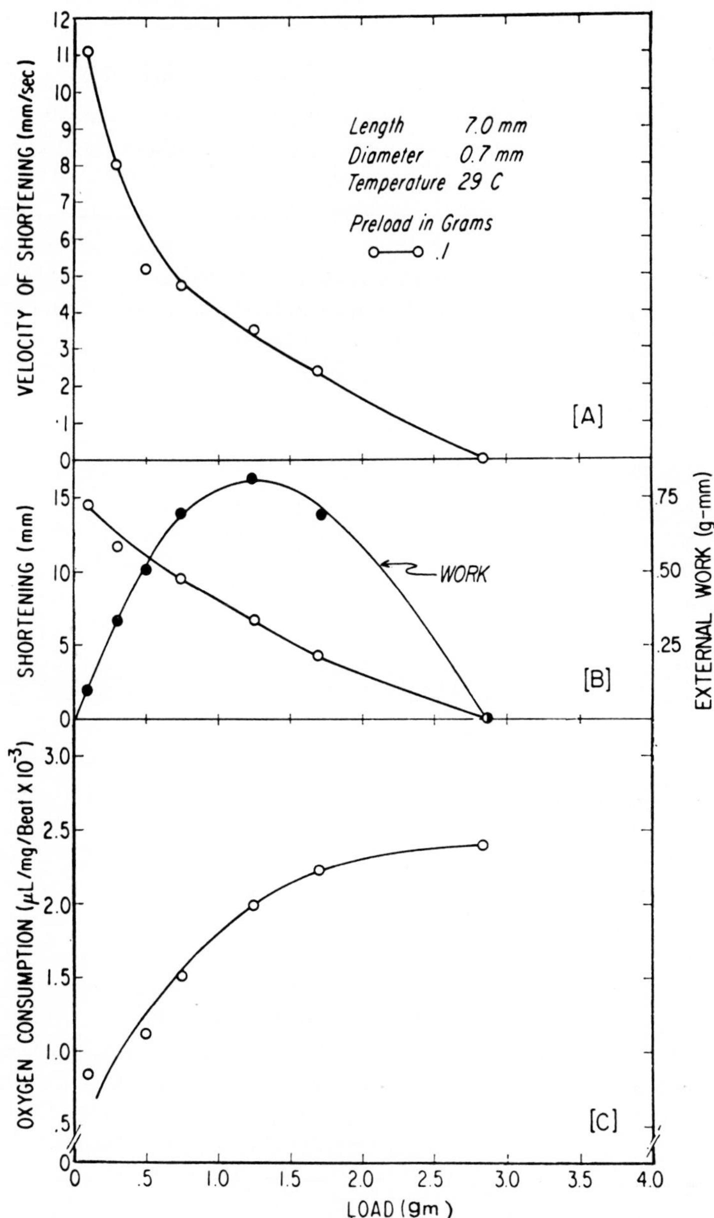

Figure 4. Effect of increasing afterload at a constant preload on myocardial mechanics and VO_2. Ordinates: A. Velocity of shortening; B. Shortening and external work; and C. oxygen consumption. Abscissa: total load. (From Coleman, H.N., Sonnenblick, E.H. and Braunwald, E.: Myocardial oxygen consumption associated with external work: The Fenn effect. Am J Physiol 217:291, 1969, by permission.)

increasing increments of afterload on velocity of contraction, degree of shortening, work done, and oxygen consumption [13]. In this study, preload was held constant, and the weight that the papillary muscle had to lift when it contracted was increased by increments (afterload). It can be seen that as one increased the weight lifted by contracting papillary muscle, the speed of contraction decreased in an almost linear fashion. Not only did the speed of shortening decrease with increasing afterload but also the amount of shortening (in millimeters) decreased. Interestingly enough, as one increased the weight lifted by the contracting muscle, the total amount of actual work done increased up to about 50 percent of isometric load. (Isometric load refers to that load which is just great enough to keep the muscle from shortening at all when a stimulus is applied.) As the weight applied as afterload continues to increase beyond the 50 percent mark, the amount of work done decreases, finally reaching zero at the isometric point. Part C of Figure 4 shows that the oxygen consumption increased with each increment in afterload. Thus, increasing the afterload against which a muscle must contract will produce progressive declines in velocity and degree of contraction and a progressive increase in the oxygen consumption of the contracting muscle. External work done increases up to about 50 percent of isometric load and decreases to zero thereafter.

Fifty years ago, Wallace Fenn [14] showed that allowing a skeletal muscle to shorten against a load increased the amount of heat liberated by the muscle in proportion to the work done. If one studies the oxygen consumption of a papillary muscle instead of heat liberated, a similar effect can be shown for cardiac muscle. A cat papillary muscle was allowed to contract against increasing increments of afterload as shown in Figure 5. Then the same muscle was released and allowed to contract isometrically in such a fashion as to develop the same amount of tension as before, but without shortening. If one studies the oxygen consumption under both circumstances, one can evaluate the cost in oxygen uptake of developing tension *and* shortening as compared to mere development of tension without shortening. It can be seen that increasing amounts of afterload results in increasing oxygen uptake directly attributable to shortening in addition to that attributable to mere tension development. At half-isometric-load, this oxygen uptake due directly to shortening in the performance of external work was equal to approximately 48 percent of the total oxygen uptake. Thus, the Fenn effect applies to cardiac muscle as well as to skeletal muscle.

The oxygen extracted from the coronary blood supply, regulated by the aforementioned factors, is required for the biochemical processes that are necessary to derive chemical energy from the substrates, that is, fuels brought to the myocardium. Published studies of substrate extraction by

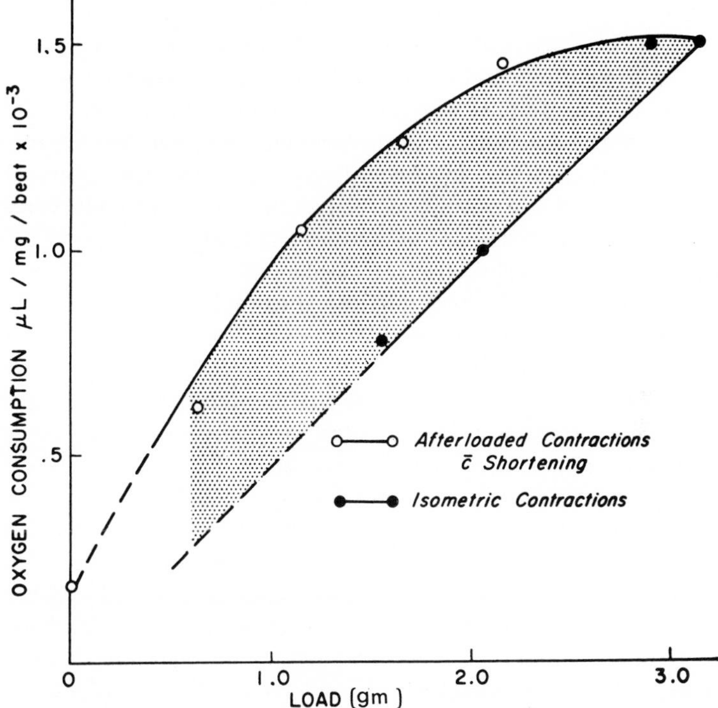

Figure 5. Comparison of VO_2 of isometric contraction (closed circles) to VO_2 of afterloaded isotonic contractions at equal levels of tension development (open circles). Dotted area is change in VO_2 associated with onset of shortening and external work in afterloaded contractions. Point on the ordinate at 0.23 ± 0.05 ml/mg per beat $\times 10^{-3}$ represents an average intercept as determined in 5 experiments. (From: Coleman, H.N., Sonnenblick, E.H., and Braunwald, E.: Myocardial oxygen consumption associated with external work: the Fenn effect. Amer J Physiol 217:291, 1969, by permission.)

the myocardium are numerous, indeed, and the literature is voluminous. For a more extensive discussion than is possible here, the reader is referred to two comparatively recent reviews of the subject that are broad in coverage and extensive in bibliography [15, 16, 17, 18]. In this part of this chapter, we will attempt to present an overview of what is known at the present time of the use of fuels by the myocardium.

Much is made of the respiratory quotient of the contracting myocardium so we will first present a brief review of this concept. The respiratory quotient is a useful figure in this context because it can serve as an index to what type of fuel is being used by a given tissue. The respiratory quotient itself is merely the ratio of the volume of carbon dioxide produced divided by the volume of oxygen consumed in the metabolism of a given substrate [19]. Carbohydrate substrates contain comparatively large amounts of oxygen in relationship to the number of carbon atoms in the molecule (i.e., glucose-$C_6H_{12}O_6$) and when they are oxidized to CO_2 and water by a living tissue, they will produce one molecule of CO_2 for every molecule of oxygen taken up. Accordingly, the respiratory quotient of a tissue that is exclusively burning carbohydrate will be 1.0. When the substrate is fat, the oxygen content of the fuel molecule is comparatively much less. For example, a typical triglyceride containing 2 molecules of stearic and 1 of palmitic acid will have a chemical formula of $C_{55}H_{106}O_6$. To convert 2 molecules of this tryglyceride to CO_2 and water will require the uptake of 157 molecules of oxygen with a production of 110 molecules of CO_2. The ratio of 110/157 is 0.701 so that the respiratory quotient of the tissue exclusively burning this particular triglyceride would be about 0.7. The technique of coronary sinus catherization has made it possible to very precisely measure the respiratory quotient and the extraction rates of various substrates in the beating intact heart. The values are derived from measurement of the content of arterial and coronary sinus venous blood of oxygen, CO_2, lactate, pyruvate, glucose, fatty acids, and triglycerides. When one combines the AV differences obtained in this fashion with measurements of the flow of blood through the myocardium, it is possible to determine the precise metabolic characteristics of the myocardium.

Bing's data, derived from coronary sinus catheterization studies in man have shown that, in the fasting state, the relationship between the contribution of carbohydrates and noncarbohydrates to total energy production in the myocardium is about 1 to 3 [20]. He used these observations to estimate the respiratory quotient of the beating heart in the fasting state at 0.82. Comparing the oxygen use of the beating heart with the oxygen use of the nonbeating heart has established a figure of 0.806 as the fraction of oxygen used in the contractile work of the heart only. The use of the respiratory quotient of 0.82 makes it possible to assign a theoretical work equivalent of 2.059 kg-m of work capable of being done per milliliter of oxygen taken up if the heart were 100 percent efficient. If one knows the cardiac output and the resistance against which the blood must be ejected, it is possible to calculate the actual work of the heart in kilogram-meters per minute. Bing used the following equation:

$$\text{Efficiency of heart} = \frac{\text{work of heart in kg} - \text{m/minute}}{\text{O}_2 \text{ consumption/minute} \times 2.059 \times 0.86}$$

to arrive at a value of approximately 37 percent efficiency in the dog and 39 percent in man. This is an interesting figure, indeed, when one realizes that the standard thermodynamic efficiency of an internal combustion engine is approximately 25 percent, and the finest steam turbines approach a value of 40 percent [21]!

With these catheter techniques, it has been possible to measure the exact amounts of all substrates taken up by the heart in both humans and experimental animals. The amount of glucose extracted by the heart is governed by several factors. One important factor governing the amount of glucose extracted is the amount of glucose in the blood. Several workers agree that the threshold for glucose extraction from arterial blood is approximately 60 to 80 mg per 100 ml. Below this level, little or no glucose is extracted. As the level rises in the arterial blood, the extraction of glucose does also, reaching a maximum when the blood glucose level is greater than approximately 200 mg per 100 ml. Insulin lack sharply decreases the glucose uptake by the heart at any level, and insulin administration increases it. The amount of lactate extracted by the myocardium is likewise affected by the concentration of the substance in the blood. Hence, the AV difference of lactate in blood that has crossed the myocardium can range from 0.16 to 9.2 mg/100 ml and the total use of lactate by the myocardium can range from 11.5 to 135 mg/100 gm of heart muscle per minute. It has been estimated that the human heart uses approximately equal quantities of glucose and lactic acid as carbohydrate substrates, and these amount to a total of approximately 11 gm of glucose and 10 gm of lactic acid per day. When one calculates the amount of oxygen required to oxidize these substrates completely to carbon dioxide and water and compares this with the total amount of oxygen extracted by the myocardium, it becomes apparent that carbohydrate substrates, on the average, account for only about 35 percent of the total amount of oxygen taken up in the fasting state.

That the heart takes up lactate has been known since 1928 [22] when Himwich and his coworkers found that the venous drainage from the perfused heart contained less lactic acid than arterial blood. The extent of lactate use by the heart depends on several factors such as the levels of lactate and glucose in the blood, the amount of work being done by the heart, and the oxygen supply of the heart. The interrelationship of glucose and lactate use is such that if one increases the use of one substance by raising its level in the blood, one will depress the use of the other. The working heart will take up lactate until the amount of oxygen extracted from the coronary blood supply decreases to the point where it is inadequate to support the work being done. At this point, lactate use will stop and lactate production will become evident.

Studies of the dog heart [15] showed that acidosis and alkalosis are both capable of affecting myocardial metabolism. Acidosis appears to decrease coronary blood flow and to interfere with myocardial uptake of glucose despite a secondary elevation in arterial blood glucose levels. Alkalosis appears to cause increase in coronary blood flow with an accompanying elevation in arterial lactate and pyruvate levels. These elevated lactate and pyruvate levels lead to an increased uptake of these substrates.

In a landmark paper published in 1959 [23], Goodale and his colleagues presented data derived from studies of myocardial metabolism by catheter techniques in normal and diabetic humans. From these studies, it appears that the heart has a remarkable capability of selecting its substrates in a fashion appropriate to the nutritional climate in which it finds itself. In the fasting state, for example, in which the rest of the body has diminished its carbohydrate utilization and is relying on adipose tissue stores as a major energy source, the heart does likewise. Hence, a normal fasting person who has blood sugar levels in a range of 60 to 80 mg/100 ml extracts a small amount of glucose from arterial blood which will account for between 10 and 32 percent of the oxygen uptake. Below the glucose level of 60 mg/100 ml, no extraction occurs. In the nonfasting state, as the blood glucose is rising the heart increases its glucose extraction asymptotically, approaching a maximum of 25 to 30 mg/100 ml at arterial blood levels above 250 mg/100 ml. In this postprandial state, then carbohydrate metabolism accounts for 90 percent of the total oxygen use. The thresholds for lactate and pyruvate use are very much lower than those for glucose, 2.5 and 0.6 mg/100 ml, respectively. As alluded to earlier, the extractions of these substrates rise as the arterial levels rise. The impact of diabetes mellitus on carbohydrate use is profound. Fasting subjects with mild diabetes extract no glucose, and the extraction of lactate and pyruvate is markedly reduced despite increased arterial blood levels of glucose and normal levels of lactate and pyruvate. The myocardial respiratory quotient of diabetic patients is 0.70, consistent with exclusive fat oxidation to meet the energy requirements of the heart. When glucose or food was given to diabetic subjects, increasing their arterial blood glucose levels, some increase in myocardial glucose extraction resulted but not nearly as much as in the normal person. Only simultaneous administration of insulin restored myocardial extraction of glucose and pyruvate to normal.

Bing and his associates [20] found that the human myocardium in the fasting state derived an average of 67 percent of its energy from fatty acids. These observations, combined with those of Goodale et al. [23] indicate that the myocardium is capable of deriving a majority, and sometimes all, of its energy from fat when the nutritional or endocrine climate precludes carbohydrate use. When the adipose tissue depots are called on to sustain the body in periods of fasting, they do so in the form of nonesterified fatty acids (NEFA) carried in the plasma, solubilized by a loose physical-chemical bonding to plasma albumin. NEFA, however, are not the sole lipid substrates for the heart that is using fat as fuel. Fatty acids esterified as triglycerides also play a very significant role. Several workers have studied the percentages of total lipid calories supplied to the heart by non-esterified and triglyceride fatty acids and precise agreement does not appear to be forthcoming. It would appear that at least half the lipid calories come from triglyceride fatty acids, and perhaps somewhat more. This large myocardial extraction of esterified fatty acids is consistent with the finding that more than half of the chylomicron triglycerides are directly oxidized on passage through that tissue.

Not only is the heart capable of using varying amounts of carbohydrate and lipid substrates, depending upon the nutritional milieu with which it is presented but also it is capable of using ketone bodies as well. It has been documented that both acetoacetic acid and beta-hydroxybutyric acid can be used as substrates by the heart when they are present in the blood stream in large quantities, as in uncontrolled diabetes mellitus. The data even suggest that acetoacetate may be the preferred substrate in that the heart presented with high blood levels of this substance will use it for fuel at the same time that it is decreasing its use of both carbohydrate and lipid substrates. The selection of substrates by the heart can also be affected by insulin administration in the case of ketone bodies. Though acetoacetate can be shown to be a preferred fuel, the administration of insulin will shift the fuel used to endogenous substrates and away from ketone bodies.

The role of amino acids as fuel for the myocardium is in dispute at the present time. Data have been published, ranging from no use at all up to use sufficient to account for 40 percent of the oxygen uptake. It is this author's opinion that when agreement is finally reached, it will be found that the myocardium generally extracts amino acids primarily to use as building blocks in the constant turnover of its own muscle tissue, and uses amino acids as fuel only in states of extreme stress.

In summary, it is safe to say that of all the substrates used by the heart, the level of oxygen supply is the most critical. The truly amazing ability of the heart to shift its substrate dependence in accordance with the nutritional and hormonal environment in which it finds itself protects it from harm by fuel deprivation. It presently appears that fuel deprivation is seldom, if ever, a problem of sufficient magnitude to produce clinical disease. It is known to all, however, that there is no substitute for oxygen in the biochemical scheme, and the heart is no exception. Ischemic injury is oxygen-lack injury and not fuel deprivation injury.

THE PROCESSING OF SUBSTRATES

With an overview of the patterns and regulation of acquisition of substrates by the cells of the heart behind us, the next step is to consider the transformations they undergo inside the cell in the orderly series of reactions under the general heading of intracellular metabolism. The overall object of the processing of fuel substrates is to extract chemical energy from them. These chemical reactions will not be discussed in detail here as they are available in the excellent review by Opie [16, 17, 18] and in any one of several modern textbooks of biochemistry. Herein, we will attempt to outline the general pathways involved in such a fashion as to provide the cardiologist with a clear conceptual understanding of them without a burdensome weight of details.

The overall aim of the step-wise transformation of substrates is to extract chemical energy from them and trap it in a chemical compound that can be tapped, as needed, by the energy-requiring parts of the cell. It is the adenine nucleotides that provide the chemical medium for such an energy exchange. The purine base, adenine, is linked to ribose and 2 molecules of phosphate to form adenosine diphosphate. A large amount of energy is required to link a third phosphate to this moiety (approximately 7,000 calories per mole.) and form adenosine triphosphate (ATP). In reactions catalyzed by the proper enzymes, this third phosphate molecule can be hydrolyzed off in such a fashion as to yield a large part of the chemical energy stored in that bond to drive other chemical or even mechanical reactions. Hence, energy is stored by the reactions:

$$\text{ADP} + \text{phosphate} + \text{energy} \rightarrow \text{ATP}$$

Energy is made available to the cellular economy by the reactions:

$$\text{ATP} \rightarrow \text{ADP} + \text{phosphate} + \text{energy}$$

The first set of reactions that glucose undergoes inside the cell has as its ultimate aim the splitting of this 6-carbon aldehyde sugar into two 3-carbon acid molecules, pyruvic acid. This process is known as glycolysis, or the Embden-Meyerhof pathway. All of the reactants in this set of reactions are phosphorylated; that is, they have a phosphate molecule attached to them. Therefore, glucose cannot begin to enter this pathway until a phosphate is attached to it. This reaction is catalyzed by the ubiquitous enzyme hexokinase and the phosphate moiety is provided by a molecule of ATP. This is a high-energy phosphate; therefore, at this point, the metabolism of glucose shows a net input of 1 high-energy phosphate unit. The resulting compound, glucose-6-phosphate, forms a ring around an oxygen molecule that is not symmetrical and, therefore, not easily amenable to splitting into even halves. The next step then is to rearrange the molecule to produce fructose 6-phosphate which is a symmetrical ring structure. Since our aim is going to be that of splitting this symmetrical ring compound into two 3-carbon compounds that are both phosphorylated, we now have to introduce another phosphate molecule. This is done at the 1- position and the product is known as hexose diphosphate, and it has a phosphate at both the 1- and the 6- position. The enzyme that catalyzed this step is called phosphohexokinase and is presently considered very important as a possible rate-limiting step, as is the first phosphorylating enzyme, hexokinase. Our energy balance at this point shows that we have had to invest another molecule of high-energy phosphate so that we now have an energy input of two such units.

The next step is the splitting, alluded to earlier. This is catalyzed by the enzyme aldolase, which is *never* rate limiting because it is present in very large amounts. The products are two 3-carbon fragments, each one having a phosphate attached. They are dihydroxyacetone phosphate and glyceraldehyde-3-phosphate. If the heart were going to make triglycerides (about which there is some doubt), some of the dihydroxyacetone phosphate could be diverted at this point to provide the glycerol part of triglyceride. In energy production, however, the dihydroxyacetone phosphate is isomerized into another molecule of glyceraldehyde-3-phosphate. Each of these two halves of the original glucose molecule is now oxidized. This process requires several steps and is the first one in which energy release is seen. The glyceraldehyde-3-phosphate reacts with inorganic phosphate and another coenzyme which is a derivative of nicotinic acid. Here, of course, we refer to nicotinamide adenine dinucleotide, and it is an energy trapper in its own fashion. Two hydrogens are removed from the glyceraldehyde-3-phosphate, and an inorganic phosphate molecule is attached to it. In addition, 2 electrons are released. These electrons and 1 of the hydrogens are used in the formation of the reduced form of nicotinamide adenine dinucleotide, abbreviated as NADH. The other removed hydrogen enters the medium as the hydrogen ion. The original glyceraldehyde-3-phosphate now becomes an acid and has 2 phosphates attached to it, 1, 3-diphosphoglyceric acid. The NADH that is produced contains a very great deal of useable chemical energy. If properly processed in the series of reactions known as oxidative phosphorylation, the reconversion of NADH to NAD can cause 3 molecules of ADP to react with 3 molecules of inorganic phosphate to produce 3 molecules of ATP. If we assume that this is to be the fate of the NADH, our energy score now shows an output of 3 ATPs for each half of the original glucose molecule or a total of 6. When balanced against our input of 2 high-energy phosphates our net gain at this point is 4 molecules of high-energy phosphate.

The high-energy phosphate put on the one position of the 1,3-diphosphate glyceric acid is also a high-energy phosphate which then reacts with a molecule of ADP to give another ATP. This raises our total net energy output to 6 high-energy phosphates, and 3-phosphoglyceric acid is then changed into the 2-phosphoglyceric acid, and a molecule of water is extracted yielding phosphoenol pyruvic acid. This is likewise a high-energy phosphate compound. It then reacts with yet another molecule of ADP, producing another ATP. Since both halves of the original glucose molecule have met this fate, our total high-energy balance shows a net yield of 8 high-energy phosphates. The other product of this reaction is pyruvic acid, signaling that we have come to the end of glycolysis. One must remember that the positive balance of 8 high-energy phosphates contains 6 such molecules derived from the oxidation of 2 molecules of NADH. This step is oxygen dependent and, therefore, will only yield 8 high-energy phosphates in a cell adequately supplied with oxygen. In the absence of oxygen, the energy contained in the NADH cannot be extracted for the cell's use. Instead, it is used to convert the pyruvic acid to lactic acid which then either accumulates or is lost from the cell. Thus, in anaerobic glycolysis the final results will be the conversion of 1 molecule of glucose to 2 molecules of lactic acid, and a positive energy balance of only 2 molecules of ATP.

The above series of reactions takes place in the soluble fraction or cytoplasm of the cell. The further oxidation of pyruvic acid to water and 3 molecules of CO_2 is accomplished in the mitochondria. As we will see later, the final pathway of the energy-yielding aspects of fat metabolism transpires in this organ also. The mitochondrion is, in a very real sense, the "power-supply" of the cell. It is here that the majority of the oxygen-dependent oxidative energy-yielding reactions of the cell take place. The energy that is freed from substrates is trapped in the form of high-energy phosphate bonds as ATP, hence the term oxidative phosphorylation.

Figure 6 shows that the mitochondrion is a roughly rod-shaped organelle from 0.5 to 2 micra in length [24]. It has thick walls that are thrown up into cristae that project into the lumen. In the lumen the enzymes catalyze the reactions that we know as the Krebs cycle, and organized structures in the walls and cristae accomplish the stepwise derivation of energy in an oxygen-dependent system yielding high-energy phosphate, the so-called electron-transport chain.

In the mitochondrion, pyruvic acid is completely degraded, yielding 3 molecules of CO_2 and 15 molecules of ATP. The first step is a complex, multireaction sequence. It involves the cofactors thiamine pyrophosphate, NAD, lipoic acid, and coenzyme A. The terminal CO_2 is removed in a

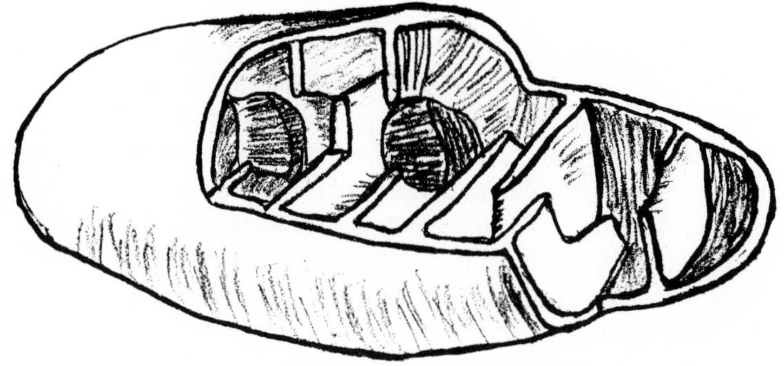

Figure 6. A mitochrondrion sketched to show inner chambers as well. (From Vester, J.W.: The cell. Scientific Clinician 1966, New York, McGraw-Hill, Ch. I, p. 23, by permission.)

thiamine-dependent decarboxylation step, and the remaining 2-carbon fragment bonds to coenzyme A to yield acetyl coenzyme A. Two hydrogens are removed from the original pyruvic acid and 1 of them is used to convert NAD to NADH, and the other one is released as hydrogen ion. The NADH is reoxidized to NAD by reacting with the front end of the electron-transport chain. NADH and H^+ react with flavin adenine dinucleotide (FAD) to produce $FADH_2$ and regenerate NAD which is then available to serve as a coenxyme in further dehydrogenation reactions. The 2 hydrogen ions that were originally removed from the pyruvic acid and the 2 electrons transferred in the process are then used to convert the flavine adenine dinucleotide to the reduced form $FADH_2$. In the reduction of FAD and the reoxidation of NAD, energy is tapped off in a fashion not completely understood to drive a reaction between ADP and inorganic phosphate and produce a molecule of ATP, high-energy phosphate. The $FADH_2$ now reacts with the next member of the chain, a coenzyme known as ubiquinone. Ubiquinone is converted to its reduced form, dihydroubiquinone, and the $FADH_2$ is reoxidized to FAD. This reduced cofactor now reacts with the first of the cytochromes, heme-containing structures that are capable of being reduced by accepting electrons and oxidized by giving them up. The 2 electrons from the dihydroubiquinone are transferred to cytochrome b, and the 2 hydrogens enter the medium as hydrogen ions, producing a net excess of 2 H^+. The electrons are then passed on down the chain from cytochrome b through cytochromes c and $a(a_3)$. This last cytochrome-$a(a_3)$-transfers its electrons to an atom of oxygen, making possible a reaction with the 2 excess hydrogens in the medium to form a molecule of water, H_2O. This eliminates the 2 excess hydrogen ions resulting from the entry of the 2 hydrogen ions from dihydroubiquinone into the medium, and completes the electron-transport system. Thus, it will be seen that the final acceptor for the 2 electrons originally removed from pyruvic acid is molecular oxygen, with the formation of water. In addition to the ATP formed at the NADH step, there are two other sites where most scientists agree that a similar process occurs. They appear to be somewhere between ubiquinone and cytochrome b as the second one, and somewhere between cytochrome c and a (a_3), as the third one. Hence, for every molecule of pyruvate that is oxidized, 1 molecule of water will be formed and 3 molecules of high-energy phosphate will be generated. Thus for every atom of oxygen used by the mitochondrion as an electron acceptor, 3 molecules of high-energy phosphate will be generated, giving rise to the standard P/O ratio of 3.

At the outset, we stated the aim of the oxygen-dependent degradation of pyruvic acid in the mitochondrion is the production of 3 molecules of CO_2 and the generation of a maximum amount of high-energy phosphate. At this point, we have converted the pyruvic acid to acetyl coenzyme A with the loss of 1 carbon atom as CO_2, and we have generated 3 molecules of ATP. Acetyl coenzyme A then combines with oxaloacetic acid to generate citric acid which is the beginning of the citric acid or Krebs cycle. In the series of reactions to follow, this 6-carbon citric acid molecule will be converted, finally, to oxaloacetic acid again to provide the starting place for another cycle. In this process, there will be the generation of 2 more molecules of carbon dioxide, accomplishing the aim of the net production of 3 molecules of carbon dioxide for every molecule of pyruvic acid degraded in the mitochondrion.

In one turn of the citric acid cycle in which the citrate formed from oxaloacetic acid and acetyl coenzyme A is degraded to oxaloacetic acid again with the generation of 2 molecules of CO_2, a total of 12 molecules of ATP are generated by the process of oxidative phosphorylation. Hence, when one adds together all of the high-energy phosphate produced in the overall transformation of 1 molecule of pyruvic acid to 3 molecules of CO_2, the total yield will be 15 molecules of ATP. When one reflects that every molecule of glucose can give rise to 2 molecules of pyruvic acid, this oxygen-dependent part of the glucose degradation scheme yields a total of 30 molecules of ATP. When one remembers that the maximum amount of ATP that can be generated by the formation of 2 molecules of pyruvic acid from glucose is 8 (it may be only 6), then it is apparent that the mitochondrial processing of 2 pyruvates yields somewhere between three and five times as much useable chemical energy as the glycolytic degradation of glucose.

The magnitude of the importance of oxygen to the energy economics of the cell is even greater than these figures would imply. In the above-described scheme proceeding from glucose to 6 molecules of CO_2 in water, a probable maximum total of 38 molecules of ATP would be yielded. The breakdown of 30 molecules from the mitochondria and 8 from glycolysis could only be achieved if the oxygen supply were adequate. If the cell were deprived of oxygen, oxidative phosphorylation would cease, and the 30 molecules so derived would be missing. Even the yield of 8 molecules of ATP from glycolysis would be altered because 6 of the 8 are dependent on the oxygen-dependent reoxidation of NADH. If oxygen is absent, this cannot occur, and the net yield of high-energy phosphate for the glycolytic breakdown of glucose drops to 2. The pyruvic acid generated under these circumstances will accumulate until it reacts, under the enzymic catalysis of lactic dehydrogenase, with the NADH generated during glycolysis to yield lactic acid. The lactic acid would then be lost from the cell in this anaerobic lactate-producing state. Thus, the deprivation of oxygen would change the total yield of ATP from glucose metabolism from 38 molecules to only 2. In addition, since the final path of fat metabolism is through the Krebs cycle, energy derivation from fat would also cease. Thus, our clinical awareness of the absolute dependence of the myocardium on oxygen is biochemically underscored. Even though the uptake and glycolytic processing of glucose are accelerated in the anaerobic as compared to the aerobic state, the rate increase is in no way adequate to overcome the profound decrease in ATP yield resulting from assuming an anaerobic stance.

The processing of lipid substrates can safely be said to be oxygen dependent from start to finish. The first step is the formation of a coenzyme-A derivative which requires the energy from ATP, as well. The fatty acyl Co-A compound then undergoes a four-step reaction that requires the participation of both FAD and NAD, finally yielding an acyl coenzyme-A derivative that is shorter than the original by 2 carbon atoms. The 2 carbons that have been removed are now in the form of acetyl coenzyme A. The reoxidation of the NADH and $FADH_2$ requires linkage to the electron transport system and is therefore oxygen dependent. The acetyl coenzyme A produced enters the Krebs cycle as previously described for carbohydrates and is processed in an identical fashion.

We must remember that the oxidation of fatty acids takes place in the mitochondria. This requires a potentially rate-limiting transfer step in the transport of mitochondria of fatty acids from the cytoplasm to the interior of the mitochondria. The previously mentioned acyl-CoA derivative of the fatty acid reacts with carnitine to form a carnitine derivative, and it is this substance that is rapidly transported into the mitochondria. The acyl-CoA is metabolised in the fashion previously described. Considering the potentially large portion of the oxidatively derived energy of the heart that comes from fatty acid metabolism, it would appear obvious that a process that interferes with this carnitine transfer step could potentially be a serious biochemical hazard to the heart. We shall see that this is indeed so when we discuss diphtheritic myocardial involvement.

If the lipid substrate is triglyceride, a preliminary step must be inserted before those mentioned above. This is a lipase activity which will split the fatty acid molecules from the glycerol. The glycerol can then phosphorylated and enter the Embden-Meyerhof system. The nonesterified fatty acids released are metabolised as described above.

If amino acids are used as substrates, the first step is an oxidative deamination releasing the nitrogen probably as ammonia. The carbon skeleton that remains is then variously altered so that 2 carbon fragments can enter the Krebs cycle as acetyl coenzyme A moieties.

CONVERSION OF CHEMICAL TO MECHANICAL ENERGY

Now that we have reviewed the extraction and processing of substrates with the trapping of chemical energy as ATP, it is appropriate to consider the present understanding of the mechanism whereby this chemical energy can be transformed into the mechanical energy necessary for the pumping action of the heart. For more extensive coverage of this subject, the reader is referred to two recent articles by Sonnenblick [25] and Davies [26]. Figures 7 and 8 are taken from Sonnenblick's article and emphasize that the primary mechanism of the contraction of muscle is the shortening of the individual units of the muscle cells, the sarcomeres. Each sarcomere is bounded on each end by the dark Z band and the filaments of actin are attached to these Z bands. The other ends of the actin filaments which extend toward the center of the sarcomere are free to slide to and fro as the sarcomere shortens and lengthens. In the more central portion of the sarcomere there are thick bands of myosin. These myosin bands are surrounded by actin filaments as the cross section in Figure 7 shows. As the muscle shortens, the actin filaments from the Z bands at either end slide in over the myosin fibers thus pulling the 2 Z bands closer to each other and shortening the length of the sarcomere. Figure 9 graphically shows how this process takes place. The biochemical events involved in this process are best explained, at the present time, by the theory of Davies [26]. The sarcolemma is the wall of the muscle cell, and it not only holds the cell together but also provides pathways of lower electrical resistance between cells. Inside the cell and surrounding the contractile elements is a system of fine membranous tubules that abut the sarcolemma and its ramifications (L system and T system). The sarcoplasmic reticulum is capable of binding calcium ions and can release them in response to electrical stimuli. If the

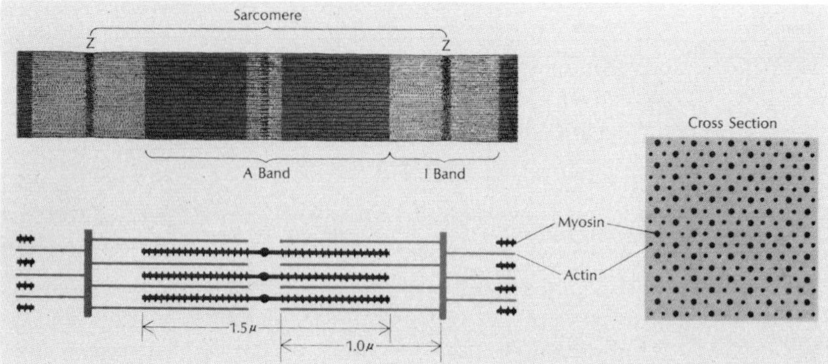

Figure 7. Within the sarcomeres, thick filaments of myosin, confined to the central dark A band, alternate with the filaments of actin which extended from the Z lines (delimiting the sarcomere) through the I band and into the A band where they overlap the myosin filaments. These landmarks are seen in detail drawings (bottom). On activation a repetitive interaction between the sites shown along these filaments displaces the filaments inward so that the sarcomere, and hence the whole muscle, shortens with maximum overlap at 2.2μ. (From Sonnenblick, E.H.: Myocardial ultrastructure in the normal and failing heart. Hosp Pract 5:35, 1970, by permission.)

calcium concentration within the sarcomere in the sarcoplasm is very low (10^{-7} to 10^{-8} *M* or less), the muscle will not contract and will remain at rest. When an electrical stimulus travels through the sarcolemma and its ramifications and reaches the sarcoplasmic reticulum, calcium is released and diffuses rapidly into the sarcoplasm. The concentration of calcium rises to 10^{-6} *M* or more, and this concentration is sufficient to allow the next steps which will involve the conversion of the chemical energy of ATP to the mechanical energy of shortening.

This release of calcium from the sarcoplasmic reticulum into the sarcoplasm in response to an electrical stimulus is graphically demonstrated in Figure 8. The figure shows Professor Davies' concept of the chemical events that ensue when calcium is released from the sarcoplasm reticulum into the sarcoplasm. There are foot processes on myosin that can be seen with an electron microscope and are considered to be the means whereby the myosin fiber can cause the actin filaments to slide over it. In Figure 8, No. 1 shows that the resting muscle has an ATP molecule attached to the foot process. This produces electrical repulsion from a negatively charged molecule at the base of the attachment of the foot process, and the foot process is accordingly stretched to its maximum. When calcium is released from the sarcoplasmic reticulum, it is capable of forming a molecular bond between the ATP on the end of the foot process and ADP that is part of the adjacent actin filament. The formation of this chemical bond neutralizes the negative charge on the terminal ATP of the foot process so that it is

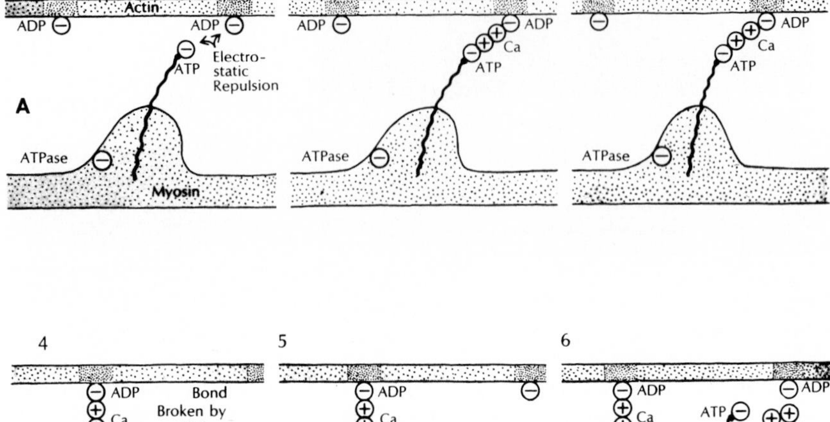

Figure 8. A. The sliding mechanism of contraction in the sarcomere is believed to operate in the stepwise fashion. In the absence of calcium (1), the ATP attached to the myosin filament and the ADP attached to the actin filament both have negative charges and repel each other. With the entry of positively charged calcium ions, an electrostatic link is formed (2). An alpha helix is formed that pulls the actin filament along the myosin filament (3). *B.* The ATP is now exposed to the ATPase of the heavy meromyosin (4). The link is broken as the ATP is cleaved to ADP and inorganic phosphate. CP in the sarcoplasm then rephosphorylates the ADP to ATP (5). The ATP attached to the myosin then repeats the attachment at the next site on the actin filament (6). (From Davies, R.E.: Biochemical processes in cardiac function. Hosp Pract 5:49, 1970, by permission.)

no longer caused to be extended by electrical repulsion of like charges. In the absence of electrical repulsion, the elasticity of the foot process is able to shorten it. This shortening pulls the actin fiber along the myosin fiber. When the shortened foot process contracts sufficiently, the terminal ATP comes in contact with an enzyme, ATPase in the base of the attachment of the foot process, and this breaks the bond holding the terminal phosphate leaving ADP. When the ADP on the foot process is rephosphorylated, the negative charges are restored, and the foot process is extended to a position where it is now capable of bonding in a similar fashion with the next integral

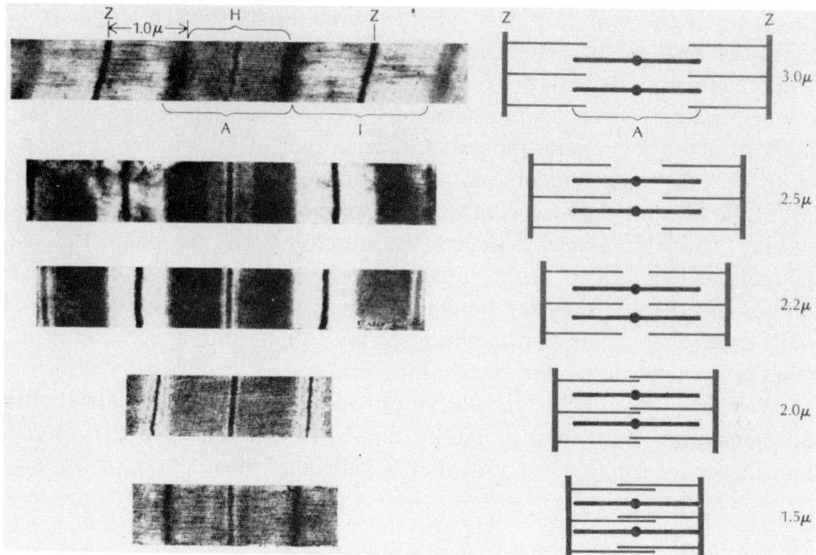

Figure 9. The way in which altering sarcomere length changes band pattern is shown in actual frog sartorius muscle sarcomeres (*left*) and in correlated diagrams. The middle sarcomere is at $L_{max.}$ (2.2 μ), at which length maximum contractile force is produced. (From: Sonnenblick, E.H.: Myocardial ultrastructure in the normal and failing heart. Hosp Pract 5:35, 1970, by permission.)

ADP molecule of the adjacent actin molecule if sufficient calcium ions are present. When electrical activation ceases, the calcium is quickly pumped back into the vesicles of the sarcoplasmic reticulum, and the muscle is once again in an inactive state. If one measures the amount of ATP in the heart at any given time, one finds that its concentration is much lower than the concentration of creatine phosphate. This suggests that creatine phosphate is present in large quantities to regenerate the foot process ATP under the enzymic catalysis of creatine phosphokinase.

Not all authorities agree that this theory explains the events of contraction of muscle, but it is the one that is most popular at this time. It does fit nicely into an older concept governing cardiac function, namely, Starling's law. The reader will remember that as the heart dilates, the force of contraction increases up to a point where further dilatation causes weakening of the force of contraction. If the Davies theory has validity, then it is apparent that the maximum force of shortening will be developed when the largest number of foot processes on the myosin are able to form bonds with the actin. A look at Figure 9 will show the direction of this line of reasoning. If the muscle is not extended and the sarcomere length is 1.5 micra, the ends of the actin that overlap in the center will not be able to form effective bonds with the foot processes on the adjacent myosin fibers. As one gradually stretches the fiber, less and less overlap occurs until at a length of about 2.2 micra, the maximum number of myosin foot processes can reach attachments on adjacent actin. This would represent the ascending part of the Starling curve as contractile force increases with the stretching of the fiber. If one continues to stretch the muscle beyond the point, the actin filaments will be pulled further apart and would then present a decreased number of effective sites for binding with myosin foot processes. At that point, then, decrease in contractile force with increasing elongation occurs as in the descending part of the Starling curve.

We have now reached the end of our survey of myocardial metabolism and mechanics. With these points in mind, we now turn our attention to abnormal myocardial states and what is known of them.

CARDIAC FAILURE

A complete review of the literature relating to cardiac failure is far beyond the scope of this text. For more extensive discussion and bibliography, the reader is referred to three reviews: Bing's treatise in *Physiological Reviews* which has already been cited [15]; the American Heart Association's English translation of a monograph by Meerson [27]; and a symposium containing a number of papers related to hemodynamic and metabolic changes in cardiac failure, edited by Evans [28].

For the purpose of this brief review, we will use the definition of heart failure as presented by Meerson [27]. He describes heart failure as that condition in which the load on the heart exceeds its work capacity. As he points out, two possibilities follow from this basic definition. The first of these is that cardiac failure may arise as a result of an excessive load on the myocardium (as in hypertension or valvular disease) and the second is that the condition may result from disease of the myocardium itself. These two states have been referred to as secondary and primary cardiac failure, respectively, and reviewed at some length in another noteworthy publication [29].

The ultimate hemodynamic consequences of overload of the myocardium are similar whether the overload is of the pressure type as in hypertension and aortic stenosis or of the volume type as in valvular incompetence and anemia. Nonetheless, it should be remembered that there is a difference in the cardiac response to the early stages of these two types of load.

In the early stages of compensation for a volume load, a true physiologic preload occurs. In this circumstance, the volume of blood in the ventricle increases during diastolic filling so that the individual muscle fibers are stretched prior to the initiation of contraction. This initiates the Frank-Starling effect and up to a point, enables the myocardium to increase its force of contraction without the consequence of a decrease in velocity. There is a geometric advantage to dilatation of a volume-overloaded ventricle which arises because the larger a hollow sphere becomes, the greater the ejection volume will be with a constant degree of shortening of the circumference of the sphere. The pressure type of load is an afterload. In the early stages of afterload, the heart simply encounters increased resistance to ejection of blood. Contraction is slowed in rate; increased contractile force is developed. Therefore, the volume-loaded heart, having a preload, achieves increased force of contration without diminution in velocity of contraction, whereas the afterloaded heart, facing a pressure load, always shows a decrease in the velocity of contraction as a consequence of the development of increased force.

Whether from preload or afterload, the failing heart has a number of fairly constant characteristics:

1. End-diastolic blood volume is increased which leads to increased end-diastolic pressure.
2. Increased end-diastolic pressure. One of the consequences of an increase in end-diastolic pressure is cardiac dilatation.
3. Cardiac dilatation enables the heart to take advantage of the Frank-Starling law.
4. The duration of systole and of the isovolumic period of tension generation in the heart is increased. This occurs because the *failing* heart always has a decrease in contractile velocity. As stated above, the afterloaded heart has a decrease in contractile velocity throughout the course of the hemodynamic evolution of heart failure. The preloaded heart will be able to increase its contractile force up to about 45 percent without any decrease in velocity. As conditions worsen and the load increases one passes over the hump, so to speak, of the Starling curve and decrease in velocity of contraction is seen.*
5. Except in such high-output states as beriberi and thyrotoxicosis, cardiac output is diminished. In the early stages, *resting* cardiac output may be normal in the presence of heart failure, but the failing heart is unable to increase cardiac output to a sufficient degree to meet all the needs imposed by stress, exercise, and so forth. One of the immediate consequences of

* *Editorial note:* It should be stated that there is no good evidence that the descending limb of the Starling curve, relating diastolic fiber tension to work, exists in man.

inadequate cardiac output is an increase in the arteriovenous oxygen saturation difference in the blood, which is considered to be an important sign of heart failure.

6. When a ventricle fails and end-diastolic pressure rises, so will the pressure in those parts of the circuit proximal to the failing ventricle.

The biochemistry of secondary heart failure (related to heart muscle disease) has likewise been extensively studied and will be summarized here. For more extensive reviews, the reader is referred to the lengthy treatises by Bing [15], Opie [16, 17, 18], Meerson [27], and Evans [28].

The changes in myocardial oxygen consumption resulting from cardiac overload are entirely predictable. Oxygen uptake increases in proportion to the amount of work demanded of the myocardium. When hypertrophy occurs, there is a further increase in oxygen consumption directly related to this increase in muscle mass. Levine and Wagman [30] studied myocardial oxygen consumption in normal patients as well as in patients with overt secondary heart failure. The oxygen consumption per 100 gm of heart muscle was identical in both groups. However, the presence of marked cardiac hypertrophy in the patients with heart failure caused the total myocardial oxygen consumption to be three times greater in the cardiac failure patients than in those who were normal.

Substrate use is similarly devoid of significant abnormalities. As long ago as 1951, Olson and Schwartz [31] summarized their own and others' studies that indicated that oxygen extraction and substrate use per 100 gm of left ventricle were normal or slightly increased in patients with radiographic evidence of left ventricular enlargment. These workers also pointed out that since the cardiac outputs were reduced in the patients studied, the thermodynamic efficiency of the failing heart is low. There seems to be general agreement, then, that uptake of fuel and oxygen by the failing heart does not depart from normal when related to unit weight of the heart. Increase in muscle mass, of course, leads to increased total uptake of oxygen and fuel.

Since the failing heart appears to have adequate uptake of oxygen and fuel, there has to be an explanation elsewhere for the diminished amount of work done. The breakdown can occur at one or both of the two subsequent steps. The first is the conversion of the chemical energy derived from substrate oxidation to high energy phosphate compounds, ATP, and creatine phosphate (CP). The other possible site of breakdown is, of course, the conversion of the chemical energy from these compounds to mechanical energy by the contractile machinery. In the literature, it is on this point that disagreement exists as to which of these two possible sites of breakdown is responsible for the low thermodynamic efficiency of the failing heart. The large number of studies directed at this point have been summarized and reviewed extensively and well by both Bing [15] and Meerson [27]. In his review, Meerson tends to emphasize those studies suggesting that there is a defect in the generation of high-energy phosphate compounds. Bing, on the other hand, points out that the experimental data must be viewed from the point in time at which the experimentally failing heart preparation is examined. It appears that several models of experimental heart failure can be shown to have decreased rates of formation of ATP and CP in the acute stages of cardiac failure. If as in the human clinical state, one waits until a stable state of congestive failure is produced, one finds that the rates of production of ATP and CP are entirely normal. Olson's data [32] clearly indicate normal levels of high-energy phosphate compounds in stable congestive failure dog hearts whether of valvular or thyrotoxic origin. This reviewer is inclined to favor the position that the defect in the failing heart represents an as yet unidentified breakdown in the conversion of high-energy phosphate energy to mechanical energy.

THE CARDIOMYOPATHIES

In reviewing the hemodynamic and myocardial metabolism studies in primary myocardial diseases, we shall follow the general classification of the cardiomyopathies as published by Fowler [33]. He classifies these numerous disorders under two main headings: idiopathic and secondary. The idiopathic is further subdivided into nonobstructive and obstructive cardiomyopathy. In discussing these groups of disorders and in touching on each of these headings as much as possible, we shall follow the general format of the earlier part of this chapter. Matters to be considered will include hemodynamic studies of cardiac function, myocardial blood flow, oxygen and substrate extraction and use when such data are available.

Nonobstructive Idiopathic Cardiomyopathy

At the outset, it is safe to say that the hemodynamic findings in idiopathic nonobstructive cardiomyopathy are ordinarily nonspecific, as Fowler states. In 1964, Goodwin [34, 35] studied 8 patients with congestive cardiomyopathy and found a low or low-normal cardiac output in all patients. In addition, there was radiologic evidence of considerable cardiac dilation (cardiomegaly) without increased thickness of the ventricular wall. The data suggested poor contractile function with little evidence of muscular hypertrophy. He found elevated right atrial pressure in 6 of the 8 patients. The right ventricular end-diastolic pressure was less than 10 mmHg in 5 of 6 patients studied, and the maximum was 12 mmHg in 1 patient. In addition, pulmonary arterial "wedge" pressure was elevated in only 1 patient.

In 1966, Pietras [36] and his coworkers published their studies of 21 adult male patients with presumed idiopathic congestive (nonobstructive) cardiomyopathy. This group also found cardiomegaly in all patients. They stated that the left atrium, left ventricle, right ventricle, and right atrium were dilated in decreasing order of frequency. In evaluating hemodynamics, they divided their patients into groups I and II. Group I consisted of 9 patients who had normal left ventricular end-diastolic pressures at rest, 6 of whom had normal and 3 had low resting cardiac indices. Five of the 9 had low cardiac indices on exercise, and 4 of these showed abnormal increases in pulmonary arterial wedge pressure on exercise. Group II consisted of 12 patients with abnormal left ventricular end-diastolic pressures at rest. Four of these had normal and 8 had low-cardiac indices at rest. Of the 12, 9 were studied during exercise, and all had low exercise cardiac indices. In the 9 so studied, the pulmonary arterial wedge pressures were elevated at rest and rose further on exercise.

In 1966, Yu and his coworkers [37] published a description of extensive studies of 15 patients with idiopathic cardiomyopathy. Of these 15 patients, there were 5 men and 1 woman who were called "the congestive group," and probably represented examples of primary cardiomyopathy with decompensation. There was electrocardiographic and radiographic evidence of left ventricular enlargement in all patients. In addition, fluoroscopy of the chest showed left atrial enlargement in all and probable right ventricular enlargement in 4. Angiocardiographic studies were performed in 2 patients and demonstrated an increased thickness of the left ventricular wall. Cardiac index was diminished in all 5 patients, and the arteriovenous O_2 difference was increased from a normal of 24 to 44 ml/liter to 54 to 83 ml/liter with an average of 68.4. Stroke index, which normally ranges between 34 and 60 ml per beat, ranged from 17 to 26 with a mean of 23. Right ventricular end-diastolic pressure was elevated in 2 of the 5, and pulmonary arterial mean pressure was elevated in 4 of the 5. Left atrial mean pressure was elevated in each, ranging from 15 to 31 mmHg. The pulmonary arterial wedge pressure was studied in 3 patients and was elevated in all. The left ventricular end-diastolic pressure was elevated in each of the 4 patients studied, ranging from 20 to 32 mmHg. Left ventricular stroke work normally ranges between 40 and 80 gm-meters per beat per square meter of body surface. In the 6 patients, left ventricular stroke work was between 12 and 29 with a mean of 21 gm-meters per square meter. This last observation is a clear demonstration of loss of contractile power of the left ventricular musculature in primary cardiomyopathy. In

1968, Burch and DePasquale summarized the literature concerning the hemodynamic alterations in nonobstructive cardiomyopathy [38]. They listed the following findings for this disorder:

> Right atrial pressure was usually elevated; there was moderate elevation of right ventricular systolic pressure; there was little or no elevation of right ventricular end-diastolic pressure; pulmonary artery pressure was normal or slightly elevated; consistent elevation of pulmonary arterial wedge pressure; low cardiac index; poor *x* descent and steep *y* descent of right atrial pressure pulse, suggesting tricuspid regurgitation; absence of hemodynamic evidence of significant valvular obstruction.

Another hemodynamic finding seen in nonobstructive cardiomyopathies was first described by Braunwald and Aygen [39]. These investigators described giant A waves that may occur in the right or left atrium in patients with this disorder.

Hamby [40] and his colleagues published two extensive reviews of studies conducted on patients with primary myocardial disease. In reporting the hemodynamic observations of these patients, the authors divided them into two groups. Group I had normal left ventricular end-diastolic pressure. Also included in group I (listed as group IB) were patients who did have an elevation of left ventricular end-diastolic pressure, but the elevation was merely that due to the transmitted prominent A wave mentioned above. Group II had true elevated left ventricular end-diastolic pressure. The first of the two studies cited by Hamby and his group [37] contains data derived from a study of 100 patients. Of the 26 patients in group IA (patients with normal left ventricular end-diastolic pressure), the mean resting values of the variables studied were generally within normal limits. However, in 6 of these patients one or two of the following measurements were abnormal; cardiac index in 4, mean systolic ejection rate in 3, and right ventricular end-diastolic pressure in 3. Though some of the patients in this group had a prominent atrial A wave, the mean atrial pressures were normal. There were 20 patients in group IB, and they all had prominent transmitted A waves that elevated left ventricular end-diastolic pressure. Even though the mean left atrial end-diastolic pressure was elevated as compared to normal, it was still much lower than the left ventricular end-diastolic pressure. Sixty percent of the patients in group IB had an elevated right ventricular end-diastolic pressure, as well. Of the 20 patients in group IB, 4 had both a low cardiac index and a low mean systolic ejection rate. Group II was distinctly abnormal in all variables studied. Right and left atrial mean pressure, and right and left ventricular end-diastolic pressures were elevated. Arteriovenous O_2 differences were increased, and both cardiac and stroke index were decreased. Mean systolic ejection rate and left ventricular stroke work were likewise both decreased. The response of these patients to a standard exercise clearly revealed that all the patients had definite abnormalities of the myocardium. As one would expect, the abnormalities were least in group IA and progressed through group IB with the most severe derangements in group II. Though each group increased myocardial oxygen consumption during exercise, none had a significant increase in cardiac index, mean systolic ejection rate, or left ventricular stroke work. In addition, exercise resulted in elevations of left and right ventricular end-diastolic volumes in each group. One other point made by Hamby in his paper is that 13 of the 54 patients in group II had a ventricular pressure curve pattern suggestive of diminished compliance of the left ventricular wall (restrictive cardiomyopathy). This pattern is characterized by an early diastolic dip followed by a plateau, and is similar to that seen in constrictive pericarditis and in some patients with hemochromatosis, amyloidosis, and myocardial fibrosis.

The second of the two cited publications by Hamby and his colleagues [41] essentially confirmed the above findings. This study of 50 patients, grouped as in the previous paper, added some additional data. Using angiocardiographic techniques described by other workers [42, 43], they were able to determine the thickness of the left ventricular free wall, left ventricular end-diastolic volume, and end-diastolic circumferential stress and tension. The circumferential stress is defined as the force present in a wall per unit cross-sectional area and is expressed as dynes per square centimeter. Since the tension in the wall is expressed as in the following equation—Tension = stress × wall thickness—tension is the product of the stress times the left ventricular free wall thickness and is expressed as dynes per centimeter. In both groups, calculated left ventricular weight was more than twice normal. End-diastolic volume was normal in group I, and the left ventricular free wall thickness was almost twice normal. In group II, however, end-diastolic volume was almost twice normal, and left ventricular wall thickness was only slightly above normal. The ejection fraction was diminished in both groups, more so in group II than in group I. End-diastolic volume was increased in both groups, again more so in group II than in group I. Calculated left ventricular weight was elevated in both groups, more so in group I than in group II. This latter finding reflected that the wall thickness was almost twice normal in group I, whereas in group II there was only a mild-to-moderate increase in wall thickness. The end-diastolic stress was normal in group I and elevated in group II. As a result of the relationship between stress, tension, and wall thickness expressed in the equation above, end-diastolic tension was increased in group I because of the increased wall thickness. With both stress and wall thickness increased in group II, the end-diastolic tension was increased in these patients, as well. The authors conclude that their data suggest that primary myocardial disease of the nonobstructive type passes through an early, latent, asymptomatic stage, followed by a symptomatic, hypertrophic stage (group I) which progresses to an irreversible stage of dilatation (group II).

The extensive data cited in the preceding paragraph indeed lend themselves to the construction of a continuum of physiologic deterioration of the affected myocardium which is at first compensatory and then inadequate. As the affected myocardium begins to be unequal to the tasks demanded of it, compensatory mechanisms are called on. The atrial kick, allowing for increased ventricular end-diastolic volume, increased ventricular end-diastolic volume itself (Frank-Starling law), and hypertrophy are all such evidences. At this stage, best represented by group I, the heart is able to meet the body's metabolic demands at rest but not during exercise. When further deterioration takes place, the result is excessive dilatation, at which point the heart is unable to meet even the demands of rest and all the measured variables become abnormal.

Badeer [44] has recently reviewed the published studies of myocardial blood flow and metabolic data in a number of types of cardiomegaly. The data relating to primary idiopathic cardiomyopathy of the nonobstructive type are generally unremarkable. In 1962, Wendt and his colleagues [45] studied 8 such patients. Cardiac index and myocardial blood flow were somewhat decreased at rest and showed slight elevation with exercise. Oxygen consumption of the myocardium was also within normal limits at rest and increased slightly on exercise. The oxygen consumption of the heart per 100 gm left ventricular weight was within normal limits at rest and rose slightly on exercise. Pyruvate and lactate extractions were essentially normal.

In 1967, Brink and Lewis [46] reported a similar study in 14 patients with South African idiopathic mural endomyocardiopathy. These workers found coronary blood flow in their patients to be essentially within normal limits. In addition, the increase with exercise was not statistically different from that reported in normal patients. Oxygen consumption per unit weight of myocardium was normal at rest and did not change significantly upon exercise. Extraction of glucose, pyruvate, lactate, and free fatty acids were likewise normal at rest. Of the substrates studied, only pyruvate showed a statistically significant increase in myocardial extraction with exercise.

Though there is some conflict in the above two reports, it would appear safe to summarize the myocardial data as follows: If the left ventricle that is affected with nonobstructive idiopathic cardiomyopathy is unable to increase its cardiac output with exercise, then there will be no concomitant increase in extraction of oxygen or fuel substrates.

IDIOPATHIC CARDIOMYOPATHY OF THE OBSTRUCTIVE TYPE

There are several excellent overall reviews of this topic to which the reader is referred for extensive coverage and bibliography [34, 47, 48]. Braunwald points out that this particular disorder is unique in that the first report of the disease by Schmincke [49] contained conjectures by the author concerning the relationship between the pathologic changes and the pathophysiology that were strikingly close to the mark. The problem appears to be, as Schmincke conjectured, that there is muscular hypertrophy of the outflow tract that, as has been shown later, in combination with a late systolic opening movement of the anterior mitral leaflet, leads to obstruction to left ventricular ejection. This obstruction, in turn, leads to further hypertrophy, a sequence of changes which would continue to intensify the obstruction. In some cases, the hypertrophy bulges through the septum resulting in obstruction to the right ventricular outflow tract as well.

Identifying hemodynamic changes in idiopathic hypertrophic subaortic stenosis (IHSS) extends to the peripheral pulses, and we will begin with these. In valvular aortic stenosis and in most patients with discrete subaortic stenosis, the obstruction to the ventricular outflow reduces the velocity of ventricular ejection. As a consequence, the arterial pulse rises slowly to a delayed peak and the total ejection period is prolonged. In 1959, Brachfeld and Gorlin pointed out that the pulse rise rate is different in patients with IHSS. As a consequence of the often extensive ventricular hypertrophy, the arterial pulse first rises more rapidly than normal, during the first portion of left ventricular ejection [50, 51]. As the isotonic phase of contraction continues, however, the outflow tract constricts and the result is a late systolic pressure gradient between the left ventricle and the aorta. The pulse-wave contour produced by this series of events is unique to this condition. The arterial pulse wave shows a very abrupt rise to a rapid peak. Then, when the hypertrophic muscle in the outflow tract obstructs outflow, there is an equally abrupt drop. As the ventricular muscle continues to shorten, the pressure in the ventricle overcomes the obstruction, and there is then a further rise in the pulse wave that is much lower in amplitude than the first one, and it is much slower in rise. This latter phenomenon represents the slowing of cardiac muscle contraction due to the imposition of an afterload late in the systolic ejection period. In some patients, this can be so marked as to produce a carotid pulsus bisferiens. The time from the onset of the carotid pulse rise to its peak has been reported to range between 0.06 and 0.11 second (mean 0.088 ± 0.013 second) in 30 normal individuals [52]. Forty-seven patients with IHSS, studied by Braunwald

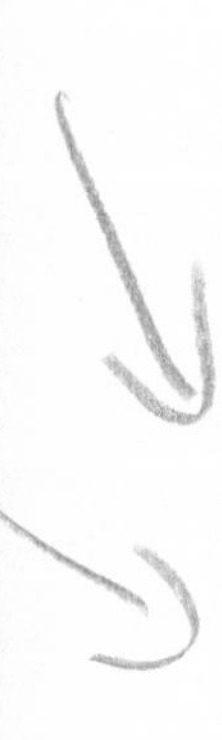

[48], showed times ranging between 0.04 and 0.12 second (mean 0.062 ± 0.019 second).

Braunwald's observations have led to a clinically useful extrapolation of these hemodynamic findings. Thirty-five of the 47 patients he studied with IHSS had a bifid indirect carotid pulse contour and 12 showed only a single peak. Catheter measurement of the maximum systolic pressure gradient across the subaortic muscular stenosis in patients with a bifid carotid pulse contour showed a gradient of 76.4± 38.7 mmHg. In the 12 patients with a single peak recorded on indirect carotid pulse contour recording, the systolic pressure gradients averaged only 9.9 mm Hg. Thus, inspection of the contour of the carotid pulse can provide a useful prediction of the hemodynamic state. A single peak pulse strongly suggests that little if any obstruction will be found at rest; whereas a double-peaked pulse suggests that significant obstruction is present. Since Benchimol's paper, cited above, pointed out that patients with valvular stenosis had a slower than normal rise of arterial pulse pressure from time of onset to peak, the arterial pulse-wave contour is useful in distinguishing between valvular stenosis and IHSS. Calculation of the first and second derivatives of the rise time of the brachial artery pressure pulse wave makes possible complete or nearly complete separation of patients with IHSS from patients with either valvular stenosis or discrete subvalvular stenosis, and from normal patients as well.

Another consequence of the imposition of an obstruction to outflow late in systole is prolongation of the ejection period. In 19 of 47 patients studied by Braunwald [48], the ejection time exceeded 0.34 second which was the longest period observed among normal subjects.

The resting cardiac index in 56 patients studied by Braunwald averaged 3.3 liters per minute per square meter of body surface. The range was 1.6 to 5.5 liters per minute per square meter body surface. The majority of the patients in each of the 4 cardiac functional classifications (New York Heart Association) had values within the normal range, but 10 patients who were either asymptomatic or only mildly symptomatic had elevated cardiac indices. Three patients who were in functional class IV had markedly reduced cardiac indices. Pulmonary hypertension does occur but is not a constant finding. Pulmonary artery mean pressure exceeded 30 mm Hg in 16 of Braunwald's 59 patients and was over 40 mm Hg in 9 [48]. A systolic pressure gradient within the right ventricular outflow tract ranging between 10 and 62 mm Hg was recorded in 10 of the 59 patients studied. In his report, he summarized a number of reports of other workers calling attention to the fairly common occurrence of this phenomenon in patients with IHSS. Twenty-one of the 59 patients studied also had right ventricular end-diastolic pressure greater than 7 mm Hg, and 6 of these were patients with significant obstruction to right ventricular outflow. Though the mean right atrial pressure was within normal limits in most patients, the A wave was the most prominent one in the atrial pressure pulse curve and exceeded the height of the V wave and the mean atrial pressure. About one-fourth of the patients had A waves with peaks greater than 8 mm Hg.

Left heart catheterization of patients with IHSS has been carried out by a large number of workers and has been summarized in the references alluded to earlier. The left atrial pressure pulse was likewise characterized by tall A waves. In addition, the mean left atrial pressure was above 12 mm Hg in approximately one-third of the patients studied. One-fourth of the patients had giant left atrial A waves (equal to or greater than 20 mm Hg). The single finding on left ventricular catheterization was the peak systolic gradient across the hypertrophic subaortic stenosis region. In well over 100 patients studied by a number of investigators, the gradient ranged from zero to a maximum of 175 mm Hg. The average was somewhere between 55 and 70 mm Hg. Most of the workers call attention to the variation in the peak systolic pressure gradient from beat to beat. Left ventricular end-diastolic pressure also varied widely, ranging from 0 to 55 mm Hg, and averaged approximately 20 mm Hg. Another characteristic in patients with IHSS is a notch on the ascending limb of the left ventricular pressure curve. This has been shown to be coincident with the opening of the semilunar valves.* It therefore occurs at the end of the isovolumic phase and at the beginning of left ventricular ejection. The mechanism of this notch is not known, but Braunwald [48] speculates that it may represent a release of the obstruction of the closed semilunar valve followed by a further rise in pressure inside the ventricular cavity as the outflow tract narrows, producing ever-increasing obstruction to outflow.

Another interesting aspect of ventricular function in IHSS is that 75 to 85 percent of the total ejection occurs during the first half of systole, as compared to a normal value of about 57 percent. Though left ventricular end-diastolic pressure tends to be elevated in these patients, the end-diastolic volume tends to be low. Brachfield and Gorlin summarize the work of their group in the Ciba symposium [51, 52] and point out that the end-diastolic volume is not only lower than in aortic valvular stenosis but is lower than that seen in normal patients as well. The response of left ventricular function to a wide variety of physiologic and pharmacologic interventions has sufficient diagnostic and therapeutic implications as to merit a brief review here.

* *Editorial Note:* Other investigators find that the notch on the ascending limb of the left ventricular pressure curve corresponds to the end of the percussion wave of the aortic pulse (See Chapter 12 by Wigle.)

Under most circumstances, the ventricular contraction after an extrasystole is more forceful than regularly occurring ones. This appears to be related to both an intrinsic characteristic of cardiac muscle and to prolongation of ventricular filling time. In the patient with IHSS, this augmentation of force of contraction appears to be capable also of increasing the degree of constriction of the outflow tract. As a consequence, the postextrasystolic contraction in these patients may show no increase in brachial artery systolic pulse pressure or even a decrease, though in some patients (12 of 57 of Braunwald's study) a normal response is seen. Therefore, a decrease or lack of augmentation of postextrasystolic arterial pulse pressure is of diagnostic significance. Remember that recordings of intraventricular pressure in these patients show marked augmentation of the force of contraction. Hence, those patients who do not show postextrasystolic augmentation of the arterial pulse can be assumed to have postextrasystolic increase in outflow obstruction.

Digitalis glycosides are likewise capable of augmenting ventricular contractility and have been shown to produce augmentation of the obstruction to outflow. Thus, for patients without atrial fibrillation (for which digitalis may be necessary to control rate) digitalis not only may not be helpful but instead may be harmful.

Another agent capable of positive inotropic effect on the myocardium is isoproterenol, a drug which stimulates only the beta adrenergic receptors. It has been shown that administration of this drug is capable of narrowing the outflow tract and producing an increase in the peak systolic gradient in most patients with IHSS. This obstruction to outflow as a consequence of isoproterenol injection may be so severe as to produce transient mitral regurgitation.

Alpha adrenergic stimulators such as methoxamine and phenylephrine tend to diminish the systolic pressure gradient and Braunwald [48] suggests that this is due to an increase in left ventricular filling and elevation of left ventricular systolic pressure which can prevent the apposition of the septum and anterior mitral leaflet of the left ventricular outflow tract.

Nitroglycerine is capable of causing small vessel dilatation and also has been shown to reduce the size of the left ventricle throughout the entire cardiac cycle. When Braunwald et al. [53] administered 0.45 to 0.60 mg nitroglycerine to 10 patients with IHSS, it always increased the systolic pressure gradient and reduced the effective orifice of the left ventricular outflow tract. In addition, those patients who had no significant obstruction in the basal state developed a pressure gradient when treated with nitroglycerine. No such increasing of gradient was seen when nitroglycerine was administered to patients with discreet valvular aortic stenosis. Thus, there may be distinct diagnostic value in determining the effect of nitroglycerine on patients suspected of having IHSS, and it is theoretically possible that clinical use of this drug could be harmful to such patients. Thus, Braunwald warns that if nitroglycerine is used at all in the treatment of patients with IHSS, it should be used with considerable caution.

Amyl nitrite is another drug with pronounced circulatory effects that has been studied in relationship to IHSS. Because this drug increases cardiac output, the increased flow across the obstructing orifice induces or exaggerates pressure gradients in patients with IHSS and in those with discrete forms of obstruction, as well. Since Wigle and his group [54] have shown that amyl nitrite is capable of reducing the size of the outflow tract in patients with muscular subaortic stenosis, it is not surprising that the elevation of the pressure gradient produced by this drug would be greater in patients with IHSS than in those with valvular disease.

One of the effects of exercise on the heart results from profound sympathetic stimulation, and a number of studies [48] indicate that exercise in patients with IHSS tends to produce markedly abnormal left ventricular responses. Failure to increase cardiac output is commonly seen, as is elevation of the left ventricular end-diastolic pressure. Another consequence of muscular exercise is an increase of venous return to the heart. This would tend to diminish the deleterious effects of the sympathetic stimulation of the heart during muscular exercise by interfering with the apposition of the ventricular walls in the outflow tract. At the cessation of exercise, this increased venous return diminishes abruptly and sympathetic stimulation appears to persist for some time. As a consequence, the majority of patients with IHSS showed an even greater worsening of left ventricular function in the period immediately following exercise than that during exercise.

The Valsalva maneuver is also of diagnostic value in differentiating IHSS from valvular aortic stenosis. The Valsalva maneuver abruptly diminishes venous return to the heart and, as an immediate consequence, cardiac output as well. For purely hydraulic reasons, this diminution in cardiac output diminishes the gradient across discrete valvular obstructions to left ventricular outflow. On the other hand, the diminished venous return tends to decrease the ventricular volume and, therefore, to allow close apposition of the ventricular septum and anterior mitral leaflet, and thus narrow the left ventricular outflow tracts in patients with IHSS. The result is that the Valsalva maneuver will cause a fall in the transvalvular systolic pressure gradient in patients with discrete aortic valvular stenosis, but an increase in the gradient across the obstruction in patients with IHSS.

As in the review cited above [48], Braunwald likewise calls attention to the value of beta adrenergic blockade in patients with IHSS. Pronethalol was found to be very helpful in diminishing the deleterious effects of exercise in patients with IHSS. Patients treated with this drug showed a diminution of the peak systolic left ventricular pressure during exercise. In addition, the increase in gradient across the left ventricular outflow tract that occurs as a consequence of exercise was also markedly diminished by pronethalol therapy.

Gorlin and his associates reported metabolic observations on 6 patients with IHSS in 1964 [55]. Coronary blood flow, expressed in milliliters per 100 gm of left ventricle muscle per minute was normal at rest in all patients and was elevated as a consequence of exercise or administration of isuprel, norepinephrine and neosynephrine. Myocardial oxygen consumption, expressed in milliters per 100 gm per minute was likewise normal. Gorlin et al. points out that though the values were normal when expressed per 100 gm of left ventricular muscle, the total oxygen consumption by the heart was greater than normal in view of the hypertrophy known to occur in patients with IHSS. Another consequence of this hypertrophy is the increased amount of systolic pressure time generated in relationship to myocardial oxygen consumption as compared to normal. They cite normal coronary AV-oxygen differences across the heart and absence of lactic acid production as indications that ischemia is not an important aspect of IHSS.

Brink and his colleagues reported myocardial metabolic studies in a patient with IHSS, in 1967 [56]. In this patient at rest coronary blood flow and myocardial AV-oxygen difference were both somewhat above normal. The arterial content of both pyruvate and lactate was elevated as was the extraction and use of these substrates by the myocardium. On the other hand, free fatty acid extraction and use was below normal at rest. Since there is not only no production of lactate but rather increased uptake of lactate, it is difficult to conceive of ischemia being present in this myocardium. From their oxidation-reduction calculations, Brink and his coworkers suggested that ischemia might nevertheless be present, but admitted that this concept should perhaps be viewed with some reservation.

Beta adrenergic blockade with pronethalol produced the same hemodynamic improvement as noted by Braunwald. The myocardial oxygen extraction was altered little by such treatment, but total oxygen consumption was somewhat reduced, as was left ventricular work. There were metabolic alterations as a consequence of pronethalol treatment, as well. Arterial blood levels and extraction and consumption of pyruvate and lactate returned to normal. In addition, fatty acid extraction and consumption increased definitely toward normal levels. It appears then, that the muscle hypertrophy in patients with IHSS leads to increased total myocardial oxygen use that is, however, normal when considered on the basis of use per unit weight. Furthermore, it is difficult to interpret published data to support a case for the presence of ischemia in these patients. The untreated patient with IHSS would appear to place a greater reliance on pyruvate and lactate substrates and less on free fatty acid. The administration of a beta adrenergic blocker appears to produce a hemodynamic improvement as well as a reversion toward normal of substrate extraction patterns.

THE SECONDARY CARDIOMYOPATHIES

The major hemodynamic types of cardiomyopathy have been outlined in the previous sections. They are sharply divided into the obstructive and nonobstructive varieties, and the nonobstructive varieties are either purely congestive or have restrictive overtones. The nonobstructive cardiomyopathy that is purely congestive represents a situation in which the sole disorder is loss of myocardial contractility. Restrictive overtones develop when the process begins to interfere with ventricular compliance. Under these circumstances, ventricular filling is resisted and hydraulic features reminiscent of constrictive pericarditis occur. Fowler [33] defines these restrictive features in his recent monograph:

> The right ventricular diastolic pressure in one-third or more of the systolic pressure. The right ventricular pressure pulse displays an early diastolic dip, and the right atrial, right ventricular diastolic, and pulmonary arterial wedge pressures are approximately equal. One is apt to see these restrictive features in patients with amyloidosis, scleroderma, or the endocardial fibrosis syndromes.

Some of the secondary cardiomyopathies have been studied extensively and are sufficiently unique as to deserve some further comment.

Alcoholic cardiomyopathy. This subject is covered in detail in Chapter 7, but a few words are not out of order here. Alcoholic cardiomyopathy would appear to be generally hemodynamically indistinguishable from nonobstructive idiopathic primary cardiomyopathy. This is implied by Hamby [40] in his study of 100 patients with primary (idiopathic) myocardial disease, in that 50 percent of his patients had a history of a high alcoholic intake. In addition, Burch and DePasquale [57] directly state that hemodynamic studies of patients with alcoholic cardiomyopathy do not differ from those in other cardiac states associated with congestive heart failure.

On the other hand, Wendt and his colleagues [58] published the results of extensive studies of 17 patients with alcoholic cardiomyopathy. They state that their cardiomyopathy patients were only able to increase cardiac output as a function of rate, with no change in stroke volume. They also point to a significant increase in oxygen extraction by the myocardium that did not change with exercise.

Beriberi heart disease. An excellent study of 4 chronic alcoholic patients with beriberi heart disease was published by Akbarian and his colleagues in 1966 [59], and it is recommended to the reader as a basic reference work not only for its data but also for its literature review. Four chronic alcoholic patients with well-documented beriberi heart disease were studied. They each showed tachycardia, elevated stroke index and cardiac index, and low peripheral vascular resistance. There was a narrow arteriovenous oxygen difference and increased right and left ventricular filling pressures. Cardiac output was increased to such an extent that, despite the lowered peripheral vascular resistance, ventricular work was significantly increased in each case, and arterial blood pressure was raised to an abnormal level in 2. In 1 patient, exercise produced only a moderate rise in cardiac index, and this was accomplished only as a consequence of increase in heart rate because stroke volume actually decreased. Another patient showed no increase in peripheral vascular resistance as a consequence of administration of 1.8 times the average amount of methoxamine needed to produce 23 percent increase in total peripheral resistance in normal patients. This latter finding is particularly interesting in that the same drug has been found capable of abolishing the high output states secondary to chronic anemia.

Administration of thiamine was followed by improvement when the patients were studied after 3 to 37 days of treatment. In 1 patient, peripheral vascular resistance markedly increased toward normal in only 37 minutes after administration of thiamine. Cardiac function did not return entirely to normal in any patient. One can not escape the speculation that the administration of thiamine abolished the signs of beriberi heart disease only to unmask the underlying congestive cardiomyopathy of chronic alcoholism. In contradistinction to the earlier literature, these observers noted a strong positive inotropic response to digitalis in 1 of the patients studied.

The same laboratory has recently published the study of another alcoholic patient with beriberi heart disease [60]. In this patient, the diagnosis was confirmed by blood transketolase measurement and was characterized by marked elevations of arterial blood lactate and pyruvate levels, well known in thiamine deficiency but not specific for this disorder. This patient showed similar hemodynamic indices of high-output cardiac failure and diminished peripheral resistance. After 7 days of therapy, hemodynamic and metabolic data were entirely normal.

THYROID HORMONE AND THE HEART

Though excesses or deficiencies of thyroid hormone are capable of exerting profound influences on cardiac function, the question whether abnormal thyroid states can produce congestive failure in the otherwise normal heart remains moot. As far as this writer is concerned, the question remains open and no position will be taken. It is admitted, however, that large doses of thyroid hormone are capable of producing congestive cardiac failure in the experimental animal, as shown by Olson (32). It is noteworthy that this same study clearly indicated that the myocardial abnormalities associated with excesses of thyroid hormone could not be traced to uncoupling of oxidative phosphorylation nor decreased myocardial levels of ATP nor creatine phosphate.

Excesses of thyroid hormone have been studied extensively regarding their hemodynamics and metabolic effect [61, 62]. Thyrotoxic patients tend to show increased cardiac output, cardiac work, coronary blood flow and myocardial oxygen consumption, and diminished peripheral vascular resistance. Animal and human studies suggest that these effects are due to the ability of the thyroid hormone to augment the effects of catecholamines. Sympathetic blockade in experimental animals was capable of completely reversing the physiologic effect of excesses of thyroid hormone. On the other hand Goldstein and Killip [63] in humans, found that guanethidine markedly diminished the physiologic effects of thyrotoxicosis without necessarily completely abolishing them. Careful studies of urinary excretion of catecholamines and their metabolites in abnormal thyroid states did not indicate any change in their level, adding further support to the concept that thyroid hormones act by augmenting the effect of catecholamines rather than increasing the amount produced or present [64].

In a recent review DeGroot and Leonard [65], took a somewhat different position than the above. They cite their own work and that of others that casts doubt on the catecholamine mediation of the circulatory effects of thyroid hormone. They found that reserpine-induced catecholamine depletion and beta-adrenergic blocking agents did not significantly alter the cardiac output of thyrotoxic patients. In further support of their position, these authors cited evidence that thyroid hormone can be shown, in vitro, to possess strong positive chronotropic properties even in the absence of autonomic innervation. Coinciding with these observations are others that show that myocardial force-velocity relationships, which are dramatically altered by thyroid hormone, are essentially the same before and after catecholamine depletion. A point of great interest is the role of periphereal vascular resistance in the circulatory alterations seen in thyrotoxicosis. Theilen and Wilson [66] have shown that administration of the selective alpha-adrenergic stimulant, phenylephrine, to a group of atropinized thyrotoxic patients reduced the cardiac output to a level somewhat below that of a comparably treated euthyroid group. These latter data suggest that the major circulatory effects of thyroid hormone excess may be traceable to a diminution in peripheral resistance.

In summary, it is safe to take the position that these authors do [66] and regard thyrotoxicosis as a high cardiac output state. There would appear to be at least three major determinants contributing to this state, and it is difficult to assign roles of correct relative importance to them at this time. The increased oxygen demand of all the tissues as a consequence of the hypermetabolic state is certainly one such determinant. It must be remembered that sole responsibility cannot be attributed to this factor because the increase in cardiac output is far in excess of that required to supply the demand of the periphery for oxygen. Another such determinant is the effect of the thyrotoxic state on the myocardium itself. The velocity of contraction of the myocardium is markedly accelerated by thyroid hormone excess, and this does not appear to be mediated by increased catecholamine sensitivity. On the other hand, the arrhythmias frequently seen in thyroid storm or prestorm are ameliorated by beta-adrenergic blocker administration. Thus, it is safe to take the position that the increased myocardial contractility is a direct effect of thyroid hormone on the myocardium, but the increased cardiac automaticity would appear to be due, in a major degree, to increased sensitivity to catecholamines. The third of the major determinants referred to above is the diminished peripheral vascular resistance. Very important in this aspect of the circulatory changes in thyrotoxicosis is the marked increase in blood flow through the skin, seen as a mechanism for dissipation for the increased amount of heat generated in this hypermetabolic state.

Though deficiencies of thyroid hormone produce diminution in cardiac output and myocardial contractility in proportion to the degree of depression of basal metabolism, it is uncertain that a true cardiomyopathy is produced.

In either event, restoration of levels of circulating thyroid hormones toward normal, whether abnormally high or low, restores cardiac function to or toward normal.

Diphtheritic cardiomyopathy. Though a tremendous amount of research has been done to define the hemodynamic and metabolic characteristics of the cardiomyopathies, understanding of the pathophysiology at the molecular level has not as yet been achieved. Recent observations [68] with experimental administration of diphtheria toxin in animals, however, suggests that the realization of such a goal is not totally outside the realm of possibility.

In 1964, Wittels and Bressler [68] put forth a hypothesis that could explain some of the findings in diphtheritic cardiomyopathy. Diphtheria toxin is capable of producing a cardiomyopathy that results in arrhythmia and myocardial failure. Microscopically, triglyceride accumulation is seen in addition to inflammatory changes and loss of myofibers. Wittels and Bressler suggested that diphtheria toxin may cause a depletion of myocardial carnitine. Since the final site of oxidation of fatty acids in the myocardium is intramitrochondrial, any molecular change that interferes with transport of fatty acids into these organelles would block their oxidation. It was pointed out in the early pages of this chapter that formation of a carnitine derivative is necessary for the normal rate of transport of fatty acids into the mitochondria. The depletion of carnitine suggested by these two investigators would interfere with the transport of the major fuel substrate of the myocardium and cause accumulation of fatty fuels outside the mitochondria.

The carnitine depletion has been documented in human beings and guinea pigs, and it has been shown that oxidation of palmitic acid by myocardial homogenates of diphtheritic guinea pigs is diminished. It was further shown that the addition of carnitine to these homogenates restored fatty acid oxidation to normal.

Challoner and his colleagues [67] have recently shown that carnitine injection exerts a very marked protective effect against LD_{50} doses of diphtheria toxin in guinea pigs. In addition, dogs were given diphtheria toxin until cardiovascular impairment, manifested by hypotension and low cardiac output, developed. Carnitine injection restored cardiac function to or toward normal in all animals treated.

The results of these studies is that, in diphtheritic cardiomyopathy at least, the central locus of the biochemical defect has been identified. In addition, the animal studies now published suggest that carnitine injection may represent a valuable mode of treatment.

Because of the obvious problems inherent in sampling the diseased myocardium, progress of this sort in the other cardiomyopathies will necessarily be slow. These very promising strides in the understanding of diphtheritic cardiomyopathy, however, give promise that the vast amount of work already done in other cardiomyopathic states may ultimately lead to studies that will give understanding of the disease processes at the molecular level and may even lead to new therapeutic modalities.

REFERENCES

1. Eckenhoff, J.E., Hafkenshiel, J.H., Harmel, M.H., Goodale, W.T., Lubin, M., Bing, R.J., and Kety, S.S.: Measurement of coronary blood flow by the nitrous-oxide method. Am J Physiol 152: 356, 1948.

2. Coffman, J.D.: The coronary circulation. In, The Physiological Basis of Medical Practice, 8th ed. Best, C.H. and Taylor, N.B. (Eds.): Baltimore, Williams & Wilkins, 1966, p 813.
3. Bove, K.E., Rowlands, D.T., and Scott, R.C.: Observations on the assessment of cardiac hypertrophy utilizing a chamber partition technique. Circ 33: 558, 1966.
4. Stone, W.E.: Uptake and delivery of the respiratory gases. In, Best, C.H. and Taylor, N.B. (Eds.): The Physiological Basis of Medical Practice, 8th ed. Baltimore, Williams & Wilkins, 1966, p 965.
5. Braunwald, E.: Control of myocardial oxygen consumption-physiological and clinical considerations. Am J Cardiol 27: 416, 1971.
6. Ross, J., Sonnenblick, E.H., Kiser, G.A., Frommer, P.L., and Braunwald, E.: Electroaugmentation of ventricular performance and oxygen consumption by repetitive application of stimuli. Circ Res 16: 332, 1965.
7. Sonnenblick, E.H., Ross, J., Jr., Covell, J.W., Kaiser, G.A., and Braunwald, E.: Velocity of contraction as a determinant of myocardial oxygen consumption. Am J Physiol 209: 919, 1965.
8. Covell, J.W., Braunwald, E., Ross, J., and Sonnenblick, E.H.: Studies on digitalis XVI. Effects on myocardial oxygen consumption. J Clin Invest 45: 1535-1542, 1966.
9. Graham, T.P., Jr., Covell, J.W., Sonnenblick, E.H., Ross, J., Jr., and Braunwald, E.: Control of myocardial oxygen consumption: Relative influence of contractile state and tension development. J Clin Invest 47:375, 1968.
10. Boerth, R.C., Covell, J.W., Pool, P.E., and Ross, J.: Increased myocardial oxygen consumption and contractile state associated with increased heart rate in dogs. Circ Res 24: 725, 1969.
11. Klocke, F.J., Kaiser, G.A., Ross, J., and Braunwald, E.: Mechanism of increase of myocardial oxygen uptake produced by catecholamines. Am J Physiol 209: 913, 1965.
12. Sonnenblick, E.H.: Series elastic and contractile elements in heart muscle: Changes in muscle length. Am J Physiol 207: 1330, 1964.
13. Coleman, H.N., Sonnenblick, E.H., and Braunwald, E.: Myocardial oxygen consumption associated with external work: The Fenn effect. Am J Physiol 217: 291, 1969.
14. Fenn, W.O.: A quantitative comparison between the energy liberated and the work performed by the isolated sartorius muscle of the frog. J Physiol 58:175, 1923.
15. Bing, R.J.: Cardiac metabolism. Physiol Rev 45: 171, 1965.
16. Opie, L.H.: Metabolism of the heart in health and disease. Part I. Am Heart J 76:685, 1968.
17. Opie, L.H.: Metabolism of the heart in health and disease. Part II. Am Heart J 77:100, 1969.
18. Opie, L.H.: Metabolism of the heart in health and disease. Part III. Am Heart J 77: 383, 1969.
19. West, E.S., Todd, W.R., Mason, H.S., and VanBruggen, J.T.: Textbook of Biochemistry, 4th ed. New York, McMillan, 1966, p. 972.
20. Bing, R.J., Michal, G.: Myocardial efficiency. Ann N.Y. Acad Sci 72:555, 1959.
21. Schleef, D.J., Ph.D., Univ Cincinnati, College of Engineering: Personal Communication.
22. Himwich, H.E., Koskoff, Y.D., and Nahum, L.H.: Changes in lactic acid and glucose in the blood on passage through organs. Am J Physiol 85: 379, 1928.

23. Goodale, W.T., Olson, R.E., and Hackel, D.B.: The effects of fasting and diabetes mellitus on myocardial metabolism in man. Am J Med 27: 212, 1959.
24. Vester, J.W.: The cell. Scientific Clinician, New York, McGraw Hill, 1966, Ch. I, p 23.
25. Sonnenblick, E.H.: Myocardial ultrastructure in the normal and failing heart. Hosp Pract 5(4):35, 1970.
26. Davies, R.E.: Biochemical processes in cardiac function. Hosp Pract 5(6):49, 1970.
27. Meerson, F.Z.: Myocardium in hyperfunction, hypertrophy and heart failure. Circ Res 25 (No. 26, Suppl II): Circ 1969.
28. Evans, J.R.: Structure and function of heart muscle. Circ Res 15 (Suppl II):, 1964.
29. Gorlin, R. and Vester, J. W.: The myocardium in health and disease. Scientific Clinician. Thoroughfare, N.J., Charles B. Slack, 1970, Ch. I.
30. Levine, H.J. and Wagman, R.J.: Energetics of the human heart. Am J Cardiol 9:372, 1962.
31. Olson, R.E. and Schwartz, W.B.: Myocardial metabolism and congestive heart failure. Medicine 30:21, 1951.
32. Olson, R.E.: Abnormalities of myocardial metabolism. Circ Res 15 (Suppl II): 109, 1964.
33. Fowler, N.O.: Differential diagnosis of cardiomyopathies. Prog Cardiovasc Dis 14:113, 1971.
34. Goodwin, J.F.: Cardiac function in primary myocardial disorders. Part I. Br Med J I: 1527, 1964.
35. Goodwin, J.F.: Cardiac function in primary myocardial disorders. Part II. Br Med J I: 1595, 1964.
36. Pietras, R.J., Meadows, W.R., Fort, M., and Sharp, J.T.: Hemodynamic alterations in idiopathic myocardiopathy including cineangiography from the left heart chambers. Am J Cardiol 16: 672, 1965.
37. Yu, N., Schreiner, B.F., Cohen, J., and Murphy, W.: Idiopathic cardiomyopathy. A study of left ventricular function and pulmonary circulation in fifteen patients. Am Heart J 71: 330, 1966.
38. Burch, G.E. and DePasquale, N.P.: Heart muscle disease. Disease-a-Month. Chicago, Year Book, 1968.
39. Braunwald, E. and Aygen, N.: Idiopathic myocardial hypertrophy without congestive heart failure or obstruction to blood flow. Am J Med 35:7, 1963.
40. Hamby, R.I.: Primary myocardial disease. Medicine 49:55, 1970.
41. Hamby, R.I., Catangay, P., Apiado, O., and Kahn, A. H.: Primary myocardial disease. Am J Cardiol 25:625, 1970.
42. Rackley, C.E., Dodge, H.T., Coble, Y.D., and Hay, R.E.: A method for determining left ventricular mass in man. Circulation 29:666, 1964.
43. Sandler, H. and Dodge, H.T.: Left ventricular tension and stress in man. Circ Res 13:91, 1963.
44. Badeer, H.S.: Myocardial blood flow and oxygen uptake in clinical and experimental cardiomegaly. Am Heart J 82: 105, 1971.
45. Wendt, V.E., Stock, T.B., Hayden, R.O., Bruce, T.A., Gudbjarnason, S., and Bing, R.J.: The hemodynamics and cardiac metabolism in cardiomyopathies Med Clin N Am 46:1445, 1962.
46. Brink, A.J. and Lewis, C.M.: Coronary blood flow, energetics, and myocardial metabolism in idiopathic mural endomyocardiopathy (14 patients). Am Heart J 73:339, 1967.

47. In, Wolstenholme, G.E.W. (Ed.): Ciba Found Symposium Cardiomyopathies. Boston, Little, Brown, 1964.
48. Braunwald, E., Lambrew, C.T., Rockoff, S.J., Ross, J., and Morrow, E.G.: Idiopathic hypertrophic subaortic stenosis, I. A description of the disease based upon an analysis of sixty-four patients. Circulation 30 (Suppl IV):3, 1964.
49. Schmincke, A., Ueber linkseitige muskulöese conusstenosen. Dtsch Med Wochschr 33: 2082, 1907.
50. Brachfeld, N. and Gorlin, R.: Subaortic stenosis: A revised concept of the disease. Medicine 38:415, 1959.
51. Brachfeld, N. and Gorlin, R.: Functional subaortic stenosis. Ann Intern Med 54:1, 1961.
52. Benchimol, A., Dimond, E.G., and Shen, Y.: Ejection time in aortic stenosis and mitral stenosis. Cardiol 6:728, 1960.
53. Braunwald, E., Oldham, H.N., Jr., Ross, J., Jr., Linhart, J.W., Mason, D.T., and Fort, L.: The circulatory response of patients with idiopathic hypertrophic subaortic stenosis to nitroglycerine and to the Valsalva maneuver Circulation 29: 422, 1964.
54. Wigle, E.D., Lenkei, S.C.M., Chrysohou, A., and Wilson, D.R.: Muscular subaortic stenosis: The effect of peripheral vasodilation. Can Med Assoc J 89:896, 1963.
55. Gorlin, R., Cohen, L.S., Elliott, W.C., Klein, M.D., and Lane, F.J.: Hemodynamics of muscular subaortic stenosis (obstructive cardiomyopathy). In, Wolstenholme, G.E.W. (Ed.): Ciba Foundation Symposium Cardiomyopathies. Boston, Little, Brown, 1964, p 76.
56. Brink, A.J., Lewis, C.M., and Van Heerden, P.D.: Coronary blood flow and myocardial metabolism in obstructive cardiomyopathy. Am J Cardiol 19:548, 1967.
57. Burch, G.E. and DePasquale, N.P.: Alcoholic cardiomyopathy. Am J Cardiol 23:723, 1969.
58. Wendt, V.E., Wu, C., Balcon, R., Doty, G., and Bing, R.J.: Hemodynamic and metabolic effects of chronic alcoholism in man. Am J. Cardiol 15:175, 1965.
59. Akbarian, M., Yankopoulos, N.A., and Abelmann, W.H.: Hemodynamic studies in beriberi heart disease. Am J Med 41: 197, 1966.
60. Jeffrey, F.E. and Abelmann, W.H.: Recovery from proved Shoshin beriberi. Am J Med 50:123, 1971.
61. Rowe, G.G., Huston, J.H., Weinstein, A.B., Tuchman, H., Brown, J.F., and Crumpton, C.W.: The hemodynamics of thyrotoxicosis in man with special reference to coronary blood flow and myocardial oxygen metabolism. J Clin Invest 35:272, 1956.
62. Brewster, W.R., Isaacs, J.P., Osgood, P.F., and King, T.L.: The hemodynamic and metabolic interrelationships in the activity of epinephrine and norepinephrine and the thyroid hormones. Circulation 13:1, 1956.
63. Goldstein, S. and Killip, T., III.: Catecholamine depletion in thyrotoxicosis effect of guanethedine on cardiovascular dynamics. Circulation 31:219, 1965.
64. Wiswell, J.G., Hurwitz, G.E., Coronho, V., Bing, O.H., and Child, D.L.: Urinary catecholamines and their metabolites in hyperthyroidism and hypothyroidism. Clin Endocrinol Metabol 23:1102, 1963.
65. DeGroot, W.J. and Leonard, J.J.: Hyperthyroidism as a high cardiac output state. Am Heart J 79: 265, 1970.
66. Theilen, E.O. and Wilson, W.R.: Hemodynamic effects of peripheral vasoconstriction in normal and thyrotoxic subjects. J Appl Physiol 22:207, 1967.

67. Challoner, D.R., Mandelbaum, I., and Elliott, W.: Protective effect of 1-carnitine in experimental intoxication with diphtheria toxin. J Lab Clin Med 77: 616, 1971.
68. Wittels, B. and Bressler, R.J.: Biochemical lesion of diphtheria toxin in the heart. J Clin Invest 43: 630, 1964.

Radiologic Features of Myocardial Diseases

The radiographic diagnosis of cardiomyopathy cannot be made from the plain chest film alone because of the lack of specific diagnostic criteria. However, the various radiologic features to be discussed are helpful when correlated with the clinical findings. The plain film and angiographic manifestations of the major categories of cardiomyopathy [1] are listed in Tables I and II.

IDIOPATHIC CARDIOMYOPATHY

Nonobstructive Cardiomyopathy

Nonobstructive cardiomyopathy includes the following cardiomyopathies: alcoholic, postinfectious, familial, peripartal, and cardiomyopathy without an identifiable antecedent.

Cardiac size. There is usually generalized enlargement of the cardiopericardial silhouette (Fig. 1). Of the 59 patients with this type of cardiomyopathy reported by Hill et al. [2], 56 had biventricular enlargement. In 29 patients reported by Gotsman et al. [3], 3 who had mild cardiomyopathy

From the Departments of Radiology and the Cardiac Research Laboratory, University of Cincinnati College of Medicine, Cincinnati, Ohio.

Table I
Radiographic Features of Cardiomyopathy: Plain Film and Fluoroscopy

Type	*Heart Size*	*Heart Shape*	*Aorta*	*Lungs, Pleura*	*Fluoroscopy*
Nonobstructive cardiomyopathy	Enlarged (generalized)	Globular or spherical; all chambers usually enlarged	Normal to small	Pulmonary venous hypertension, pulmonary edema, and pleural effusion occur frequently	Generalized decreased pulsations
Obstructive cardiomyopathy	Normal or enlarged	Normal or left ventricular configuration; LA usually enlarged, RV often enlarged	Normal	Usually normal	Normal, increased or decreased pulsations

Table II
Radiographic Features of Cardiomyopathy: Angiography

Type	*LV Enlargement*	*LV Cavity*	*LV Contractility*	*LV Septum*	*LV Outflow*	*LV Trabecular Pattern*	*Mitral Insufficiency*	*Coronary Arteries*
Nonobstructive cardiomyopathy	Dilated	Large but normal contour	Poor	Normal	Normal	Normal	Minimal to severe	Normal
Obstructive cardiomyopathy	Hypertrophied	Small	Normal or hyperkinetic	Greatly hypertrophied	Obstructed during systole	Markedly hypertrophied	Often present, minimal to severe	Normal or enlarged

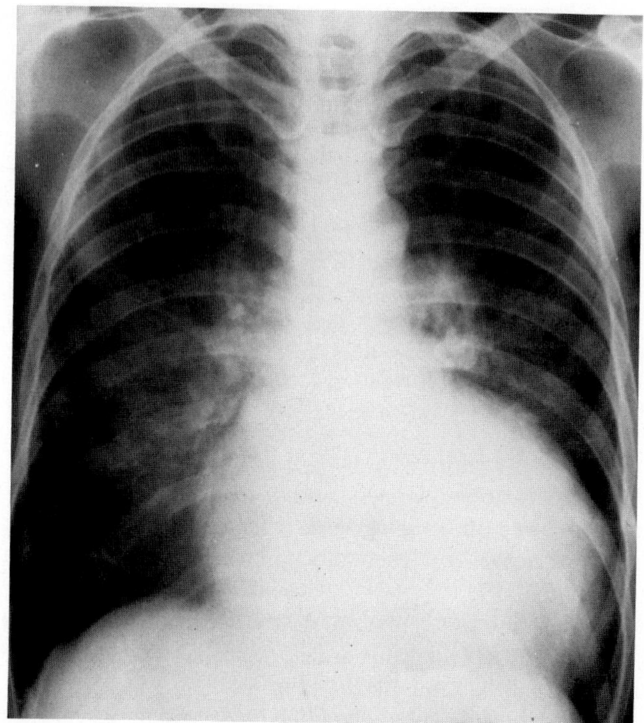

Figure 1. Nonobstructive Cardiomyopathy. This 46-year-old man's disease is probably due to alcoholism. There is cardiomegaly, predominantly left ventricular. The left heart border has a sharp outline. The interstitial edema is best seen in the right midlung field.

without heart failure had a mean cardiothoracic ratio (C/T) of 54 percent (range 49-58 percent). The mean C/T ratio of 18 patients in heart failure or recently recovered from it was 64 percent (range 54-75 percent); 6 patients with associated mitral insufficiency had a C/T ratio of 68 percent (range 54-84 percent).

Frequently in patients with cardiac enlargement, there is a rapid decrease in heart size after bed rest, digitalis, and diuretic therapy; this pattern of response to treatment may recur many times in the course of illness. This so-called *accordion effect* (Fig. 2) may be helpful in suggesting the diagnosis [2].

Cardiac shape. The generalized cardiac enlargement often results in a globular or spherical configuration. The left ventricle (LV) may be more

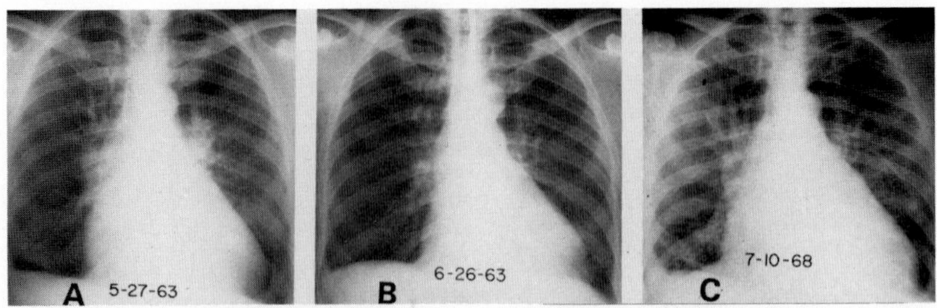

Figure 2. Nonobstructive Cardiomyopathy. Accordion effect shown in 66-year-old man. A. Cardiomegaly, predominantly left ventricular with left atrial enlargement as well. Dilated upper lobe veins are evident. B. Rapid decrease in heart size and regression of the congestive heart failure. C. The heart is now larger than on the original study. The congestive changes are more severe, and there is right-sided pleural effusion.

prominent and occasionally is so disproportionately enlarged as to impart an appearance more in keeping with aortic valve disease, hypertensive cardiovascular disease, or rheumatic mitral insufficiency than cardiomyopathy [4] (Fig. 1).

Bridgen described the margin of the heart as stenciled or etched, implying an exquisitely sharp border, perhaps secondary to decreased movement of the cardiac muscle [5] (Fig. 1).

Symmetrical biventricular chamber enlargement is very common in nonobstructive cardiomyopathy [2]. The LV is usually dilated, its size depending on the severity of the disease. In the more advanced cases, mild-to-moderate enlargement of the left atrium (LA) accompanies the LV enlargement (Fig. 3).

The atria usually become dilated when incompetence of the atrio-

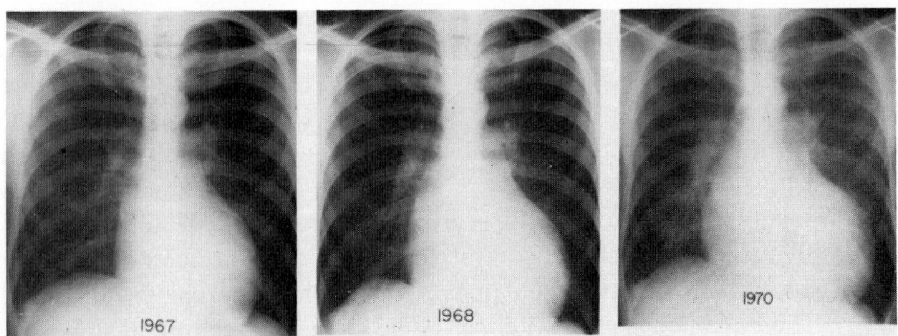

Figure 3. Nonobstructive Cardiomyopathy. Progression of the disease for 3 years in a 41-year-old man. There is cardiomegaly with an enlarged left ventricle and left atrium. The prominent pulmonary arc segment and pulmonary arteries suggest associated right ventricular enlargement. The left heart border is etched. The aorta is small.

ventricular valves occurs. There is often moderate increase in the size of the right ventricle (RV), recognized, in the presence of LV enlargement, by prominence of the pulmonary arc segment (Fig. 3).

Aorta. The aorta was normal or small in 48 of the 59 patients in Hill's study [2]. This is apparently related to the poor contractility of the LV resulting in decreased cardiac output (Fig. 3). It is possible, though, that these aortas are of normal size but appear small in relation to the enlarged heart. Aortic dilatation is more common in the older patients, apparently related to age [3]. The aortic valve does not calcify in this condition.

Lungs and pleura. Many patients with idiopathic cardiomyopathy present dilated upper lobe veins secondary to pulmonary venous hypertension. Interstitial and/or alveolar pulmonary edema, pleural effusion (Fig. 2), and dilatation of the azygos vein may also occur [2]. Pericardial effusion may coexist. These signs of cardiac failure frequently disappear rapidly with treatment. The superior vena cava may be distended, its dilatation paralleling the severity of the congestive heart failure.

Fluoroscopy. Cardiac movement is hypoactive. Decreased amplitude of pulsations is common, especially along the left heart border. Pulsations of the right border and pulmonary arteries are generally more active [6].

Angiography. The angiocardiogram reveals increased circulation time, dilated cardiac chambers, and pooling of the contrast material on both sides of the heart [7].

Left ventricular angiography shows LV dilatation. The contractility is poor, with slow emptying of the chamber. The ejection is notably reduced, causing an increase in the end-diastolic volume. There may be very little change in volume between systole and diastole(Fig. 4). Swirling of the contrast material may be seen in the LV at the end of systole, explaining the frequency of thrombus formation [3].

The ventricular septum, outflow area, and trabecular pattern are normal [8]. Thinning of the apex of the LV has been described [6]. Mitral insufficiency may be minimal or severe depending on the degree of dilatation of the mitral valve ring. The coronary arteries are normal.

Obstructive Cardiomyopathy

Both familial and nonfamilial types are included in this group.

Cardiac size. The heart size was normal in a third of the patients reported by Steiner, the remainder showing variable degrees of enlargement [9] (Fig. 5). In the series of Braunwald et al. [10], the C/T ratio ranged from

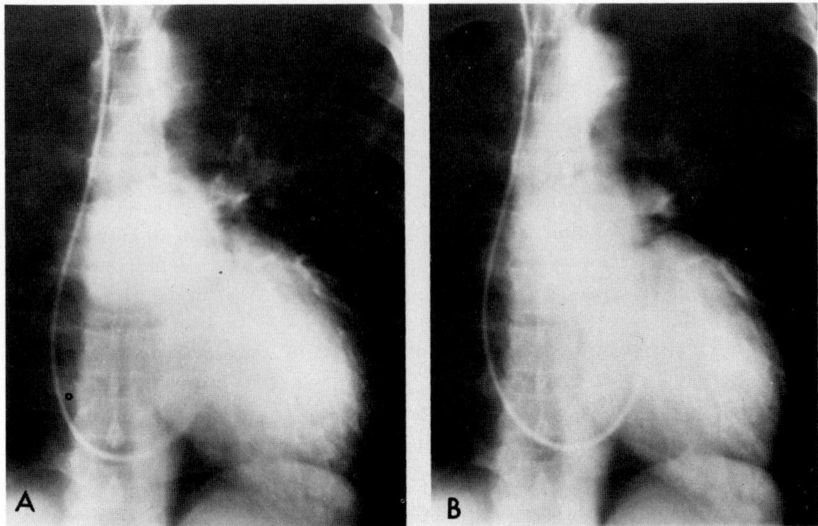

Figure 4. Alcoholic Cardiomyopathy. Same patient as in Figure 1. A. Diastolic phase following injection into the pulmonary artery reveals an enlarged left atrium and markedly dilated left ventricle. B. Systolic phase shows little change in volume of the left ventricle as compared to diastolic phase. The end-systolic volume is increased.

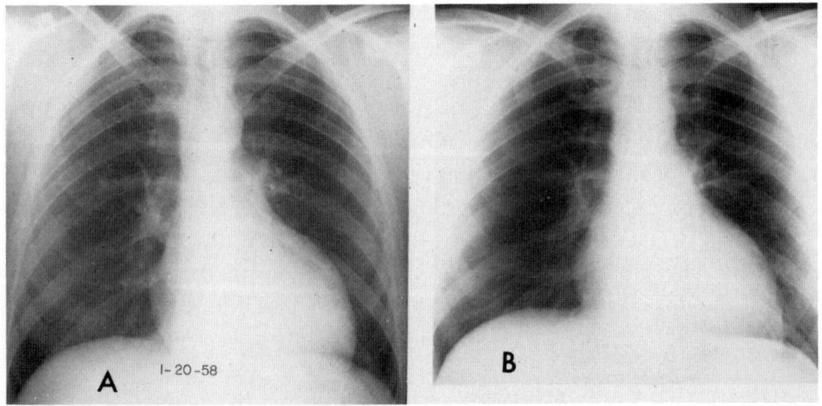

Figure 5. Obstructive Cardiomyopathy. A. Mild cardiomegaly, predominantly left ventricular, in a 37-year-old man. The aorta is normal. There was a moderate systolic pressure gradient across the left ventricular outflow tract in 1958. B. Thirteen years later, there has been little change in cardiac size or configuration. Recatheterization revealed no systolic pressure gradient in the left ventricular outflow tract at rest, with exercise, or with injected isoproterenol.

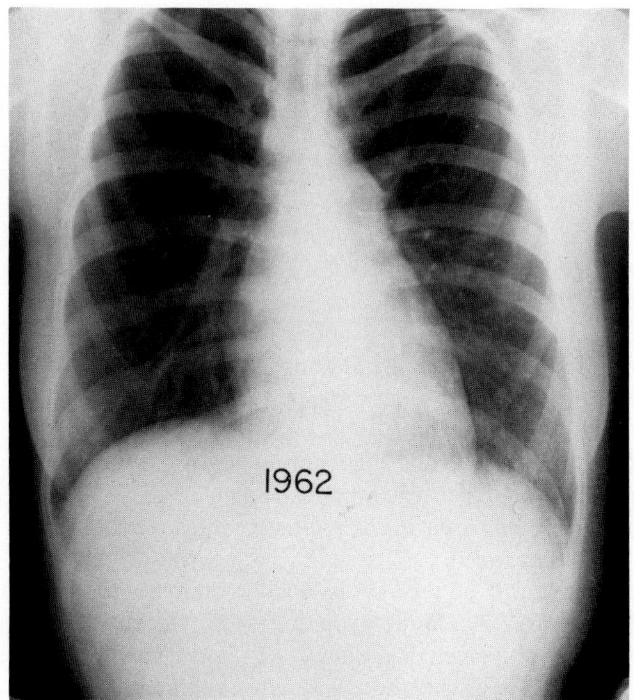

Figure 6. Obstructive Cardiomyopathy. The disease is primarily confined to the right ventricle in this 17-year-old girl. The heart is normal in size. The pulmonary arc segment is enlarged, indicating right ventricular enlargement.

40 to 67 percent, about half of the patients having a C/T ratio less than 50 percent. In this group, heart size did not correlate with peak systolic pressure gradient or with functional classification.

Cardiac shape. In those patients with a normal C/T ratio, the shape of the heart is usually normal. A left ventricular configuration is more often seen in those with cardiomegaly, since moderate-to-severe enlargement of the LV is usually present. Typical downward outward expansion generally occurs, but a more globular contour may occur, especially when there is concomitant enlargement of the right heart [10] (Fig. 5).

In one group reported [10], about three-fourths of the patients had some degree of LA enlargement, apparently secondary to mitral insufficiency. In many of these patients the LA enlargement was slight. The LA was larger in those who had severe symptoms. Some degree of RV enlargement was present in about half these patients. In 4, it was quite pronounced. Solitary RV enlargement is uncommon [4] (Fig. 6).

Aorta. The ascending aorta is normal in size. Poststenotic dilatation usually does not occur.

Lungs and pleura. Usually the lungs and pleural spaces are normal. Some patients, especially those with mitral insufficiency, may show dilated upper lobe veins and Kerley B lines.

Fluoroscopy. Cardiac pulsations may be normal, increased [11], or even decreased, especially when the myocardium is greatly thickened. Paradoxical pulsation of the left ventricular wall may be observed due to asymmetrical hypertrophy. Aortic pulsations are normal. Aortic valvular calcification usually does not occur, although it and coronary artery calcification have been reported in older patients [12].

Angiography. Left ventricular angiography gives more diagnostic information than forward angiocardiography. Biplane examination is preferred. In patients suspected of having RV disease, biplane right ventricular angiography is recommended.

The lateral wall of the LV is thicker than normal in almost every patient with obstructive cardiomyopathy (Fig. 7). In some patients, this mural thickening is greater than that seen in aortic valvular or discrete subvalvular stenosis [10]. Thus, the LV is hypertrophied in obstructive cardiomyopathy, whereas it is dilated in nonobstructive cardiomyopathy.

The LV cavity in obstructive cardiomyopathy is often narrow. The width during diastole is less than normal and even smaller than in aortic valvular or discrete subvalvular stenosis. During systole, the LV cavity is often quite small, even slitlike.

The shape of the LV cavity was normal in 8 of the 36 patients studied by Braunwald et al. [10]. In 16, the cavity in frontal view revealed an inward concavity at the midportion of the right margin; the left margin was normally convex. Two of their patients showed a biconcave configuration in this view.

In the lateral projection, the LV cavity is narrowed and tongue-shaped during systole. During diastole, there is often a deep concavity along the posterior inferior margin of the ventricle. The tongue shape of the opacified LV lumen on the lateral view and the concave indentation on its right margin in the frontal view are caused by the greatly hypertrophied interventricular septum. The lower half of the chamber may be obliterated by the approximation of the anterior and inferior borders [13]. Cavity distortion is also caused by abnormal prominence of the trabecular pattern and indentation by localized hypertrophy of myocardial and papillary muscle.

The marked muscle hypertrophy of the ventricular septum narrows

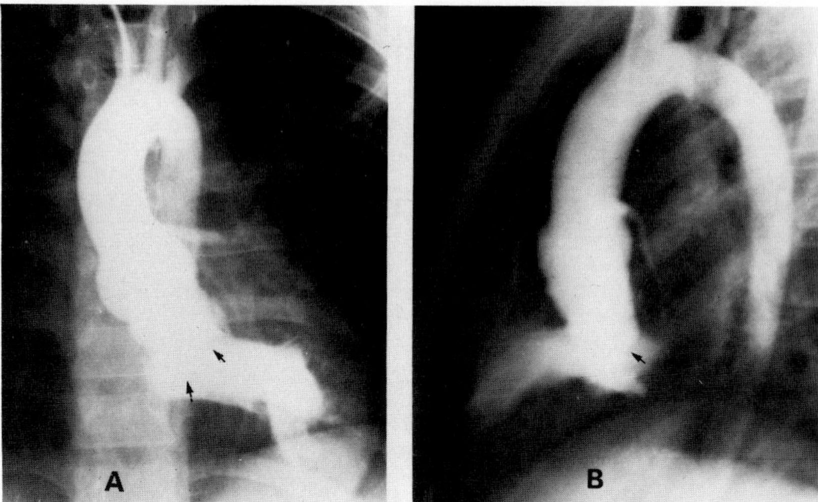

Figure 7. Obstructive Cardiomyopathy. Selective left ventricular angiogram, systole. A. Frontal view shows marked thickening of the lateral wall of the LV, narrowing of the LV lumen, and a biconcave encroachment on its cavity by the hypertrophied lateral and septal walls. A faint radiolucent line (arrows) crossing the outflow tract below the aortic valve represents the point of contact of the edge of the anterior leaflet of the mitral valve with the hypertrophied interventricular septum. B. Lateral view reveals a narrow, tongue-shaped cavity. The anterior portion of the outflow tract is narrowed by the hypertrophied interventricular septum. The mitral valve is restricted in its posterior movement and narrows the posterior portion of the outflow tract (arrow).

the anterior portion of the outflow tract of the LV. The lower portion of the septum projects along the diaphragmatic aspect of the ventricle, causing malalignment of the papillary muscles; angulation of the ventricle during contraction results in abnormal traction on the chordae tendineae. All this restricts the normal posterior displacement of the mitral valve leaflets during systole. These leaflets, held in the outflow tract during systole (Fig. 7B) comprise the posterior component of the outflow obstruction. A radiolucent line, seen across the LV outflow tract 2 to 2.5 cm below the aortic valve (Fig. 7A) at a level corresponding to the location of the intraventricular pressure change, actually represents the point of contact of the leading edge of the anterior leaflet of mitral valve with the hypertrophied muscular interventricular septum. Mitral insufficiency, found in about half the patients, varies from minimal to severe in amount. It is apparently caused by the failure of the edges of mitral leaflets to meet because of restriction of their movement posteriorly [14, 15].

Ventricular contractility is either hyperkinetic or normal. There is

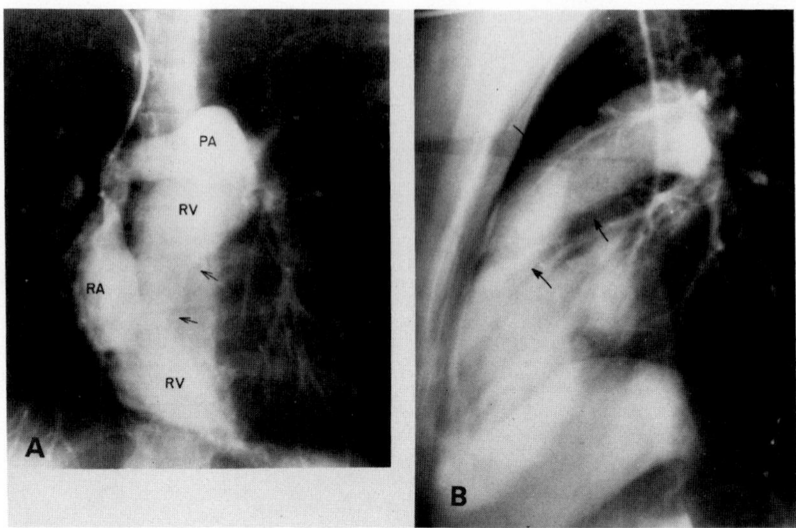

Figure 8. Obstructive Cardiomyopathy. Same patient as in Figure 6. Selective injection into the right atrium. A. Frontal view reveals narrowing of the right ventricular outflow tract with displacement of the entire right ventricle to the right (arrows) by the hypertrophied interventricular septum. B. Lateral view shows that the right ventricular cavity, especially the outflow area (lower arrow), is narrow and appears to be compressed against the sternum. The pulmonary valve (upper arrows) is normal.

rapid emptying of the chamber in striking contrast to the poor contraction and slow emptying seen in nonobstructive cardiomyopathy. The coronary arteries are usually normal or enlarged. There is often distinct separation between the left coronary artery and the cavity of the LV, caused by the hypertrophied muscle.

Right ventricular angiography (Fig. 8) reveals generalized muscular hypertrophy with filling defects produced by localized areas of extreme hypertrophy. During angiography, these muscle bulges cause pockets of contrast material which appear to be completely cut off from the main cavity in systole [9].

The RV outflow tract is narrowed and pushed anteriorly and either to the right or left by the hypertrophied interventricular septum. In the lateral projection, the RV cavity is relatively thin, appearing compressed anteriorly against the sternum. When there is a right ventricular pressure gradient, the obstruction occurs at the junction of the outflow tract and body of the RV. The apex of the RV is pointed, imparting a triangular appearance in frontal projection.

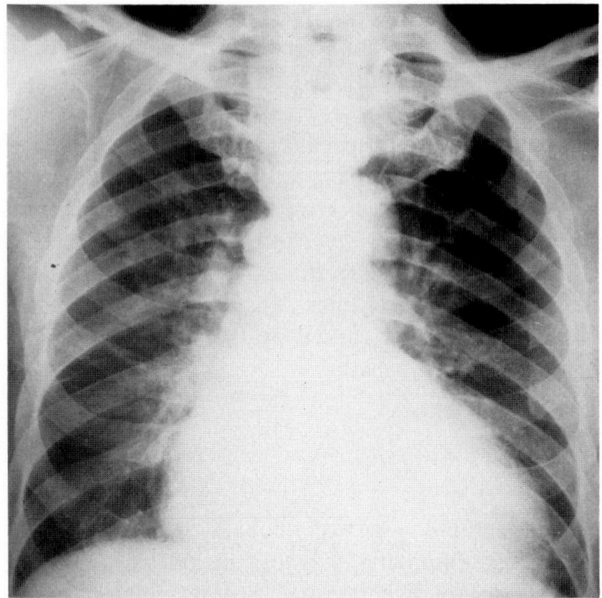

Figure 9. Cardiomyopathy, Secondary to Amyloidosis. There is cardiomegaly, predominantly left ventricular. The aorta is elongated. Mild prominence of the upper lobe veins is present.

Secondary Myocardopathy

The radiographic signs of secondary myocardopathy are similar to those of nonobstructive idiopathic cardiomyopathy (Fig. 9). Recognition of their secondary nature depends on the clinical or laboratory findings. For example, if there is a history of primary neoplasm, metastatic involvement of the heart is likely. A butterfly malar rash should raise the question of lupus myocardopathy. Elevated serum protein-bound iodine may indicate thyrotoxic myocardopathy.

However, certain radiographic signs may lead to the diagnosis of secondary cardiomyopathy. Atrophy of the chest wall muscles should suggest progressive muscular dystrophy. Pericardial or pleural effusion, infiltrate, collapse, or linear fibrosis in the lung may be seen in collagen disease, especially lupus erythematosus. Hilar adenopathy or extensive pulmonary fibrosis or nodulation suggests sarcoidosis. A localized bulge on the heart implies a primary or metastatic neoplasm.

In myxedema, the enlargement of the cardiopericardial silhouette is often due to pericardial effusion. Angiography, echocardiography, or an isotope scan may be helpful in recognizing the effusion.

Beriberi is often accompanied by considerable cardiac enlargement. Prominence of the pulmonary arc segment, predominant RV enlargement, and active cardiac pulsations may occur because of the high output state.

In thyrotoxicosis, heart size may be normal. When the heart is enlarged, the configuration is nonspecific. The pulmonary arc segment may be increased in size with pulmonary arterial overcirculation. Fluoroscopically, there are tachycardia and increased amplitude of pulsations.

Glycogen-storage disease may cause a grossly enlarged heart with heart failure. All cardiac chambers are enlarged angiographically, and the left ventricular wall is extremely thick. There may be narrowing of the LV outflow tract. The obstruction caused by the thick LV is similar to that seen in obstructive cardiomyopathy.

DIFFERENTIAL DIAGNOSIS

Since the radiographic signs of idiopathic cardiomyopathy are nonspecific, the radiologic differential diagnosis includes a wide variety of conditions, among which are hypertensive cardiovascular disease, rheumatic heart disease, pericardial effusion, coronary artery disease, and congenital aortic valvular disease.

A patient with idiopathic cardiomyopathy and associated congestive heart failure may have elevation of the systolic and diastolic blood pressure. With treatment of the heart failure, the diastolic pressure usually reverts to normal. Patients with long-standing hypertension usually have more elongation and dilatation of the aorta than those with idiopathic cardiomyopathy.

Rheumatic heart disease, especially when mitral or aortic insufficiency is the predominant lesion, may closely simulate idiopathic cardiomyopathy. Fluoroscopy is sometimes of value here since it may reveal the collapsing pulsations of the aorta in aortic insufficiency or the presence of valvular calcification.

Fluoroscopy may also be of value in pericardial effusion since a pulsating fat line may be seen on the true cardiac surface with the outer silhouette showing diminished pulsations. Complete absence of pulsations of the cardiopericardial margin is diagnostic of pericardial effusion. Angiocardiography, CO_2 angiography, cardiac radioisotope scanning, or echocardiography may be necessary to determine the presence or absence of a pericardial effusion. It is important to remember that cardiomyopathy and pericardial effusion may coexist. In such instances, pericardial effusion may result from heart failure or from pericarditis accompanying myocarditis.

Coronary artery disease as a cause of cardiac enlargement or failure may be extremely difficult to differentiate from idiopathic cardiomyopathy. Selective coronary arteriography may be necessary in resolving this dilemma.

Congenital aortic valvular stenosis usually is accompanied by post-stenotic dilatation of the aorta, a finding rarely present in obstructive cardiomyopathy. In discrete subvalvular aortic stenosis, the aorta is often normal and thus the resemblance to obstructive cardiomyopathy is quite close; left ventricular angiography may be necessary to differentiate the two.

REFERENCES

1. Fowler, N.O.: Differential diagnosis of cardiomyopathies. Prog Cardiovasc Dis 14:113, 1971.
2. Hill, C.A., Harle, T.S., and Gaston, W.: Cardiomyopathy: A review of 59 patients with emphasis on the plain chest roentgenogram. Am J Roentgenol 104:433, 1968.
3. Gotsman, M., van der Horst, R.L., and Winship, W.S.: The chest radiograph in primary myocardial disease. Radiology 99:1, 1971.
4. Meszaros, W.T.: Cardiac Roentgenology. Springfield, Ill. Charles C Thomas, 1969.
5. Brigden, W.: Uncommon myocardial diseases. The non-coronary cardiomyopathies. Lancet 2:1179, 1957.
6. Cockshott, W.P., Thorpe, G.J., and Ikeme, A.C.: Radiological aspects of heart muscle disease in Nigerian adults. Circulation 36:460, 1967.
7. Schreiber, M.H.: Radiologic investigations in idiopathic cardiomyopathy. Tex Rep Biol Med 25:468, 1967.
8. Rosenblum, R., Rubinstein, B.M., Solomon, N., and Jacobson, H.G.: Cineangiocardiographic studies of the left ventricle in idiopathic hypertrophic subaortic stenosis and other primary myocardial diseases. Radiology 87:23, 1969.
9. Steiner, R.E.: Radiology of Hypertrophic Obstructive Cardiomyopathy. In, Wolstenholme, G.E.W. (Ed.): Ciba Foundation Symposium Cardiomyopathies. Boston, Little, Brown, 1964, pp. 233-249.
10. Braunwald, E., Lambrew, C.T., Rockoff, S.D., Ross, J., Jr., and Morrow, A.G.: Idiopathic hypertrophic subaortic stenosis. 1. A description of the disease based upon an analysis of 64 patients. Circulation 30 (Suppl 4): 3, 1964.
11. Steiner, R.E.: The roentgen features of the cardiomyopathies. Sem Roentgenol 4:311, 1969.
12. Whiting, R.B., Powell, W.J., Jr., Dinsmore, R.E., and Sanders, C.A.: Idiopathic hypertrophic subaortic stenosis in the elderly. New Eng J Med 285:196, 1971.
13. Bourdarias, J.P., Ourbak, P., Ferrane, J., Sozutek, Y., Scebat, L., and Lenègre, J.: Obstructive cardiomyopathy: Cineangiocardiographic study of 50 cases. Am J Roentgenol 102:853, 1968.
14. Simon, A.L., Ross, J., Jr., and Gault, J.H.: Angiographic anatomy of the left ventricle and mitral valve in idiopathic hypertrophic subaortic stenosis. Circulation 36:852, 1967.
15. Simon, A.L.: Angiographic diagnosis of idiopathic hypertrophic subaortic stenosis. Radiol Clin N Am 6:423, 1968.

Electrocardiographic and Vectorcardiographic Features of Myocardial Diseases

The discussion in this chapter will be confined to surface potential alterations occurring in diseases which mainly attack cardiac muscle. The comments relating to primary myocardial disease will indicate the *idiopathic* nature of the process in contrast to secondary myocardial disease which will indicate myocardial involvement with systemic disease of specific etiology [1]. It should be understood that this, too, is an artificial separation. In the category of primary (idiopathic) myocardial disease, there are undoubtedly a number of individual diseases with common clinical manifestations, each awaiting the discovery of its unique origin in order to move it into the category of secondary myocardial disease.

We wish to state at the outset that there are no classic electrocardiographic or vectorcardiographic patterns that warrant out-of-context pronouncement of a categoric diagnosis for any of the primary or secondary myocardial diseases. There are, however, clues and some circumstantial evidence available which may be extremely helpful when viewed in clinical context.

This chapter includes a report and summary of the findings in over 1200 cases collected from our review of the English literature. When either

From the Section of Cardiology, Medical Service, FHD, Veterans Administration Hospital, and the Department of Medicine, Medical College of Georgia, Augusta, Georgia.

This study was supported by an award from the Veterans Administration, U.S. Public Health Services grant No. HE-11667, grant No. 69 783 from the American Heart Association, and a Grant-in-Aid from the Tennessee Heart Association.

the electrocardiogram or vectorcardiogram was illustrated and thus available for interpretation, or when the original author's description was clear enough to warrant accepting his diagnosis, the findings were tabulated and catalogued (see Table I). Such a review must contain instances of incompleteness and inaccuracy. It is hoped, however, that by the scope of the review and the effort toward validation that it will provide an overall accurate, if not precise, picture.

We have tried to provide both accuracy and precision in reporting additional information in 80 patients with primary (idiopathic) myocardial disease studied at the University of Tennessee College of Medicine and the Medical College of Georgia, their associated Veterans Administration Hospitals, and the Eugene Talmadge Memorial Hospital (see Tables II, III). In addition to complete histories and physical examinatons, every patient classified as Obstructive Cardiomyopathy, all of whom had idiopathic hypertrophic subaortic stenosis (IHSS), had the diagnosis confirmed at cardiac catheterization. Twenty-four patients with nonobstructive disease had complete hemodynamic studies. Seventy-five patients had standard electrocardiograms, vectorcardiograms, and high-frequency electrocardiograms. Two more had only electrocardiograms and 3 had only vectorcardiograms. Seven patients had 142-lead body surface isopotential maps recorded, and 7 had the diagnosis confirmed at postmortem examination. No patient was included in this study in whom there was any ambiguity regarding the etiologic classification. No patient with dual etiologies was included. Vectorcardiograms were recorded by the McFee-Parungao system [2], the Helm system [3], or the Frank system [4]. Because the abnormalities were judged in the context of the normal parameters of the specific system used in this discussion we will refer to the vectorcardiographic diagnostic conclusion (as opposed to degrees, angles, and magnitudes which do vary for each system). The normal values for the Frank system are those reported by Chou and Helm [5], by Witham and Lahman in the case of the Helm system [6, 7], and our modification of the Frank data for the McFee system.

In Table I the electrocardiographic findings from our review are grouped in categories which represent 3 fairly distinct clinical presentations of electrophysiological and hemodynamic alterations [8-11]. Under the Nonobstructive Familial heading, patients are included with family histories of cardiomegaly occurring in childhood or young adulthood but without outflow tract obstruction, without valvular, hypertensive, or large coronary vessel disease, without known systemic etiology, and without strong etiologic association. In this group, we have not included familial IHSS since these patients seem to have more clinical kinship to nonfamilial

Table I
From Literature Review of 1218 Patients with Primary (Idiopathic) Myocardial Disease:
Percent of Abnormality in Each Group

	Nonobstructive		*Obstructive*
Abnormality	*Familial Group (169 Patients) (%)*	*Nonfamilial Group (631 Patients) (%)*	*Familial and Nonfamilial (418 Patients) (%)*
Abnormal P waves	24.2	14.4	25.3
Atrial flutter or fibrillation	9.4	17.5	2.6
Supraventricular tachycardia	4.7	4.5	—
Atrial or junctional premature beats	3.5	9.6	0.7
All premature beats reported together	0.5	8.3	—
Ventricular premature beats	1.1	11.7	1.6
Atrioventricular dissociation and junctional rhythm	2.3	0.6	—
Ventricular tachycardia	4.7	1.5	—
Incomplete atrioventricular block	4.1	14.4	2.6
Complete atrioventricular block	7.1	0.7	0.7
Left ventricular enlargement	20.1	33.4	53.5
Right ventricular enlargement	*	*	0.4(?)*
Biventricular enlargement	*	*	*
Anomalous atrioventricular excitation	15.3	0.6	8.6
Pathologic Q waves	18.3	6.6	20.0
Left bundle branch block	8.2	8.8	3.5
Right bundle branch block	3.5	3.8	1.9
Intraventricular conduction defect	7.1	4.9	4.3

* See text for details.

obstructive patients than to familial cases which manifest themselves primarily by conduction system abnormalities, defects in contractility, or a combination of both [12-34].

The Nonobstructive Nonfamilial columns include patients who have cardiomegaly and congestive heart failure or documented evidence of significantly decreased contractility, but who have no evidence of ventricular outflow obstruction, valvular, hypertensive, or large coronary vessel disease, familial occurrence or known systemic etiology. Because we currently are unable to separate the clinical course and the electrophysiologic manifestations of patients with alcoholic cardiomyopathy from those with nonfamilial primary myocardial disease (with or without a history of regular, moderate-to-heavy alcohol ingestion), we have classified these patients together under the Nonfamilial heading. Indeed, the relative

Table II
From Author's Study of 77 Patients with Primary (Idiopathic) Myocardial Disease: Percent of Abnormality in Each Group

	Nonobstructive	*Obstructive*
Abnormality	*Nonfamilial (58 Patients) (%)*	*Nonfamilial and Familial (19 Patients) (%)*
Abnormal P waves	25.8	33.3
Atrial flutter or fibrillation	6.8	5.5
Supraventricular tachycardia	1.7	0
Atrial or junctional premature beats	3.4	0
All premature beats reported together	3.4	0
Ventricular premature beats	22.4	5.5
Atrioventricular dissociation and junctional rhythm	0	0
Incomplete atrioventricular block	18.9	16.6
Complete atrioventricular block	1.7	0
Left ventricular enlargement	67.2	61.1
Right ventricular enlargement	3.4	5.5
Biventricular enlargement	25.0(?)*	*
Anomalous atrioventricular excitation	0	0
Pathological Q waves	1.7	33.3
Left bundle-branch block	8.6	0
Right bundle branch block	0	0
Intraventricular conduction defect	0	0
Absent septal Q waves	39.6	0

* See text for details.

etiologic role of host factors versus alcohol per se remains unsettled [8, 9, 12, 13, 35-75] (Tables I, II, III).

The columns headed Obstructive include all patients with left ventricular outflow tract obstruction. This also includes those with and without a family background [29, 30, 76-113]. In the succeeding discussion, then, references to nonfamilial and familial will indicate a category of *nonobstructive* disease only, whereas the *obstructive* group includes patients with and without family histories of obstructive heart disease (Tables I, II, III).

Some of the patients in the Nonfamilial and Familial columns may represent myocardial reflection of disease processes of the smaller branches of the coronary arteries [114]. However, we have not included those patients with cardiac manifestations of known systemic disease such as Friedreich's ataxia or progressive muscular dystrophy. Rather, we have chosen to comment on these later as Secondary myocardial diseases.

Table III
Vectorcardiograms in 75 Patients with Myocardial Disease: % of Abnormality in Each Category

Abnormality	*Primary (Idiopathic) Myocardial Disease* *Nonobstructive Nonfamilial (56 Patients)*		*Obstructive Nonfamilial and Familial (19 Patients)*		*Other* *(3 Patients)*	
		(%)		*(%)*		*(%)*
Group I: Frontal plane QRS $_{max}$ vector inferior to transverse plane		*60.71*		*84.21*		*66.66*
A. LV enlargement	19.64		47.37		33.33 (postpartal)	
B. Posterior orientation without voltage criteria for LVE	12.5		31.58		33.33 (thyroid)	
C. Left BBB	5.36					
D. Right BBB	0.0					
E. Not subclassified	23.21		5.26			
Group II: Frontal plane QRS $_{max}$ vector superior to transverse plane		*35.71*		*15.79*		*33.33*
A. LV enlargement	5.36		5.26			
B. Posterior orientation without voltage criteria for LVE	5.36		10.53			
C. Left BBB	3.57				33.33 (acromegalic)	
D. Right BBB						
E. Not subclassified	21.43					
Group III: Unclassified		*3.57*				
1. Anterior loop, biventricular enlargement, inferior frontal loop	1.79					
2. Anterior loop, no ventricular enlargement, inferior frontal loop	1.79					
Additional findings in the above patients with primary (idiopathic) myocardial disease						
1. Slowing $\geq$ 24 msec	10.0		33.3			
2. Infarct pattern	1.7		33.3			
3. Left atrial enlargement	10.0		30.0			
4. Absent rightward initial vector	40.0		52.6			

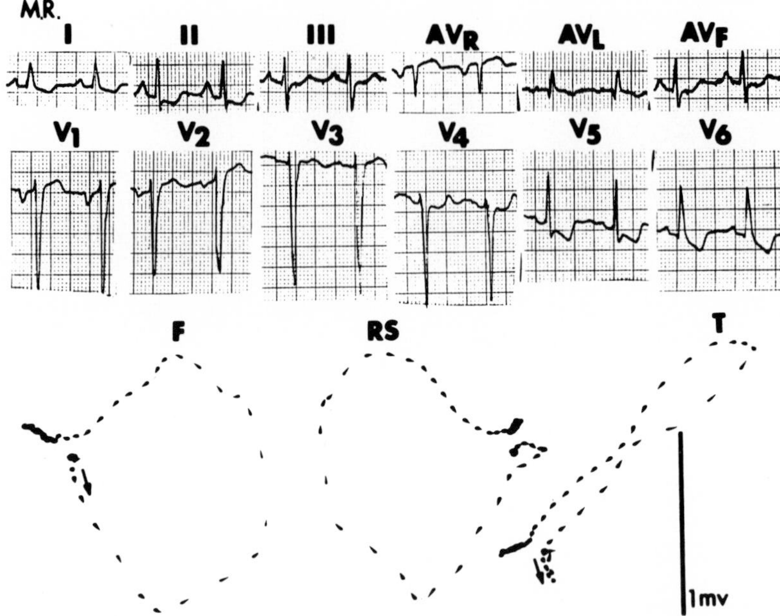

Figure 1. IHSS. MR is a 46-year-old White man. P waves of 0.3 mv in lead II suggest atrial abnormality or right atrial enlargement, whereas the 120 msec duration in lead II and the deep negative component and duration of about 60 msec in V_1 suggest left atrial enlargement. Criteria of Romhilt and Estes for left ventricular enlargement are also met. In the vectorcardiogram, recorded by the Helm system, the sharp end of the 4 msec time mark indicates the direction of inscription. Note the prominent slowing of inscription, best seen in the right sagittal and transverse projections. Such slowing lasts for at least 28 msec. The loop and maximum vector are displaced posteriorly. The narrow transverse loop is in contrast to the large rounded one usually seen. The maximum leftward vector in the frontal plane is abnormally superiorly oriented. This system's criteria for LVE are met.

PRIMARY (IDIOPATHIC) MYOCARDIAL DISEASE

Atrial Activation

Abnormalities of atrial activation are common in all 3 groups. Because many authors fail to specify right or left in reporting "atrial abnormalities," the realistic incidence of each is unclear. We have found when right or left specification was made that left atrial enlargement was more frequent in all groups [8]. Over 75 percent of atrial abnormalities in our study were also of the left (Figs. 1-4), and, indeed, many may represent atrial conduction defects.

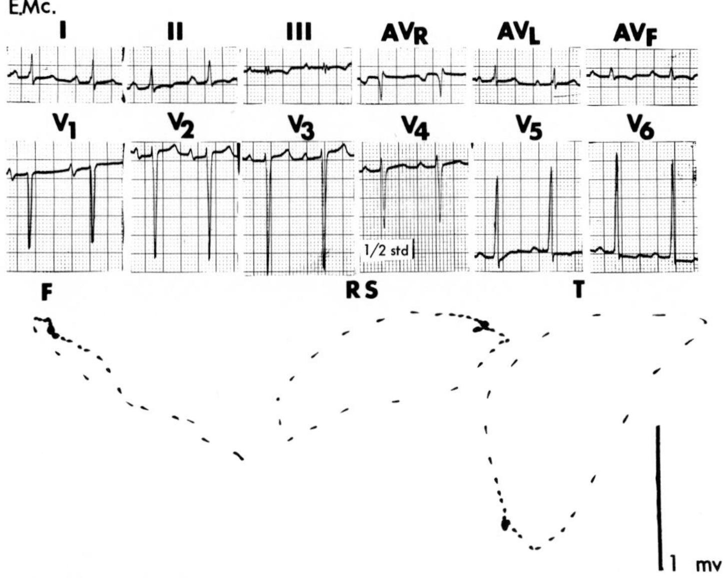

Figure 2. Nonobstructive Idiopathic Cardiomyopathy. EMc. This is a record from a 37-year-old Black woman, whose electrocardiogram demonstrates left atrial enlargement in V_1 by the 0.15-mv negative component of at least 40 msec duration, and left ventricular enlargement. Note the absence of a septal Q wave in leads I, aVL, V_5, and V_6. The sharp end of the 4-msec time marker indicates the direction of inscription in the vectorcardiogram. Though less impressive than in Figure 1, slowing of the initial inscription is again seen in all projections lasting for about 28 msec. Initial leftward vectors reflect the frequent absence of left-to-right septal activation seen in these patients. The characteristically large, oval, posteriorly oriented transverse loop is seen with the characteristically narrow frontal and somewhat narrow right sagittal loops.

A pattern of right atrial enlargement may be found with obstruction of the right ventricular outflow tract in some cases of IHSS, or when biventricular heart failure or pulmonary embolization has occurred in nonobstructive diseases. A pattern of left atrial enlargement is usually associated either with regurgitation through a dilated mitral annulus or with increased atrial mass associated with filling a poorly compliant or failing left ventricle. Abnormalities of rhythm and conduction will be discussed later.

Ventricular Activation

Early abnormalities. In over 40 percent of our patients with nonfamilial disease, there was lack of electrocardiographic and vectorcardiographic evidence for early left-to-right spread of activation across the interventricular

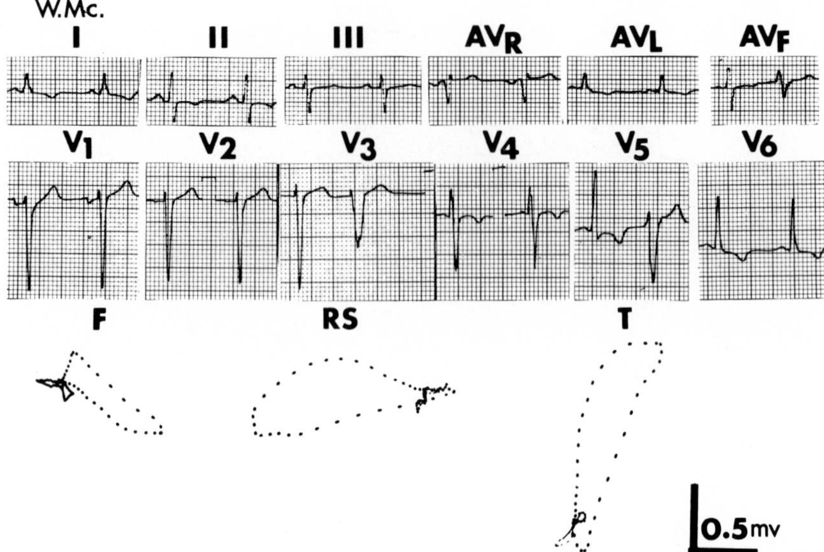

Figure 3. Nonobstructive Idiopathic Cardiomyopathy. WMc is a 59-year-old black man whose electrocardiogram demonstrates left ventricular enlargement, failure of early left-to-right septal activation by the absence of a septal Q, further faltering illustrated by the slurred upstroke of the R wave in leads I, aVL, V_6, and premature ventricular beats. The vectorcardiographic time markers are at 2.5 msec with the blunt end leading. Note the posterior orientation of the right sagittal and the transverse loops, the wide QRS-T angle in the frontal and transverse planes, and the prominent P wave, best seen in the frontal and the transverse planes. The extreme posterior orientation of the P loop suggests left atrial enlargement, though its magnitude is borderline.

septum [115]. This failure manifested as an absent septal Q wave in lead I, aVL, V_5, and V_6, or early direction of the vectorcardiographic loop absolutely anteriorly or anteriorly and to the left. In half of these nonfamilial cases, there was also evidence of slowing of the QRS loop in 2 planes for a duration of at least 24 msec after onset. Over half of our cases with obstructive disease also demonstrated such early slowing (Fig 1 and 2; Tables II and III).

Q waves greater than .03 second and Q waves to the right of transition in the precordial leads except V_1 were considered pathologic. Specific vectorcardiographic criteria for infarction patterns were applied for the system used [2-6]. These positive findings occurred with almost equal frequency in the familial category and the obstructive group, and less frequently in the nonfamilial category. In our own experience, pathologic Q waves were rare in the nonobstructive category, but occurred in about one-third of our obstructive patients (Fig. 5). In another study of 25 patients

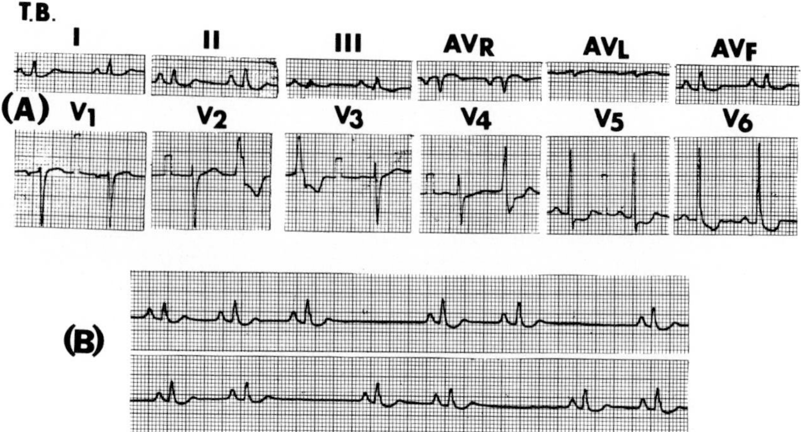

Figure 4. Nonobstructive Cardiomyopathy. TB is a 42-year-old White man with cardiomyopathy with unknown antecedent. A. Atrial enlargement is suggested by P-wave amplitude in lead II. Left ventricular enlargement is suggested by voltage of $SV_2 + RV_5$, the fact RV_6 greater than RV_5, and the ST-T1[n] morphology V_5. B. An example of 3:2 SA block with probable simultaneous SA and AV-Wenckebach periods.

with IHSS, the incidence was also 34 percent. These authors suggested that perhaps we do not see evidence of "septal hypertrophy" more often in cases of IHSS because of either hypertrophy of the left ventricular free wall or because of septal fibrosis [108] (Table II).

We still lack the electrophysiologic detail of the faulty left-to-right activation across the septum necessary to explain these abnormal findings in the early part of the QRS complex and in the early part of the vector loop. There are various hypotheses as to their genesis. Septal fibrosis has been offered as an explanation in absent septal Q waves. It is recognized that activation of the septum from left to right by branches of the left bundle predominates in normal man, but it is also well known that there is concomitant right-to-left activation generated from twigs of the right bundle branch. In examples of nonfamilial disease, body surface isopotential maps have been remarkably consistent* (Fig. 6A). At 20 msec in the normal, patient, we expect to see an anterior bulge in the map which represents primarily left-to-right septal activation, early anteroseptal free wall activation, and some right ventricular free wall activation prior to major right ventricular breakthrough to the epicardial surface. In patients with myo-

* *Editorial note:* Only a small number of patients have been studied by body surface mapping. Since the conventional electrocardiograms are not consistent in this group, isopotential body surface maps can be expected to show variations when larger numbers of patients are studied by this method.

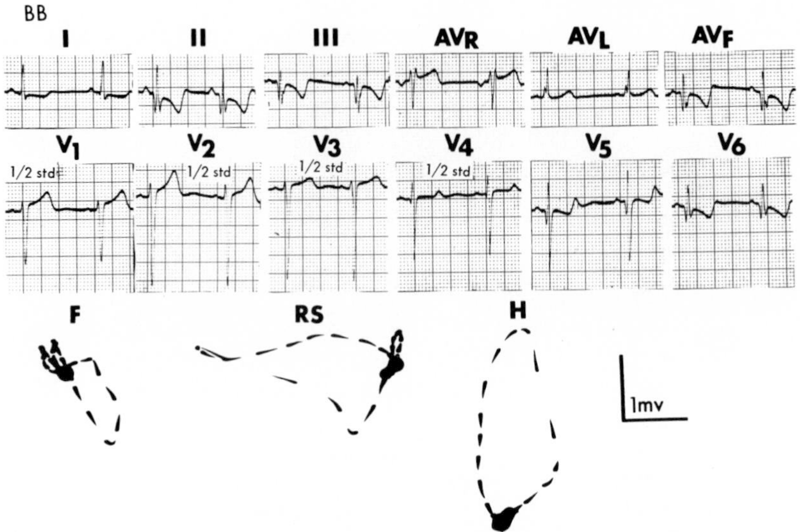

Figure 5. IHSS. BB is a 44-year-old-man in whom Q waves well over 30 msec in duration are seen in inferolateral leads II, III, aVF, V_5, and V_6. A pretransition small pathological Q is also seen in V_4. The initial forces move slightly to the right superiorly and very slightly anteriorly, but almost immediately proceed toward the back. There is a superior orientation of the vectorcardiogram through at least 24 and probably through 28 msec. Criteria, thus, are fulfilled electrocardiographically and vectorcardiographically for inferior as well as anterolateral myocardial infarctions. The patient had nothing to suggest atherosclerotic heart disease clinically, had classic hemodynamic findings of IHSS, and had normal coronary arteriograms. The electrocardiogram suggests left ventricular enlargement by the exceptionally high voltage in the S wave of the right precordial leads and the ST-T morphology in V_6. However, there are certain signs suggestive of concomitant right ventricular enlargement: The S wave in V_5 well over 7 mm, the drop in R/S ratio between V_2 and V_3, the presence of $S_1S_2S_3$, SV_5 and V_6, and the S_1Q_3 pattern suggest this possibility which is quite apparent radiographically.

cardial disease, instead of this relatively uniform mound of positive potential, there is a distinct sink of negativity beginning just to the left of the sternum and extending across to the right of the sternum. At 30 msec. though apical epicardial breakthrough has occurred, predominant activation is still anterior and to the left in the normal patient, whereas in patients, with nonobstructive cardiomyopathy negativity is seen very early and progresses frequently past 40 msec. with increasing magnitude. Early in ventricular depolarization normal left-to-right septal activation is either absent or attenuated, and the usual vectorially obscure right-to-left activation is relatively unopposed. The persistent deepening of the right and anterior negativity, however, probably relates to electrical breakthrough to the apical epicardium. Thus, the negative aspect of 2 enlarged fronts of activation are seen through the "anterior hole created." This also occurs in the normal heart but is less pronounced, which is probably due to the lesser magnitude of the right and left ventricular shell of activation in the nonhypertrophied heart and the fact that these shells are not as widely separated (see caption Fig. 6). The most striking contrast can be seen at 30 msec. Note the absence of the normal septal Q wave in lead X (Fig. 6A S.W.) and in electrocardiographic lead V_6 in the same patient seen in Figure 6B in contrast to the pattern from a normal man (B.E.) illustrated in Figures 6A and 6B.

Ventricular septal hypertrophy has been offered as an explanation when Q waves of increased duration or increased magnitude have occurred, especially in IHSS (Fig. 5). In a single-plunge electrode study of a patient with IHSS, Durrer was able to suggest that the cause for this man's deep Q wave in a lateral unipolar epicardial complex was related to synchronous excitation in over half of the thickness of the left ventricular free wall. This is in contrast to the expected outward spread of the wave of excitation seen in successive layers from endocardium to epicardium. The epicardial electrode in effect continued to "see" cavitary potential until a later-than-expected time in the QRS complex. Near to the epicardial surface after the simultaneous activation of the underlying subendocardial layers, an activation gradient could be seen to begin to falter and then to proceed to the epicardium. If this general pattern of altered subendocardial activation occurs with progressively increasing degrees of impairment, and if it obtains in septal areas as well as in the left ventricular free wall, it might explain the early slowing of the loop seen in certain subjects as well as the false infarction patterns seen in others [116] (Figs. 1, 2, 5; Tables I, II, III).

Mid- and late abnormalities and enlargement. An increase in the number of high-frequency notches in the QRS complex has been reported in patients with primary myocardial disease [117]. We have been able to separate clearly those with biventricular enlargement from normal patients on the basis of notch count alone and to identify less perfectly those with single ventricular enlargement. In X, Y, and Z summed, more than 6 notches were found only in those with single or biventricular enlargement [118].

In the 3 categories reviewed and in our own patients, the single common theme is the finding of left ventricular enlargement, both electrocardiographically and vectorcardiographically (Figs. 1, 2, 5). The incidences of right and biventricular enlargement, however, have been grossly underestimated. In our autopsied patients with myocardial disease, right ventricular enlargement uniformly accompanied left ventricular enlargement. However, the electrocardiographic indications of such concomitant

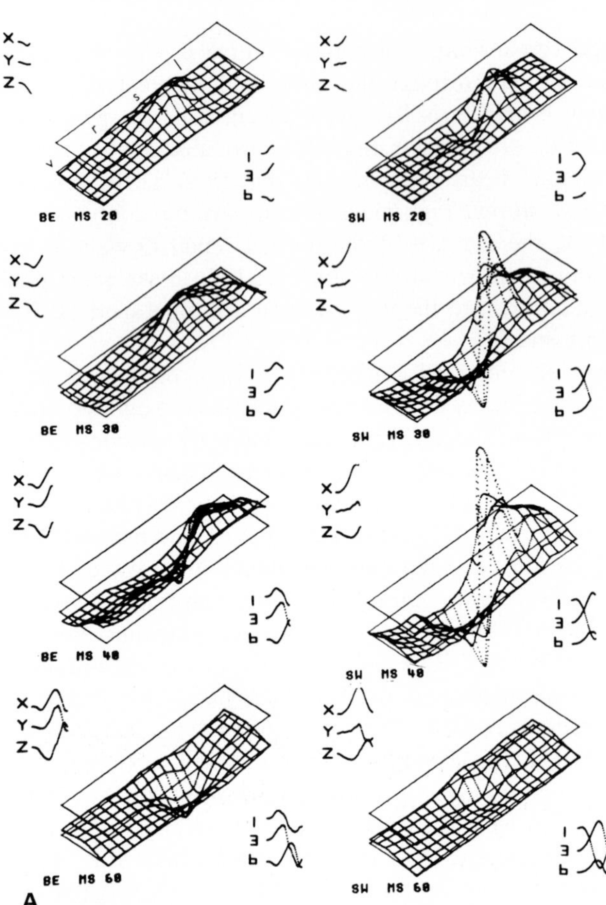

Figure 6A. Nonobstructive Idiopathic Cardiomyopathy. Scalar leads, N, Y, Z, V_1, V_3, and V_6 and body surface isopotential maps. Left. A relatively typical normal example from BE, a 24-year-old man. Right. The same data is portrayed for a 36-year-old man with nonobstructive idiopathic myocardial disease. Landmarks for the grid are seen in the first normal projection map. The midsternal lines (s), the left midaxillary line (1), the right midaxillary line (r), the vetebral line (v), and xiphoid (x) are indicated and apply to each of the successive maps. The plane inscribed above each grid represents the 1-mv level. Positive potential is represented by outward bulges, whereas negative potential is represented by sinks in the map. By 20 msec, in the normal adult a large portion of the middle of the left side of the interventricular septum is activated, activation has begun to spread toward the anterior wall of the left ventricle, and a very small amount of the right ventricular surface near the attachment of the anterior papillary muscle has been broken through by the activation front. From 10 msec, there has been some excitation of the right ventricular septal surface [116]. The net effect of this on the body surface map is an outward mound just to the right of the sternum, a larger outward mound moving anterior and leftward. This pro-

enlargement were usually subtle (Fig. 5) [119], and usually took the form of cancellation of the expected left axis shift of predominant left ventricular enlargement, of S waves greater than 7 mm in V_5 or V_6 [120], and of the presence of the 4 subtle signs of right ventricular enlargement occurring in the presence of left ventricular enlargement. These signs were (1) Presence of $S_1S_2S_3$, (2) Presence of S_1Q_3, (3) Presence of SV_5 and V_6, and, most valuable, (4) A pretransitional drop in R/S ratio in the precordial leads [119].

We have not included figures on electrocardiographic evidence of right or biventricular enlargement from the literature review because we feel that we are not able to do so with any degree of certainty. Our own work would suggest that although there is rarely pure right ventricular enlargement, there is often a suggestion of biventricular enlargement (Table II).

Other vectorcardiographic findings. A relatively consistent finding in nonobstructive disease is a spatial orientation of the mean axis of the QRS loop hovering somewhere near the equator, with little deviation along the *Y* axis. Posterior orientation is almost uniformly dominant [10, 121-124] (Table III).

Hamby et al. have seen fit to classify patients into 2 groups, based upon whether the frontal plane maximum vector lay inferior (group I) or superior (group II) to the transverse plane [122, 123]. They divided these patients further into those with left ventricular enlargement (A), those with simply posterior orientation but without the voltage criteria for left ventricular enlargement (B), those with left bundle-branch block (C), and those with right bundle-branch block (D). On applying this very useful classification, we found that in 56 of our patients with nonobstructive disease, about 61 percent fell in group I with inferiorly oriented loops while about 36 percent were categorized in group II with loops whose maximum frontal plane vector lay above the *X* axis (Table III). These figures correspond closely to those of Hamby and coworkers in a study of

---

gresses through 30 msec at which time a diffuse elevation occurs whose peak approaches the left midclavicular line at about the fourth intercostal space. By 40 msec, a large part of the epicardial surface of the left ventricle and much of the right ventricle has been activated—creating a larger hole in the wavefronts, manifested by the prominent sink. There is a maximum positivity near the left midaxillary line, and a maximum negativity that has shifted slightly to the left of the sternum. The patient with myocardial disease manifests an earlier and deeper region of negativity centered at the midsternal area. By 30 msec, this has become deeper and wider, reflecting the increasing size of the opening in the anterior electrical front as more and more of the enlarged right and left ventricular surfaces are activated.

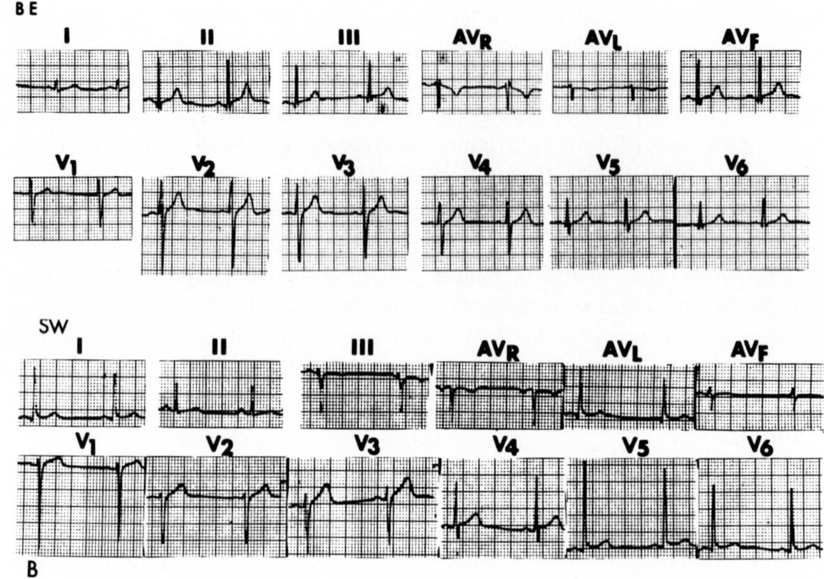

Figure 6B. Direct writer electrocardiogram. Top, the direct writer electrocardiogram of normal subject BE whose body surface map and high-frequency scalar leads are illustrated in figure 6*A*. *Bottom*, is the direct writer electrocardiogram of patient SW whose studies are also illustrated in figure 6A. Excessive voltage is noted when the amplitude of the R wave in V_5 is summed with that of the S wave in V_2, which has been recorded at half standard. After seeing the rather dramatic alterations in the body surface map of SW at the time of early septal and right and left ventricular free wall activation, retrospectively one might note that there is attenuation of the normal septal Q wave in leads 1, V_5 and V_6, though it is present. The frontal plane axis is about —20°. The major differences in the direct writer electrocardiograms of the normal subject and the patient with nonobstructive PMD is primarily QRS amplitude, frontal plane axis, and the size of Q waves relative to the size of the QRS complex in leads V_5 and V_6. More subtle differences as well as more striking differences become apparent when the body surface maps are compared in figure 6A.

125 patients [123]. Of the 25 subjects we were unable to completely subclassify, all had posterior loops but 13 lacked voltage criteria for left ventricular enlargement. Two were not classified because of failure to have a posterior orientation or LVE, (group III).

Most of our obstructive cases also fell into either group IA or B (Table III). Most of the QRS loops of the nonobstructive patients fell near the lead *X* axis and two-thirds were within ±30°. In contrast, a much larger percentage of the loops in the obstructive group had their mean spatial axes below the transverse plane and half of these centered around +50° (Table III).

A large rounded transverse loop and relatively narrow frontal and sagittal loops were again a relatively constant finding [10, 108, 121, 122] (Fig. 2).

Though Coyne noted in 19 of 33 patients with IHSS that the loops initially moved anteriorly and to the right, 13 of these had a slow inscription of the loops. Two had very large anterior and rightward vectors representing septal or right ventricular activation, and 5 had anterior and leftward initial activation. Of these 5 patients, one also demonstrated slowing of activation. Of 9 with initial posterior and leftward loops, 2 demonstrated slowing of the loop [110]. Although we are impressed with the frequency of protracted slowing in association with IHSS, we have not found it to be specific for IHSS (Table III).

Anomalous atrioventricular excitation has been discovered with increasing frequency as more cases are reviewed and as techniques of recording are improved. Fifteen percent of those reviewed with familial origins and 9 percent of those with obstructive disease manifested either classical Wolff-Parkinson-White syndrome or some variant of the preexcitation syndromes. We had no instances, however. This is, in part, accounted for because we did not study familial patients of the nonobstructive type (Table I).

Rhythm and Conduction

One of the distinguishing features of the 3 groups reviewed relates to the frequency of disturbances of rhythm. The incidence was high in the nonfamilial patients, low in the obstructive patients, and of intermediate frequency in the patients with familial backgrounds.

Atrial flutter or fibrillation and ventricular premature beats were the two most frequently encountered disturbances of rhythm in the nonfamilial group from the literature review. Ventricular premature beats (Figs. 3, 4) were followed in frequency by atrial flutter and fibrillation in our patients. Other premature beats were encountered in about 10 percent of patients reviewed and supraventricular tachycardia in about 4.5 percent. Ventricular tachycardia and atrioventricular dissociation with a junctional escape rhythm were the least frequently encountered disturbances. We encountered supraventricular tachycardia in slightly less than 2 percent of our patients, and ventricular tachycardia only in the agonal state.

In the obstructive group, isolated atrial or junctional premature beats occurred with the greatest frequency in the literature review, though in our experience, single ventricular premature beats were more frequently seen (Tables I, II).*

* *Editorial Note:* Supraventricular tachycardias are common in the experience of some investigators. (See Chapter 12 by Wigle et al.)

Because digitalis has often entered the clinical picture before the diagnosis is made, the exact incidence of sinoatrial (SA) or atrioventricular (AV) block due to the disease process alone may be only roughly estimated (Fig. 4). The etiology of block in these patients is clouded even further because patients with cardiomyopathy are particularly sensitive to the toxic effects of digitalis. However, in the literature there are a number of instances of block without digitalis. These are of a sufficient number to make it clear that blocks are not infrequent sequellae to the disease process itself. An effort was made then to eliminate cases of drug toxicity in both the authors' review and study. From the review, incomplete AV block occurred in over 14 percent of the nonfamilial and in only 4 percent of the familial patients; it occurred in 3 percent of the obstructive patients. The familial patients, on the other hand, had a higher instance of complete AV block. Complete AV block occurred in less than 2 percent of our own nonfamilial patients and not at all in the obstructive group (Tables I, II).

We have used the term "intraventricular conduction defect" specifically to mean instances in which the QRS complex was .12 second or greater and yet did not correspond to one of the bundle branch block patterns. This occurred most frequently in the familial patients in the literature, but it did not occur in our study. A previous estimate of 24 percent for the occurrence of left bundle branch block in nonobstructive patients appeared to us excessive [125]. Our review indicated an incidence of about 8, 9, and 4 percent in the nonobstructive familial, nonobstructive nonfamilial, and obstructive groups, respectively (Table I). Our own experience reflected a 9 percent incidence in the nonfamilial group, and we failed to encounter either left or right bundle branch block otherwise. Patients were classified as having AV dissociation with an escape junctional rhythm when this mechanism occurred secondary to abnormal slowing or arrest of the SA pacemaker. This is distinguished from occurrences secondary to an accelerated lower pacemaker or secondary to AV block. With this definition, we found an abnormality over 2 percent of the time in the familial, less than 1 percent in the nonfamilial, and not at all in the *obstructive* category. We did not encounter it in our patients.

Repolarization Abnormalities

We are progressively more impressed with the wide spectrum of unhelpful repolarization abnormalities. ST-T-wave morphologic change tends to parallel the degree of cardiomegaly and the level of left ventricular end-diastolic pressure, rather than to predict specific etiology.

SUMMARY: PRIMARY (IDIOPATHIC) MYOCARDIAL DISEASES

The relative sparsity of rhythm disturbances in obstructive patients provides a striking contrast with the frequent abnormalities of rhythm in the nonobstructive group, with nonfamilial incidences exceeding familial ones. Left ventricular and left atrial enlargement are frequent findings in all 3 categories. Complete AV block stands out as a manifestation encountered in familial patients. The demonstration of pathological Q waves was more frequent in patients with obstructive disease. Patients with familial origins but without obstruction also had a relatively high incidence of such abnormality. Second only to left ventricular enlargement was the absence of septal Q waves in leads I, aVL, V_5, and V_6 in our study of nonfamilial patients without obstruction.

The vectorcardiographic loop in the transverse plane most frequently hovers about the equator and is generally posteriorly oriented in the nonobstructive patients, whereas in the obstructive group, the loop is more inferiorly oriented but still assumes a position more posterior than the normal for the recording system used. The early vectors are frequently abnormal. Such abnormalities range from the mere absence of initial rightward forces to distinct early slowing (through 24 msec after onset) to loops that mimic myocardial infarction. This latter finding of abnormal initial forces was more frequent in patients with IHSS. These early abnormalities may relate to synchronous activation of a large part of the depth of the left ventricle and thus failure of an early, outwardly moving wavefront as suggested by Durrer [116]. In instances of Q waves in the right precordial leads, unmasking of the usual less dominant right-to-left septal vectors may have resulted from impaired left-to-right activation, thus, reversing the dominant direction of early ventricular activation.

MYOCARDIAL DISEASES OF QUESTIONABLE CLASSIFICATION

There are several other disease states which closely parallel those that have been catalogued in Tables I, II, and III. Perhaps postpartal heart disease should be considered as an example of primary (idiopathic) myocardial disease. We have chosen to discuss it separately as an example of myocardial disease with a strong etiologic association but with as yet undetermined cause and effect relationship. This cardiomyopathy is frequently found in late pregnancy or in the postpartal period. Its manifestations are sometimes indistinguishable from those in other patients with nonobstructive forms of primary (idiopathic) myocardial disease [126]. P-pulmonale patterns suggesting right atrial overload and QRS changes of right ventricular overload have been observed. Almost invariably electrocardiographic evidence of left ventricular enlargement has been present. In 16 of 32 patients from one series, there was no evidence of early left-to-right septal activation. Vectorcardiograms were recorded in 25 patients and of these, 18 had the posteriorly oriented loop similar to those reported above. However, in one careful study of 15 patients, there were no instances of conduction defects and only transitory premature ventricular beating, probably related to hypokalemia and digitalis sensitization [127-131].

The role of the heavy metals—especially cobalt and lead—in the genesis of myocardial disease and their interrelationship to the intake of alcohol poses an unanswered question. Therefore, we have not catalogued the electrocardiographic and vectorcardiographic findings in the Quebec beer-drinkers' cardiomyopathy patients in the tabular summary. These patients probably should be currently considered to belong to an intermediate group having a strong etiologic association but not yet clearly specified as secondary myocardial disease. These patients differ from the uniform picture presented by other patients in the nonobstructive groups in that they manifest low voltage, relatively frequent atrial premature beats, but infrequent troublesome disturbances of rhythm. They are similar to the other nonobstructive patients in their frequent manifestations of abnormal septal and early ventricular activation. This is represented either by an absent septal Q wave or by initial slowing of the upstroke of an R wave. A frequent finding has been nonspecific ST-T abnormalities which are transient and which disappear with abstinence. This is reminiscent of certain acute processes such as beriberi heart disease in which there is rather rapid electrocardiographic return to normal with therapy [132-133].

Two cases of an infantile type of myocardial disease have been reported with a previously unrecognized histiocytoid reaction. One child was found dead, and there was no electrocardiographic record. A second was found to have supraventricular tachycardia and right bundle branch block. The place of these infants in the spectrum of myocardial disease is currently unclear [134].

SECONDARY MYOCARDIAL DISEASE

In a number of heritable conditions, involvement of heart muscle has been reported. In Friedreich's ataxia, T-wave abnormalities and a relatively consistent pattern of deep, narrow Q waves, especially in inferolateral leads (II, III, aVF, and V_6) associated with very large R waves in V_1 have been noted. The vectorcardiographic findings, likewise, show a prominent early vector, representing a combination of interventricular septal activation and right ventricular free wall activation. The magnitude of this vector is frequently in excess of 1mv and the total anterior activation time may last as long as 48 msec. In spite of these findings suggestive of right ventricular or septal hypertrophy, only 1 patient has been noted to have the structural and hemodynamic changes of IHSS. The actual relationship of this pattern to the morphology of the ventricle is unknown. One very complete review indicates that electrocardiographic abnormalities occur in over 30 percent of the patients with Friedreich's ataxia [135, 136].

The electrocardiogram in a number of varieties of muscular dystrophy has been the subject of recent interest. One case of what was probably benign Duchenne's muscular dystrophy (pseudohypertrophic progressive muscular dystrophy) demonstrated atrial flutter and the cardiomyopathic syndrome. Noninflammatory degeneration of coronary arteries 1 mm or less in diameter was found, and arteries supplying the sinoatrial and atrioventricular nodes were involved [137]. An extensive review of 106 patients with Duchenne's muscular dystrophy showed electrocardiographic abnormalities in 101. The deep, narrow Q waves in leads V_5 and V_6 were similar to the findings in Friedreich's ataxia. There was prominent septal and right ventricular activation represented by tall R waves in lead V_1 and occasionally by a nonprolonged RSR′ complex. Frequently, an R/S ratio greater than 1 was found. Premature beats were rare, but heart failure associated with other electrocardiographic abnormalities was extremely common [138, 139].

Scleroderma or systemic sclerosis, is often associated with myocardial disease. ST-T abnormalities are frequent as is left ventricular enlargement. Other electrocardiographic findings include all degrees of atrioventricular block, right and left bundle branch block, atrial fibrillation and paroxysmal atrial tachycardia, all types of premature beats, and false myocardial infarction patterns [140-146].

We studied 1 case of dermatomyositis in a 35-year-old woman in whom the diagnosis was supported with a myocardial biopsy. Prior to the biopsy, she demonstrated deep, symmetrical T waves across the precordium and in II, III, and aVF. There is scant other pathologic correlation, though others have noted incomplete and complete AV block, atrial arrhythmias, and ST-T abnormalities [147-150].

Patterns indistinguishable from those of myocardial infarction have been seen with neoplastic infiltrates of the heart [151].

A single case with a peculiar polysaccharide accumulation in the heart has been reported in a patient with cardioskeletal myopathy with an associated left bundle branch block [152].

Currently, there is some question as to whether a chronic form of beriberi heart disease exists. Certainly, the classic fulminating acute variety responds readily to thiamin and is indeed a clinical entity distinct from the chronic process previously discussed. Repolarization abnormalities, particularly T-wave inversions and prominent U waves, rapidly revert to normal with treatment. A report of a number of cases called "perimyocardiopathies" has been brought to our attention which resemble fulminating beriberi to some extent. Thirteen of 17 subjects were reported to have pericardial effusion, and right atrial enlargement was a prominent feature. In a case reported of recovery from Shoshin beriberi, the patient demonstrated ST-T abnormalities, the development of a Q wave in lead III and an RSR′ pattern in V_1 which we relate to right ventricular overload [153-155]. Some believe that beriberi heart disease and heart disease associated with the excessive intake of alcohol may be phases of the same underlying process. The strongest advocate of this notion studied 100 patients, two-thirds of whom were alcoholics; one-sixth were judged to have beriberi heart disease, and one-sixth to be nonalcoholic but with myocardial disease. A spectrum of electrocardiographic abnormalities were demonstrated in these 3 groups, suggesting a spectral kinship between the beriberi patients and the alcoholic patients [156].

The relationship of other nutritional diseases to myocardial disease is even more difficult to determine. From Ceylon, there are reports of heart failure and electrocardiographic abnormalities in individuals who presumably did not have beriberi, but who did have a low serum potassium, protein deficiency, heart failure, cardiomegaly, hepatomegaly, and portal fibrosis. In 28 patients, the most frequent findings were complete AV block, atrial fibrillation, premature beats, left ventricular enlargement. Eighteen percent had biventricular enlargement. An occasional patient had paroxysmal atrial tachycardia, right ventricular enlargement, extreme left axis deviation, right bundle branch block, and left bundle branch block. We interpret the pattern reported as incomplete right bundle branch block in 4 patients as right ventricular overload when such pattern is not associated with a prolonged QRS complex and the R′ occurs earlier than 0.08 second after onset of ventricular activation [157].

Amyloid heart disease is best characterized as a large heart with low QRS voltage on electrocardiograms. Electrical alternans of the P wave, atrial fibrillation, varying degrees of AV block, and right bundle branch block have all been reported. One instance of pericollagenous amyloidosis is recorded in a patient with progressive muscular dystrophy of the limb-girdle variety who manifested paroxysmal tachycardia of an unspecified type, premature ventricular beats, and ST-T abnormalities [158-161].

Myocardial sarcoidosis has been associated with atrial fibrillation, atrial premature beats, successive ventricular premature beats, and occasionally a short burst of ventricular tachycardia. On occasion, a pattern imitative of myocardial infarction has been noted to disappear both with and without steroid therapy [162-164].*

Recently, myocardial disease in association with sickle cell disease or trait in patients who are not anemic has been reported. Large P waves, atrial fibrillation, premature ventricular beats, and intraventricular conduction defects have been noted. Left axis deviation to —60° has been seen. Biventricular and biatrial enlargement are reported [165, 166].

Fabry's disease or angiokeratoma corporis diffusum universale has been reported to cause 4-chamber enlargement in 1 patient without skin manifestations [167].

Supraventricular tachycardia, ventricular premature beats, and ST-T abnormalities have been seen in patients with pheochromocytoma [168, 169].

The reported incidence of right bundle branch block in Chagas' disease varies between 30 and 60 percent. Left bundle branch block, on the other hand, occurs very rarely in from 2 to 5 percent of the patients. This may well be a manifestation of the greater vulnerability to the panmyocarditis of the long, narrow, later branching, partially intramyocardial right bundle, in contrast to the left. The axis is frequently superiorly oriented, and some would raise the question as to whether this suggested that the most anterior ramifications of the left bundle might also be involved. Varying degrees of AV block and intraventricular conduction defects have been noted. Premature ventricular beats, atrial fibrillation, and P-wave abnormalities occur with varying frequencies, depending primarily on the stage of the disease process [170-173].

With acromegaly, extreme cardiomegaly may occur. Our patient gradually acquired left atrial enlargement and left ventricular enlargement but later developed a left bundle branch block pattern. He encountered a transient 145°-shift in axis to the right with an atrial or junctional pacemaker and 24 hours later resumed normal sinus rhythm and left bundle branch block with extreme left axis deviation. He had angina, and though these abnormalities of conduction may relate to the acromegalic hypertrophy, they may also be the result of an undocumented myocardial infarction in a heart that has literally outgrown its blood supply [174-176] (Fig. 7).

Isolated reports of myocardial involvement in many infectious disease processes and many parasitic diseases as well as in association with highly toxic substances have been noted. We have tried to limit our inclusion to

* *Editorial Note:* In our own experience, AV block, including complete AV block, has been relatively common in myocardial sarcoidosis.

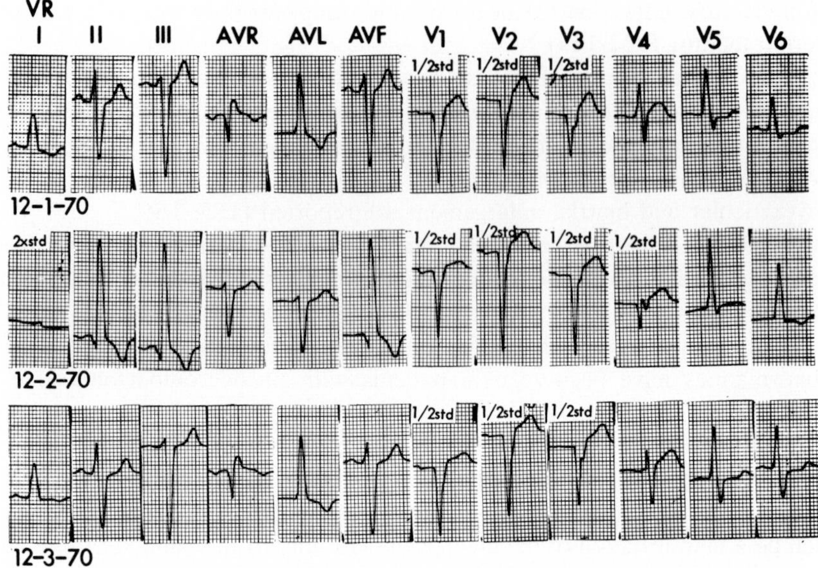

Figure 7. Acromegaly. VR is a 53-year-old White man whose electrocardiogram has progressed from one demonstrating primarily left ventricular enlargement to one meeting the criteria for left bundle branch block which was relatively constant through 12/1/70. Twenty-four hours later his pattern of conduction changed drastically with an axis shift from about $-50°$ to $+90°$ and a change in the pacemaker site at this same time. The negative P waves in leads II, III, and aVF with a P-R interval of about 150 msec would suggest a site somewhere in the low atrium or perhaps a junctional site. Twenty-four hours later, the patient had resumed his pattern of left bundle branch block and sinus rhythm.

those which were more than evanescent, which had some independent documentation, and which usually progress to develop the syndrome of cardiomegaly and heart failure.

SUMMARY: SECONDARY MYOCARDIAL DISEASE

Just as in primary (idiopathic) myocardial diseases, certain secondary myocardial diseases provide electrical clues to their existence. There are distinctive and consistent electrocardiographic patterns in Friedreich's ataxia, Duchenne's progressive muscular dystrophy, and Chagas' disease. In other instances of secondary myocardial manifestations of systemic disease, we have been unable to elucidate a diagnostically dependable pattern. It should be emphasized, however, that any patient having systemic disease which (1) is known to involve other striated muscle, (2) has frequent autoimmune associations or is known to involve connective tissue, (3) is known to infiltrate other organs, (4) is associated with metabolic dysfunction of other organs, (5) is associated with manifestations of nutritional deficiency in other organ systems, or (6) is associated with a high level of cellular toxicity of an infectious, physical or chemical nature, should be considered a candidate for possible myocardial involvement. Thus, in reality, any systemic disease may have a place somewhere in the spectrum of potential cardiac hazard. We have presented examples of some with the greatest propensity for cardiac involvement, and we have explored the electrocardiographic and vectorcardiographic hints of such involvement.

REFERENCES

1. Fowler, N.O.: Differential diagnosis of the cardiomyopathies. Progr Cardiovas Dis 14:113, 1971.
2. McFee, R. and Parungao, A.: An orthogonal lead system for clinical electrocardiography. Am Heart J 62:93, 1961.
3. Helm, R.A.: An accurate lead system for spatial vectorcardiography. Am Heart J 53:415, 1957.
4. Frank, E.: An accurate, clinically practical system for spatial vectorcardiography. Circulation 13:737, 1956.
5. Chou, T.C. and Helm, R.A.: Clinical Vectorcardiography, New York, Grune & Stratton, 1967, Ch. 5, pp 50-63.
6. Witham, A.C.: The vectorcardiogram recorded with sponge electrodes. Am Heart J 72:730, 1966.
7. Lahman, J.E. and Witham, A.C.: Vectorcardiogram past forty. Am Heart J 79:149, 1970.
8. Goodwin, J.F., Gordon, H., Hollman, A., and Bishop, M.B.: Clinical aspects of cardiomyopathy. Br Med J 1:69, 1961.
9. Braunwald, E. and Aygen, M.M.: Idiopathic myocardial hypertrophy without congestive heart failure or obstruction to blood flow. Am J Med 35:7, 1963.
10. Horan, L.G., Flowers, N.C., Thomas, J.R., and Tolleson, W.J.: The spatial vectorcardiogram in idiopathic cardiomyopathy. Progr Cardiovas Dis 7:11, 1964.
11. Marriott, H.J.: Electrocardiographic abnormalities, conduction disorders and arrhythmias in primary myocardial disease. Progr Cardiovas Dis 7:99, 1964.
12. Harris, L.C., Nghiem, Q.X., Schreiber, M.H., and Wallace, J.M.: Severe pulsus alternans associated with primary myocardial disease in children. Observations on clinical features, hemodynamic findings, mechanism and prognosis. Circulation 34:948, 1966.
13. Ohsuzu, H.: Symposium on idiopathic myocardial fibrosis and allied disease. 5. Familial cardiomegaly. Jap Circ J 30:1590, 1966.
14. Kariv, I., Sherf, L., and Solomon, M.: Familial cardiomyopathy with special consideration of electrocardiographic and vectorcardiographic findings. Am J Cardiol 13:734, 1964.

15. Schiebler, G.L., Adams, P., Jr., and Anderson, R.C.: Familial cardiomegaly in association with the Wolff-Parkinson-White syndrome. Am Heart J 58:113, 1959.
16. Westlake, R.E., Cohen, W., and Willis, W.H.: Wolff-Parkinson-White syndrome and familial cardiomegaly. Am Heart J 64:314, 1962.
17. Schraeder, W.H., Pankey, G.A., Davis, R.B., and Theologides, A.: Familial idiopathic cardiomegaly. Circulation 24:599, 1961.
18. Treger, H. and Blount, S.G., Jr.: Familial cardiomegaly. Am Heart J 70:40, 1965.
19. Gaunt, R.T. and Lecutier, M.A.: Familial cardiomegaly. Br Heart J 18:251, 1956.
20. Evans, W.: Familial cardiomegaly. Br Heart J 11:68, 1949.
21. Campbell, M. and Turner-Warwick, M.: Two more families with cardiomegaly. Br Heart J 18:393, 1956.
22. Whitfield, A.G.: Familial cardiomyopathy. Quart J Med 30:119, 1961.
23. Walther, R.J., Madoff, I.M., and Zinner, K.: Cardiomegaly of unknown cause occurring in a family. Report of three siblings and review of the literature. New Engl J Med 263:1104, 1960.
24. Soulie, P., di Matteo, J., Abaza, A., Nouaille, J., and Thibert, M.: Cardiomegalie familiale. Arch Mal Coeur 50:22, 1957.
25. Barry, M. and Hall, M.: Familial cardiomyopathy. Br Heart J 24:613, 1962.
26. Kariv, I., Szeinberg, A., Fabian, I., Sherf, L., Kreisler, B., Zeltzer, M.: A family with cardiomyopathy. Am J Med 40:140, 1966.
27. Beasley, O.C., Jr.: Familial myocardial disease. A report of three siblings and a review of the literature. Am J Med 29:476, 1960.
28. Battersby, E.J. and Glenner, G.G.: Familial cardiomyopathy. Circulation 22:721, 1960.
29. Weber, D.J., Gould, L., and Schaffer, A.I.: A family with idiopathic myocardial hypertrophy. Am J. Cardiol 17:419, 1966.
30. Nasser, W.K., Williams, J.F., Mishkin, M.E., Childress, R.H., Helmen, C., Merritt, A.D., and Genovese, P.D.: Familial myocardial disease with and without obstruction to left ventricular outflow. Clinical, hemodynamic, and angiographic findings. Circulation 35:638, 1967.
31. Allensworth, D.C., Rice, G.J., and Lowe, G.W.: Persistent atrial standstill in a family with myocardial disease. Am J Med 47:775, 1969.
32. Kariv, I., Szeinberg, A., Fabian, I., Sherf, L., Kreisler, B., and Zeltzer, M.: A family with cardiomyopathy. Am J Med 40:140, 1966.
33. Barold, S.S., Linhart, J.W., Hildner, F.J., Rywlin, A., and Samet, P.: Familial cardiomyopathy: A clinical, hemodynamic and angiographic study in one family. Chest 57:141, 1970.
34. Machida, K., Iguchi, K., Saito, Y., Sugishita, Y., Murayama, M., Mori, M., Yamaguchi, H., Ito, I., and Ueda, H.: Familial cardiomyopathy: Immunological studies and review of literature on autopsied cases in Japan. Jap Heart J 12:40, 1971.
35. Wolanskyi, B.M., Pintar, K., and Gubbay, E.R.: Alcoholic cardiomyopathy. Can Med Assoc J 93:103, 1965.
36. Evans, W.: Alcoholic cardiomyopathy. Progr Cardiovas Dis 7:151, 1964.
37. Sanders, V.: Idiopathic disease of the myocardium. Arch Intern Med 112:661, 1963.
38. Davies, H and Evans, W.: The significance of deep S waves in leads II and III. Br Heart J 22:551, 1960.

39. Forbes, G. and Bradley, A.: Idiopathic cardiomegaly. Br Med J 2:1125, 1960.
40. Sackner, M.A., Lewis, D.H., Robinson, M.J., and Bellet, S.: Idiopathic myocardial hypertrophy. Am J Cardiol 7:714, 1961.
41. Elster, S.K., Horn, H., and Tuchman, L.R.: Cardiac hypertrophy and insufficiency of unknown etiology. A clinical and pathologic study of ten cases. Am J Med 18:900, 1955.
42. Case Records of the Massachusetts General Hospital, Case 28042: New Engl J Med 266:158, 1942.
43. Dye, C.L., Rosenbaum, D., Lowe, J.C., Behnke, R.H., and Genovese, P.D.: Primary myocardial disease. Part I: Clinical features. Ann Intern Med 58:426. 1963.
44. Sommers, B.: Problems in clinical diagnosis and classification of ventricular hypertrophy in adults. 1: Idiopathic left ventricular hypertrophy. Minn Med 39:12, 1956.
45. Serbin, R.A. and Chojnacki, B.: Idiopathic cardiac hypertrophy: Report of three cases. New Engl J Med 252:10, 1955.
46. Shabetai, R. and McGuire, J.: Idiopathic cardiac hypertrophy simulating valvular heart disease. Am Heart J 65:124, 1963.
47. Speckhals, R.C., Winchell, P., Amplatz, K., Edwards, J.E., and From, A.H.L.: Clinical pathologic conference. Am Heart J 69:551, 1965.
48. Harvey, W.P., Segal, J.P., and Gurel, T.: The clinical spectrum of primary myocardial disease. Progr Cardiovas Dis 7:17, 1964.
49. Bloomfield, D.K. and Liebman, J.: Idiopathic cardiomyopathy in children. Circulation 27:1071, 1963.
50. Davies, R.R., Marvel, R.J., and Genovese, P.D.: Heart disease of unknown etiology. Am Heart J 42:546, 1951.
51. Dines, D.E.: Alcoholic cardiomyopathy. Rocky M Med J 62:32, 1965.
52. Massumi, R.A., Rios, J.C., Gooch, A.S., Nutter, D., De Vita, V.T., and Datlow, D.W.: Primary myocardial disease: Report of 50 cases and review of the subject. Circulation 31:19, 1965.
53. Fowler, N.O. and Gueron, M.: Primary myocardial disease. Circulation 32:830, 1965.
54. Segal, J.P., Harvey, W.P., and Gurel, T.: Diagnosis and treatment of primary myocardial disease. Circulation 32:837, 1965.
55. Pietras, R.J., Meadows, W.R., Fort, M., and Sharp, J.T.: Hemodynamic alterations in idiopathic myocardiopathy including cineangiography from the left heart chambers. Am J Cardiol 16:672, 1965.
56. Simkins, S.: Idiopathic cardiac hypertrophy in adults. Am Heart J 42:453, 1951.
57. Fowler, N.O., Gueron, M., and Rowlands, D.T., Jr.: Primary myocardial disease. Circulation 23:498, 1961.
58. Ware, E.R. and Chapman, B.M.: Chronic fibroplastic myocarditis. Am Heart J 33:530, 1947.
59. Smith, J.D. and Furth, J.: Fibrosis of the endocardium and the myocardium with mural thrombosis. Arch Intern Med 71:602, 1943.
60. Von Bonsdorff, B.: Myocardial disease of obscure origin. Acta Med Scand 100:403, 1939.
61. Shugoll, G.I.: Primary idiopathic myocardial disease. GP magazine 32:129, 1965.
62. Reisinger, J.A. and Blumenthal, B.: Myocardial degeneration with hypertrophy and failure of unknown cause. Am Heart J 22:811, 1941.

63. Lenz, R.L. and Rousselot, L.M.: Cardiac hypertrophy of unknown etiology in young adults. A clinical and pathological study of three cases. Am Heart J 9:178, 1933.
64. Norris, R.F and Pote, H.H.: Hypertrophy of the heart of unknown etiology in young adults: Report of four cases with autopsies. Am Heart J 32:599, 1946.
65. Levy, R.L. and von Glahn, W.C.: Cardiac hypertrophy of unknown cause. A study of the clinical and pathologic feature in ten adults. Am Heart J 28:714, 1944.
66. Doane, J.C. and Skversky, N.J.: Massive cardiac hypertrophy: A case report. Am Heart J 29:816, 1944.
67. Levin, E.B. and Cohen, S.L.: Idiopathic myocardial hypertrophy simulating rheumatic heart disease. Am Heart J 48:637, 1954.
68. Spodick, D.H. and Littmann, D.: Idiopathic myocardial hypertrophy. Am J Cardiol 1:610, 1958.
69. Naughton, J.: The myocardiopathies: Some electrocardiographic features. J Okla Med Assoc 58:50, 1965.
70. Tobin, J.R., Jr., Driscoll, J.F., Lim, M.T., Sutton, G.C., Szanto, P.B., and Gunnar, R.M.: Primary myocardial disease and alcoholism. The clinical manifestations and course of the disease in a selected population of patients observed for three or more years. Circulation 37:754, 1967.
71. Rosen, R.J., Schoonmaker, F., and Laszlo, J.: Treatment of idiopathic myocardial hypertrophy with thioguanosine. Am Heart J 76:35, 1968.
72. Castleman, B., and McNeely, B.U.: Case records of the Massachusetts General Hospital. Case 49-1967. New Engl J Med 277:1193, 1967.
73. Rothfeld, E.L., Zucker, I.R., and Alinsonorin, C.: Panconduction myocardiopathy. Dis Chest 51:541, 1967.
74. Castleman, B and McNeely, B.U.: Case records of the Massachusetts General Hospital. Case 45-1966. New Engl J Med 275:835, 1966.
75. Goldstrich, J.D. and Shapiro, W.: Abnormal Q waves and normal coronary arteriograms in primary myocardial disease. Tex Med 67:70, 1971.
76. Braunwald, E., Morrow, A.G., Cornell, W.P., Aygen, M.M., and Hilbish, T.F.: Idiopathic hypertrophic subaortic stenosis. Clinical, hemodynamic and angiographic manifestations. Am J Med 29:924, 1960.
77. Estes, E.H., Jr., Whalen, R.E., Roberts, S.R., Jr., and McIntosh, H.D.: The electrocardiographic and vectorcardiographic findings in idiopathic hypertrophic subaortic stenosis. Am Heart J 65:155, 1963.
78. Braudo, M., Wigle, E.D., and Keith, J.D.: A distinctive electrocardiogram in muscular subaortic stenosis due to ventricular septal hypertrophy. Am J Cardiol 14:599, 1964.
79. Lundquist, C.B., Amplatz, K., Palma, S.P., Raghib, G.: Angiocardiographic findings in idiopathic myocardial hypertrophy with right and left ventricular outflow tract obstruction. Am J Roentgenol 93:315, 1965.
80. Hollman, A., Goodwin, J.F., Teare, D., and Renwick, J.W.: A family with obstructive cardiomyopathy (asymmetrical hypertrophy). Br Heart J 22:449, 1960.
81. Brent, L.B., Aburano, A., Fisher, D.L., Moran, T.J., Myers, J.D., and Taylor, W.J.: Familial muscular subaortic stenosis. Circulation 21:167, 1960.
82. Bentall, H.H., Cleland, W.P., Oakley, C.M., Shah, P.M., Steiner, R.E., and Goodwin, J.F.: Surgical treatment and post-operative haemodynamic studies in hypertrophic obstructive cardiomyopathy. Br Heart J 27:585, 1965.
83. Wood, R.S., Taylor, J., Wheat, M.W., and Schiebler, G.L.: Muscular sub-

aortic stenosis in childhood. Report of occurrence in three siblings. Pediatrics 30:749, 1962.

84. Teare, D.: Asymmetrical hypertrophy of the Heart. Br Heart J 20:1, 1958.
85. Cohen, J., Effat, H., Goodwin, J.F., Oakley, C.M., and Steiner, R.E.: Hypertrophic obstructive cardiomyopathy. Br Heart J 26:16, 1964.
86. Estes, E.H., Jr., Whalen, R.E., Roberts, S.R., Jr., and McIntosh, H.D.: Electrocardiographic and vectorcardiographic findings in idiopathic hypertrophic subaortic stenosis. Circulation 26:714, 1962.
87. Moes, C.A., Peckham, G.B., and Keith, J.D.: Idiopathic hypertrophy of the interventricular septum causing muscular subaortic stenosis in children. Radiology 83:283, 1964.
88. Morrow, A.G. and Brockenbrough, E.C.: Surgical treatment of idiopathic hypertrophic subaortic stenosis. Ann Surg 154:181, 1961.
89. Tafur, E., Guntheroth, W.G., Baum, D., Blackmon, J.R.: The development of outflow tract obstruction of the left ventricle in idiopathic myocardial hypertrophy. Circulation 30:569, 1964.
90. Goodwin, J.F., Hollman, A., Cleland, W.P., and Teare, D.: Obstructive cardiomyopathy simulating aortic stenosis. Br Heart J 22:403, 1960.
91. Hollister, R.M. and Goodwin, J.R.: The electrocardiogram in cardiomyopathy. Br Heart J 25:357, 1963.
92. McIntosh, H.D., Sealy, W.C., Whalen, R.E., Cohen, A.I., and Sumner, R.G.: Obstruction to outflow tract of left ventricle. Arch Intern Med 110:312, 1962.
93. Menges, H., Jr., Brandenburg, R.O., and Brown, A.L., Jr.: The clinical, hemodynamic, and pathologic diagnosis of muscular subvalvular aortic stenosis. Circulation 24:1126, 1961.
94. Prescott, R., Quinn, J.S., and Littmann, D.: Electrocardiographic changes in hypertrophic subaortic stenosis which simulate myocardial infarction. Am Heart J 66:42, 1963.
95. Wigle, E.D., Heimbecker, R.O., and Gunton, R.W.: Idiopathic ventricular septal hypertrophy causing muscular subaortic stenosis. Circulation 26:325, 1962.
96. Braudo, M., Wigle, E.D., and Keith, J.D.: A distinctive electrocardiogram in subaortic stenosis. Presented at 13th Annual Convention of American College of Cardiology, 1964.
97. Daoud, G., Gallaher, M.E., and Kaplan, S.: Muscular subaortic stenosis. Am J Cardiol 7:860, 1961.
98. Nagle, R.E., Boicourt, O.W., Gillam, P.M.S., and Mounsey, J.P.D.: Cardiac impulse in hypertrophic obstructive cardiomyopathy. Br Heart J 28:419, 1966.
99. Hancock, E.W. and Eldridge, F.: Muscular subaortic stenosis. Reversibility with varying cardiac cycle length. Am J Cardiol 18:515, 1966.
100. Husson, G.S. and Blackman, M.S.: Aortic stenosis with marked right ventricular hypertrophy. Am J Cardiol 17:273, 1966.
101. Wigle, E.D. and Baron, R.H.: The electrocardiogram in muscular subaortic stenosis. Effect of a left septal incision and right bundle-branch block. Circulation 34:585, 1966.
102. Horlick, L., Petkovich, N.J., and Bolton, C.F.: Idiopathic hypertrophic subvalvular stenosis. A study of a family involving four generations. Clinical, hemodynamic and pathologic observations. Am J Cardiol 17:411, 1966.
103. Ewy, G.A., Marcus, F.I., Bohajalian, O., Burke, H.L., and Roberts, W.C.: Muscular subaortic stenosis. Clinical and pathologic observations in an elderly patient. Am J Cardiol 22:126, 1968.

104. Frank, S. and Braunwald, E.: Idiopathic hypertrophic subaortic stenosis. Clinical analysis of 126 patients with emphasis on the natural history. Circulation 37: 759, 1968.

105. Reeve, R.: Clues to the bedside diagnosis of mild idiopathic subaortic stenosis. JAMA 195:41, 1966.

106. Warkentin, D.L. and Korns, M.E.: Hypertrophic subaortic stenosis in the aged. Am Heart J 73:106, 1967.

107. Parker, B.M.: The course of idiopathic hypertrophic muscular subaortic stenosis. Ann Intern Med 70:903, 1969.

108. Bahl, O.P., Walsh, T. and Massie, E.: Electrocardiography and vectorcardiography in idiopathic hypertrophic subaortic stenosis. Am J Med Sci 259:262, 1970.

109. Karatzas, N.B., Hamill, J., and Sleight, P.: Hypertrophic cardiomyopathy. Br Heart J 30:826, 1968.

110. Coyne, J.J.: New concepts of intramural myocardial conduction in hypertrophic obstructive cardiomyopathy. Br Heart J 30:546, 1968.

111. Sanders, C.A., Austen, W.G., Jordan, J.C., and Scannel, J.G.: Idiopathic hypertrophic subaortic stenosis in two elderly siblings. New Engl J Med 274: 1254, 1966.

112. Bernstein, L. and Mitchell, A.S.: The acute and chronic effects of pharmacological adrenergic blockage in obstructive cardiomyopathy. Isr J Med Sci 5:803, 1969.

113. Pooya, M., Khoi, N., Sarin, R., Rios, J., and Massumi, R.A.: Clinical and hemodynamic features of idiopathic hypertrophic subaortic stenosis (IHSS) Med Ann DC 37:594, 1968.

114. James, T.N.: An etiologic concept concerning the obscure myocardiopathies. Progr Cardiovas Dis 7:43, 1964.

115. Hamby, R.I. and Raia, F.: Electrocardiographic aspects of primary myocardial disease in 60 patients. Am Heart J 76:316, 1968.

116. Durrer, D.: Electrical aspects of human cardiac activity: A clinical-pathological approach to excitation and stimulation. Cardiovas Res 2:1, 1968.

117. Reynolds, E.W., Jr., Muller, B.F., Anderson, G.J., and Muller, B.T.: High-frequency components in the electrocardiogram: A comparative study of normals and patients with myocardial disease. Circulation 35:195, 1967.

118. Flowers, N.C. and Horan, L.G.: Diagnostic import of QRS notching in high-frequency electrocardiograms of living subjects with heart disease. Circulation 44:605, 1971.

119. Flowers, N.C. and Horan, L.G.: Subtle signs of right ventricular enlargement and their relative importance. In: Hurst, J.W. and Schlant, R. (Eds.): Advances in Electrocardiography, New York, Grune & Stratton, 1972, pp. 9-18.

120. Sokolow, M. and Lyon, T.P.: The ventricular complex in right ventricular hypertrophy as obtained by unipolar precordial and limb leads. Am Heart J 38:273, 1949.

121. Banta, H.D. and Estes, E.H., Jr.: Electrocardiographic and vectorcardiographic findings in patients with idiopathic myocardial hypertrophy. Am J Cardiol 14: 218, 1968.

122. Hamby, R.I.: Vectorcardiographic aspects of primary myocardial disease in 50 patients. Am Heart J 76:304, 1968.

123. Hamby, R.I., Raia, F., and Catangay, P.: Primary myocardial disease: Vectorcardiographic findings in 125 patients. In, Hoffman, I., Hamby, R.I., and

Glassman, E. (Eds.): Vectorcardiography 2. Amsterdam, North-Holland, 1971, pp. 424-431.

124. Stein, P.D., Solis, R.M., Brooks, H.L., Matson, J.L., and Hyland, J.W.: Vectocardiogram simulating myocardial infarction in idiopathic hypertrophic subaortic stenosis. Dis. Chest 54:469, 1968.

125. Goodwin, J.F.: The nonobstructive cardiomyopathies. Acta Cardiol 21:272, 1966.

126. Benchimol, A.B., Carneiro, R.D., and Schlesinger, P.: Post-partum heart disease. Br Heart J 21:89, 1959.

127. Walsh, J.J., Burch, G.E., Black, W.C., Ferrans, V.J., and Hibbs, R.G.: Idiopathic myocardiopathy of the puerperium (postpartal heart disease). Circulation 32:19, 1965.

128. Burch, G.E., Walsh, J.J., Ferrans, V.J., and Hibbs, G.: Prolonged bed rest in the treatment of the dilated heart. Circulation 32:852, 1965.

129. Burch, G.E., McDonald, C.D., and Walsh, J.J.: The effect of prolonged bed rest on postpartal cardiomyopathy. Am Heart J 81:186, 1971.

130. Bashour, F. and Winchell, P.: "Post partal" heart disease—a syndrome? Ann Intern Med 40:803, 1954.

131. Becker, F.F. and Taube, H.: Myocarditis of obscure etiology associated with pregnancy. New Engl J Med 266:62, 1962.

132. Tetu, A. and Samson, M.: Quebec beer-drinkers' cardiomyopathy: electrocardiographic study. Can Med Assoc J 97:893, 1967.

133. Quebec beer-drinkers' cardiomyopathy. JAMA 202:1145, 1967.

134. Reid, J.D., Hajdu, S.I., and Attah, E.: Infantile cardiomyopathy: a previous unrecognized type with histiocytoid reaction. J Pediat 73:335, 1968.

135. Chaco, J.: Friedreich's ataxia with myocardial involvement and myopathy. Isr J Med Sci 2:52, 1966.

136. Gach, J.V., Andriange, M., and Frank, G.: Hypertrophic obstructive cardiomyopathy and Friedreich's ataxia. Report of a case and review of literature. Am J Cardiol 27:436, 1971.

137. James, T.N.: Observations on the cardiovascular involvement, including the cardiac conduction system in progressive muscular dystrophy. Am Heart J 63:48, 1962.

138. Slucka, C.: The electrocardiogram in Duchenne progressive muscular dystrophy. Circulation 38:933, 1968.

139. Perloff, J. K., de Leon, A.C., Jr., and O'Doherty, D.: The cardiomyopathy of progressive muscular dystrophy. Circulation 33:625, 1966.

140. Nasser, W.K., Mishkin, M.E., Rosenbaum, D., and Genovese, P.D.: Pericardial and myocardial disease in progressive systemic sclerosis. Am J Cardiol 22:538, 1968.

141. Johnson, M.L. and Ikram, H.: Scleroederma of Buschke. An uncommon cause of cardiomyopathy. Br Heart J 32:720, 1970.

142. Escudero, J. and McDevitt, E.: The electrocardiogram in scleroderma. Am Heart J 56:846, 1958.

143. Sachner, M.A., Heinz, E.R., and Steinberg, A.J.: The heart in scleroderma. Am J Cardiol 17:542, 1966.

144. Oram, S. and Stokes, W.: The heart in scleroderma. Br Heart J 23:243, 1961.

145. Roth, L.M. and Kissane, J.M.: Panaortitis and aortic valvulitis in progressive systemic sclerosis. Am J Clin Path 41:287, 1964.

146. Beigleman, P.M., Goldner, F., Jr., and Bayles, T.B.: Progressive systemic sclerosis. New Engl J Med 249:45, 1953.
147. Sheard, C.: Dermatomyositis. Arch Intern Med 88:640, 1951.
148. Walton, J. and Adams, R.: Polymyositis. Edinburgh, Livingstone, 1958, p. 269.
149. Wedgwood, R., Cook, C., and Cohen, J.: Dermatomyositis. Pediatrics 12:447, 1953.
150. Diessner, G.R., Howard, F.M., Jr., Winkelmann, R.K., Lambert, E.H., and Mulder, D.W.: Laboratory tests in polymyositis. Arch Intern Med 117:757, 1966.
151. Harris, T.R., Copeland, G.D., and Brody, D.A.: Progressive injury current with metastatic tumor of the heart; case report and review of the literature. Am Heart J 69:392, 1965.
152. Karpati, G., Carpenter, S., Wolfe, L.S., and Sherwin, A.: A peculiar polysaccharide accumulation in muscle in a case of cardioskeletal myopathy. Neurology 19:553, 1969.
153. Weiss, S. and Wilkins, R.W.: The nature of the cardiovascular disturbance in vitamin deficiency states (Beriberi). Trans Am Physicians 51:341, 1936.
154. Kesteloot, H., Terryn, R., Bosmans, P., and Joossens, J.V.: Alcoholic perimyocardiopathy. Acta Cardiol 21:341, 1966.
155. Jeffrey, F.E. and Abelmann, W.H.: Recovery from proved Shoshin beriberi. Am J Med 50:123, 1971.
156. Alexander, C.S., Idiopathic heart disease. I. Analysis of 100 cases with special reference to chronic alcoholism. Am J Med 41:213, 1966.
157. Obeyesekere, I.: Idiopathic cardiomegaly in Ceylon. Congestive cardiac failure, cardiomegaly, hepatomegaly, and portal fibrosis associated with malnutrition. Br Heart J 30:226, 1968.
158. Van Buchem, F.S.P.: Cardiac amyloidosis. Report of six cases. Acta Cardiol 21:367, 1966.
159. Pomerance, A.: The pathology of senile cardiac amyloidosis. J Path Bacteriol 91:357, 1966.
160. Brownstein, M.H.: Cardiac amyloidosis and complete heart block. N Y J Med 66:397, 1966.
161. Reichenmiller, H.E., Bundschu, H.D., Bass, L., Missmahl, H.P., and Arnold, M.: Progressive muscular dystrophy and pericollagenous amyloidosis. Ger Med Month 13:380, 1968.
162. Bashour, F.A., McConnell, T., Skinner, W., and Hanson, M.: Myocardial sarcoidosis. Dis Chest 53:413, 1968.
163. Phinney, A.O., Jr.: Sarcoid of the myocardial septum with complete heart block. Report of two cases. Am Heart J 62:270, 1961.
164. Gold, J.A. and Cantor, P.J.: Sarcoid heart disease. A case with an unusual electrocardiogram. AMA Arch Intern Med 104:101, 1959.
165. Rubler, S., Fleischer, R.A.: Sickle cell states and cardiomyopathy. Sudden death due to pulmonary thrombosis and infarction. Am J Cardiol 19:867, 1967.
166. Fleischer, R.A. and Rubler, S.: Primary cardiomyopathy in nonanemic patients. Association with sickle cell trait. Am J Cardiol 22:532, 1968.
167. Kemp, G.L.: Fabry's disease involving the myocardium and coronary arteries; without skin manifestations. Vasc Dis 4:100, 1967.
168. Sode, J., Getzen, L.C., and Osborne, D.P.: Cardiac arrhythmias and cardiomyopathy associated with pheochromocytomas. Report of three cases. Am J Surg 114:927, 1967.

169. Van Vliet, P.D., Burchell, H.B., and Titus, J.L.: Focal myocarditis associated with pheochromocytoma. New Engl J Med 274:1102, 1966.
170. Puigbo, J.J., Rhode, J.R. Nava, Barrios, H. Garcia, Suarez, J.A., and Yepez, C. Gil: Clinical and epideumiological study of chronic heart involvement in Chagas' disease. Bull World Health Organ 34:655, 1966.
171. Rosenbaum, M.B., Chagasic myocardiopathy. Progr Cardiovas Dis 7:199, 1964.
172. Feher, J., Pileggi, F., Teixeira, V., Tranchesi, J., Lima, F.X., Spiritus, O., Chansky, M., and Decourt, L.V.: The vectorcardiogram in chronic Chagas myocarditis. An analysis of the intraventricular conduction delays associated with a superiorly oriented AQRS. Am J Cardiol 5:349, 1960.
173. Schabelman, M., Rosenbaum, M.B., and Citrinovitz, A.: Alteraciones electrocardiograficas de la miocarditis cronica Chagasica: Estudios efectuados sobre 100 casos en la provincia de San Juan (Electrocardiographic changes of Chagasic chronic myocarditis: Studies carried out on 100 cases in the Province of San Juan). Prensa Med Arg 48:974, 1961.
174. Courville, C. and Mason, V.R.: The heart in acromegaly. AMA Arch Intern Med 61:704, 1938.
175. Hejtmancik, M.R., Bradfield, J.Y., Jr., and Herrmann, G.R.: Acromegaly and the heart: A clinical and pathologic study. Ann Intern Med 34:1445, 1951.
176. Herrmann, G.R. and Hejtmancik, M.R.: The heart in acromegaly: A clinical and pathologic study. Acta Med Scand 256:171, 1951.

Heritable and Familial Aspects of Myocardial Diseases

One of the more remarkable achievements of clinical genetics in the past several decades has been the separation of arbitrary, heterogeneous, and overlapping clinical syndromes into natural systems of nosology. This separation is essential for accurate prognosis, for estimation of risk, mutation rates, linkage, and other genetical variables. Most important of all, the way is paved for the discovery of the gene product. As little as 30 years ago, a typical list of gene disorders found in man comprised fewer than 100 diseases [1], whereas the best current estimate is 1876 diseases. For example, the muscular dystrophies were either all grouped together [2] or arbitrarily segregated into simple groups [3, 4] until 1953, when Walton and Nattrass [5] devised a simple classification in which genetic and clinical varieties were correlated.

The manner in which accurate classification leads to therapy is demonstrated by such well-known examples as hemophilia and gargoylism. As soon as hemophilia and Christmas disease were separated, it became possible to identify antihemophilic globulin. Similarly, the discovery of cross-complementation had to await the separation of the Hunter-Hurler syndrome into the Hunter syndrome (X-linked) and the Hurler syndrome (autosomal recessive).

We hope that in the future, an improved understanding of the genetics of myocardial disease will lead to rapid advances in understanding the fundamental mechanisms, classification, and therapy of that heterogeneous

* With the assistance of Roger Freeman, William Shuffett, Lee Coleman, and Grace Carlson, R. N.

group of cardiac disorders known as idiopathic myocardial disease. In the following pages we will review present knowledge in this area, discuss some of the practical implications, and summarize our own genetic studies of idiopathic myocardial disease.

Several forms of myocardial disease may be familial. This observation has great importance in the diagnosis of individual cases as well as for the epidemiologic and other public health aspects of the disease. The significance of such nonspecific findings as inversion of T waves in the electrocardiogram of an asymptomatic patient may become clear only after the physician has learned that several of the patient's first-degree relatives have proven myocardial disease. In patients with clinical heart disease the true significance of mild arterial hypertension, mitral or tricuspid incompetence; or a syndrome of syncope, chest pain, cardiac murmurs, or bundle branch block may not emerge until after a family history compatible with myocardial disease has been obtained.

Screening of the largest possible number of first-degree relatives of patients with known idiopathic myocardial disease yields a large number of new patients, many of whom are asymptomatic and would not have been treated for many more years. Exhaustive screening of the families of patients with myocardial disease provides the data from which the precise hereditary patterns of the various forms of myocardial disease can be determined.

Numerous pitfalls hinder the physician who would attempt to construct hypotheses concerning the genetics of a malady using only the time-honored but blunted tool of a family history obtained at the bedside or in the office. Ignorance of the whereabouts and health of close relatives, deliberate withholding of evidence to protect the secrecy of parenthood, and the variable expressiveness of hereditary disorders are the most important sources of these pitfalls. Frequently, the busy physician simply fails to obtain as accurate a family history as he should in the clinic or in the office. This failure was dramatically enacted on the occasion when two of our patients with hypertrophic obstructive cardiomyopathy, both of whom had given a negative family history, greeted each other in the foyer of the clinic as long lost cousins. A short conference rapidly uncovered the names of several affected members of the family in 4 generations. Screening of this family led to the discovery of additional members who were asymptomatic, many of whom were children.

It is now well known that the disorder variously known as hypertrophic obstructive cardiomyopathy, idiopathic subaortic stenosis, and a host of other now less popular names may be familial [6-24]. Moreover, it has been established that familial cases are transmitted as Mendelian autosomal dominants [6, 7, 10, 11, 13, 14, 15, 18, 19].

R. D. Teare [25], in his paper entitled "Asymmetrical hypertrophy of the heart in young adults," described 8 cases of idiopathic hypertrophy of the heart with principal involvement in the intraventricular septum. In an addendum to his paper, Teare states that a brother of one of his patients collapsed and died while riding a bicycle. His heart at postmortem examination was virtually identical in appearance with that of his sister, showing a localized hypertrophy affecting the anterior wall and interventricular septum. By coincidence on the day of his death, his younger sister attended the outpatient department of the hospital and was found to have signs identical to those of their sister. Teare was still uncertain of the etiology of the disease he was rather diffidently proposing as a new clinicopathological entity, but he promised to report the family in detail in a subsequent paper. Teare was as good as his word, but this paper [9] did not appear until after it had been proposed and rapidly became the consensus that idiopathic subaortic stenosis, hypertrophic obstructive cardiomyopathy, and asymmetrical hypertrophy of the heart were one and the same disease. Earlier reports such as that of Evans [26] who described familial cardiomegaly in 1949 and that of Davies [27] who reported "A familial heart disease" in 1952, and that of Campbell and Turner-Warwick [28] were considered to be examples of the same disease. In the enthusiasm which greeted, as it almost always does, the discovery of a new disease, certain awkward discrepancies were laid aside or ignored. For example, in none of Teare's [25] cases was the question of outflow tract obstruction so much as raised. The cases described by Evans [26] and by Gaunt [29] had Stokes-Adams attacks, very bizarre electrocardiograms, unusual vacuoles in the myocardium, and large abnormal deposits of glycogen in the cardiac and somatic muscle. These findings are not typical of what is usually reported in idiopathic hypertrophic subaortic stenosis.

Lord Russell Brock [30] was the first to speculate in the literature that hypertension may result in left ventricular outflow tract hypertrophy and obstruction, analogous to infundibular stenosis complicating congenital right ventricular outflow tract obstruction. This, when it was first proposed, was greeted as a fascinating new observation, but after the concept of hypertrophic obstructive cardiomyopathy had become established, it was treated with that mixture of embarrassment and disdain so often accorded a mistake made by a great man. Indeed, Brock himself in a later paper [31] rescinded this opinion of the etiology of functional outflow tract obstruction.

Considering this background, it is hardly surprising that the picture of the genetics of obstructive cardiomyopathy which emerged in the literature was unclear. The ratio of hereditary to sporadic cases varied greatly from series to series; most authors agreed that the disorder is transmitted as a

Mendelian autosomal dominant [11]. Some claimed that the clinical manifestations of the hereditary cases differed from those of the sporadic ones. Syncope and sudden death were said to be more common among hereditary cases, whereas outflow tract obstruction and the clinical course were more severe in the sporadic cases, who were also found to be older [12].

In 1961, Parē et al. [10], in their important contribution entitled "Hereditary cardiovascular dysplasia," described the familial distribution of what is now taken to be idiopathic subaortic stenosis or hypertrophic obstructive cardiomyopathy. Although this paper describes a single family, until recently it was the most complete study of the familial aspects of myocardial disease ever published. Of the 77 subjects examined, 20 were affected; inquiries suggested that an additional 10 may have died of the disease. A 95-year-old man supplied most of the early history, including that of his uncle's sudden death in 1860. In 1971, Kariv and his colleagues [11] reported on 11 families with cardiomyopathy. Of 98 persons examined, 47 were affected and the findings were considered consistent with transmission by an autosomal dominant gene with high penetrance. The genetic aspects of familial cardiomyopathy are very well covered in this important contribution to the literature.

The functional classification [21] of cardiomyopathy or idiopathic myocardial disease into congestive (systolic pump failure) hypertrophic (diastolic compliance failure) and the restrictive forms was a step forward not only toward a better appreciation of the pathophysiology and manifestations of primary myocardial disease but also in the direction of differing genetic patterns for different forms of myocardial disease.

Idiopathic myocardial disease in the sense of a disease of unknown etiology which chiefly affects the myocardium, but affects to a lesser extent the endocardium and the pericardium, is usually found in patients without evidence of other systemic disease. On the other hand, the myocardium may be severely or even principally affected in such generalized disease processes as amyloidosis, sarcoidosis, and carcinomatosis. Such are the secondary myocardial diseases. The myocardium is abnormal in certain neuromuscular and neurological disorders such as as progressive muscular dystrophy, Friedreich's ataxia, and myotonic dystrophy [32]. Indeed, in his 1949 description of familial cardiomegaly Evans [26] discussed its possible relationship with Friedreich's ataxia, and since that time clinicians have been taught to look for minor evidences of Friedreich's disease, such as pes cavus, in patients with unexplained heart failure. Usually the mode of inheritance of these forms of myocardial disease can be simply ascertained by knowledge of the mode of inheritance of the neuromuscular disorders themselves. However, the nosology and genetics of the muscular and neuromuscular disorders are themselves complex, and only in relatively recent years has some order been brought to them [5]. Furthermore, the clinical spectrum includes cases with neuromuscular manifestations in which the cardiac manifestations may be mild, moderate, or severe, and cases which present as cardiomyopathy with varying degrees of neuromuscular disease. In cases with cardiac and extracardiac manifestations, cardiomyopathy has usually been assumed to be a feature of the neuromuscular disorder. However, the possibility should at least be considered that the neuromuscular abnormalities are manifestations of what is primarily a cardiomyopathy. From the clinical point of view, this may seem a mere semantic difference, but nevertheless the distinction may be of considerable importance in genetics. Thus in situations in which the cardiac involvement is overt and the extracardiac involvement either absent or subtle, the mode of inheritance would most easily be learned by surveying the patients' families for cardiac disease.

In the summer of 1970, we surveyed the families of 21 patients in whom the diagnosis of idiopathic myocardial disease had been established by cardiac catheterization including coronary arteriography or by autopsy. In most instances there was one proband per family, but on some occasions 2 members of the family were already known to our clinic before the study was commenced. We attempted to examine all first-degree relatives of the probands. A team including a geneticist, a public health nurse trained in genetics, a cardiologist, and 3 medical students was organized to carry out the study. A large proportion of the families was scattered throughout the remote areas along the creeks in eastern Kentucky. It would have been difficult, expensive, and inconvenient for these individuals to travel to the medical center in Lexington. Besides, many of these people would not have felt particularly at home in such surroundings. Furthermore, an impersonal approach of that kind would have failed to win the confidence of these kindly, yet highly superstitious, mountain people, and it would thus have become difficult or impossible to elicit sufficient cooperation to obtain a satisfactory population study. We therefore deemed that it would be advisable to visit the patients in their homes even though we realized that, in consequence, some of the patients would be examined by less experienced and less skillful clinicians.

The cardiac and family histories were obtained, the patients were examined, and electrocardiograms were made with a portable electrocardiograph machine. Postero-anterior radiographs of the chests were obtained with the cooperation of community hospitals, the public health service, and private physicians in the area. The screening material gathered in the field was brought to the medical center, and subjects were classified into two categories; normal or affected. Subjects considered to be affected were brought to the medical center for complete cardiac evaluation

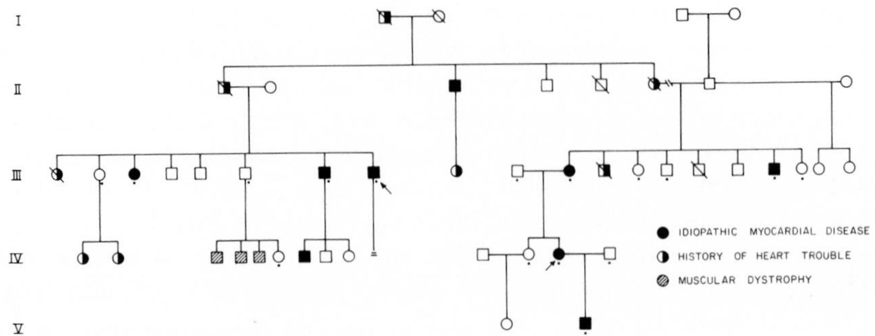

Figure 1. Hypertrophic Obstructive Cardiomyopathy. Pedigree showing autosomal dominant inheritance in which an affected man (III_7) has an affected offspring (IV_3). An affected woman in this family (IV_{11}) has an affected son (V_3). A dot under a symbol means that the patient was examined by one of the authors.

including, when appropriate, cardiac catheterization and coronary arteriography.

Of the 21 families studied, 9 were families of patients with hypertrophic cardiomyopathy, and 12 were the families of patients considered to have congestive cardiomyopathy. Seven of the 9 probands with hypertrophic cardiomyopathy were of the obstructive type and 2 were of the nonobstructive type. Our data indicate that 5 of 7 (71 percent) of patients with hypertrophic obstructive cardiomyopathy have a familial background of this disease. This figure is considerably higher than is frequently quoted in the literature. Hypertrophic cardiomyopathy without obstruction may also be inherited [33]; indeed, hypertrophic cardiomyopathy and hypertrophic obstructive cardiomyopathy may be found in members of the same family [14]. This observation indicates that these are not two diseases but are different manifestations of the same disease [11, 12, 33, 34]. In their study of 47 affected members of 11 families, Kariv et al. [11] emphasized that cardiomyopathy does not run true to a specific form in a particular family. However, idiopathic congestive cardiomyopathy has not been found to occur in families with hypertrophic cardiomyopathy either in our studies or in those of others.

Figure 1 illustrates a family with hypertrophic obstructive cardiomyopathy including 2 probands, both of whom underwent complete hemodynamic investigations. The family is interesting for several reasons. The male proband was descended from a family in which hypertrophic obstructive cardiomyopathy was frequently manifested and was an example of male-to-male transmission which is uncommon. In fact, Brigden [35] reported that this form of inheritance does not occur, and it was not illustrated in any of the 5 family trees published in Kariv's excellent study [11] of 11

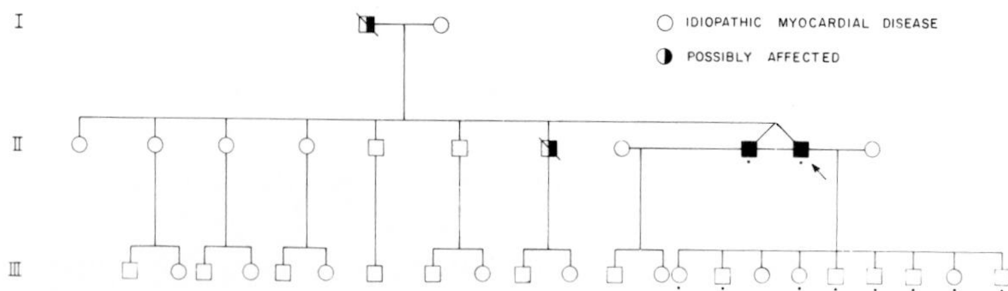

Figure 2. Hypertrophic Obstructive Cardiomyopathy. Pedigree showing monozygotic twins (II_6 and II_7) both affected. One (II_7) was severely affected; the other II_6 was minimally affected (see text). Generation III is at high risk despite negative clinical findings. A dot under a symbol means that the patient was examined by one of the authors.

families in Israel. One of our proband's brothers was the father of 3 boys and 1 girl. The 3 boys all suffered from Duchenne's muscular dystrophy without, as yet, evidence of heart disease. The female proband was also descended from a family with hypertrophic obstructive cardiomyopathy, and screening of her family indicated that her only boy, a lad of 10 years, was affected although asymptomatic.

Twins provide excellent material for genetic studies. Figure 2 depicts the family of 10 children descended from a father who had died before our study, but who may have been affected. The proband, a 51-year-old man with severe angina pectoris, was known to have had a heart murmur since discharge from the army when he was a young man. The electrocardiogram showed left ventricular hypertrophy. Hemodynamic studies showed that he had a systolic pressure gradient of 82 mm Hg across the aortic subvalvular area at rest. The left ventricular end-diastolic pressure was 35 mm Hg. The hemodynamic postextrasystolic response and the effects of isoproterenol infusion were typical of the changes seen in hypertrophic obstructive cardiomyopathy. His identical twin (substantiated by means of fingerprints and blood groups) had a normal electrocardiogram and no cardiac complaints, but he did have a nonpansystolic murmur at the left sternal border and a fourth heart sound. It is probable that idiopathic myocardial disease would not have been suspected had not the diagnosis been established in his twin brother. This pair furnishes an excellent example of the variation in expression of hypertrophic obstructive cardiomyopathy, exemplifying that the family history may be unreliable, and illustrates some of the principles and limitations of clinical genetic studies.

We have observed a "double gradient" in several patients with severe aortic valvar stenosis with marked left ventricular hypertrophy. These patients show a drop in systolic pressure as the catheter tip is pulled from the body to the outflow tract of the left ventricle and a further drop when the catheter tip is pulled across the aortic valve into the aorta. In these patients, the arterial pulse pressure was smaller in postextrasystolic beats than in normal beats; however, transseptal cardiac catheterization was not carried out, and, therefore it was difficult to be certain whether the gradient was caused by catheter entrapment or by outflow tract hypertrophy with obstruction. We did not obtain a positive family history in any of these cases, an observation which suggests that the left ventricular outflow tract obstruction in these cases was *acquired*. Others have reported double gradients in patients with aortic valvar stenosis and usually have attributed this phenomenon to the coexistence of idiopathic hypertrophic subaortic stenosis and aortic valvar stenosis [36, 37]. The evidence of this, however, is seldom convincing, and it seems more probable that most of these cases have an acquired intraventricular obstruction much as Brock originally proposed [30]. The role of systemic arterial hypertension in the pathophysiology of hypertrophic obstructive cardiomyopathy has recently been reevaluated by Hamby et al. [38] who reported 8 cases of hypertrophic obstructive cardiomyopathy secondary to systemic arterial hypertension. Goodwin, who has extensive experience with the cardiomyopathies, distinguishes clearly between a primary type without cardiovascular disease and a secondary type in which the cardiomyopathy appears to be associated with some condition causing an increased afterload on the left ventricle such as severe systemic hypertension, aortic valve stenosis, or discrete subaortic stenosis [39]. We have reported a patient with acquired intraventricular pressure gradient who had septic shock and an anatomically normal left ventricle, at autopsy [40]. Recognition of the possibility of acquired obstruction within the left ventricle further reduces the prevalence of "sporadic" hypertrophic obstructive cardiomyopathy.

Congestive cardiomyopathy embraces many different disease entities which converge to produce the common syndrome of severe biventricular congestive failure. In this syndrome the ventricles are primarily dilated and hypertrophy is inadequate [21], a situation which is in sharp contrast to that which prevails in hypertrophic cardiomyopathy. Many instances are acquired from viral infections, cobalt toxicity, alcohol ingestion, and other specific causative agents. Here, a hereditary basis is not to be anticipated. Other instances are truly idiopathic in that exhaustive studies fail to uncover the etiology. Even in these patients, it is much less common than in hypertrophic cardiomyopathies to find families in which more than one member is affected. Thus, most instances of congestive cardiomyopathy are considered to be sporadic and our own studies confirm this.

Not all familial myocardial disease, however, is of the hypertrophic variety. Our survey uncovered several families with other forms of familial myocardial disease, some with typical congestive cardiomyopathy.

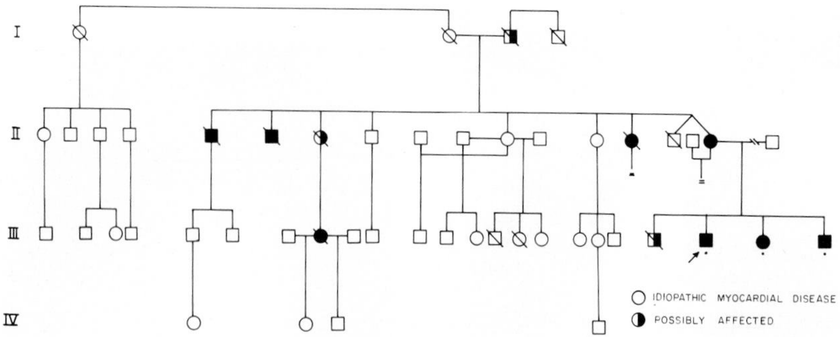

Figure 3. Nonobstructive Cardiomyopathy. Pedigree that simulated Ebstein's anomaly. The mother of the proband II_{13} has an unaffected dizygotic twin. A dot under a symbol indicates that the patient was examined by one of the authors.

Thus Figure 3 depicts a family with 2 probands. The female proband was first thought to have Ebstein's anomaly of the tricuspid valve because of the appearance of the heart on the chest radiograph (Fig. 4A), bizarre P waves (Fig. 5A), and a prominent gallop rhythm. Findings at cardiac catheterization (Fig. 6A), including intracardiac electrocardiography, were inconsistent with Ebstein's anomaly, but showed severe pulmonary hypertension and elevation of the left and right ventricular diastolic pressures without evidence of coronary arterial or valvar dysfunction. Her 16-year-old son was referred 3 years later, also with the diagnosis of Ebstein's anomaly and for the same reasons (Figs. 4B, 5B). Cardiac catheterization demonstrated pulmonary hypertension with considerable elevation of the ventricular diastolic pressures (Fig. 6B). Atrialization of the right ventricular pressure pulse and evidence of valve disease were not found. Survey of the family showed that all 3 of his younger siblings were affected, although asymptomatic (Figs. 3, 4C, 5C, 6C).

Figure 7 depicts a family with congestive cardiomyopathy. The proband was referred to us when she was 40 years old. She was descended from a family whose father was affected. Three of her 15 siblings were affected. She had 3 girls and 1 boy of whom 1 girl and 1 boy were affected. The hearts were exceedingly enlarged. The systemic venous pressures were high and gallop rhythm was present in all. The proband also had recurrent effusive pericarditis. Hemodynamic studies yielded findings typical of severe congestive cardiomyopathy. Her 18-year-old daughter was admitted to the hospital with severe congestive cardiac failure. Hemodynamic studies revealed findings virtually identical to those of her mother. Subsequently, the daughter became pregnant. The pregnancy was complicated by pulmonary embolism and intractable cardiac failure. Regrettably she was away at college when she conceived and did not return to the clinic until it

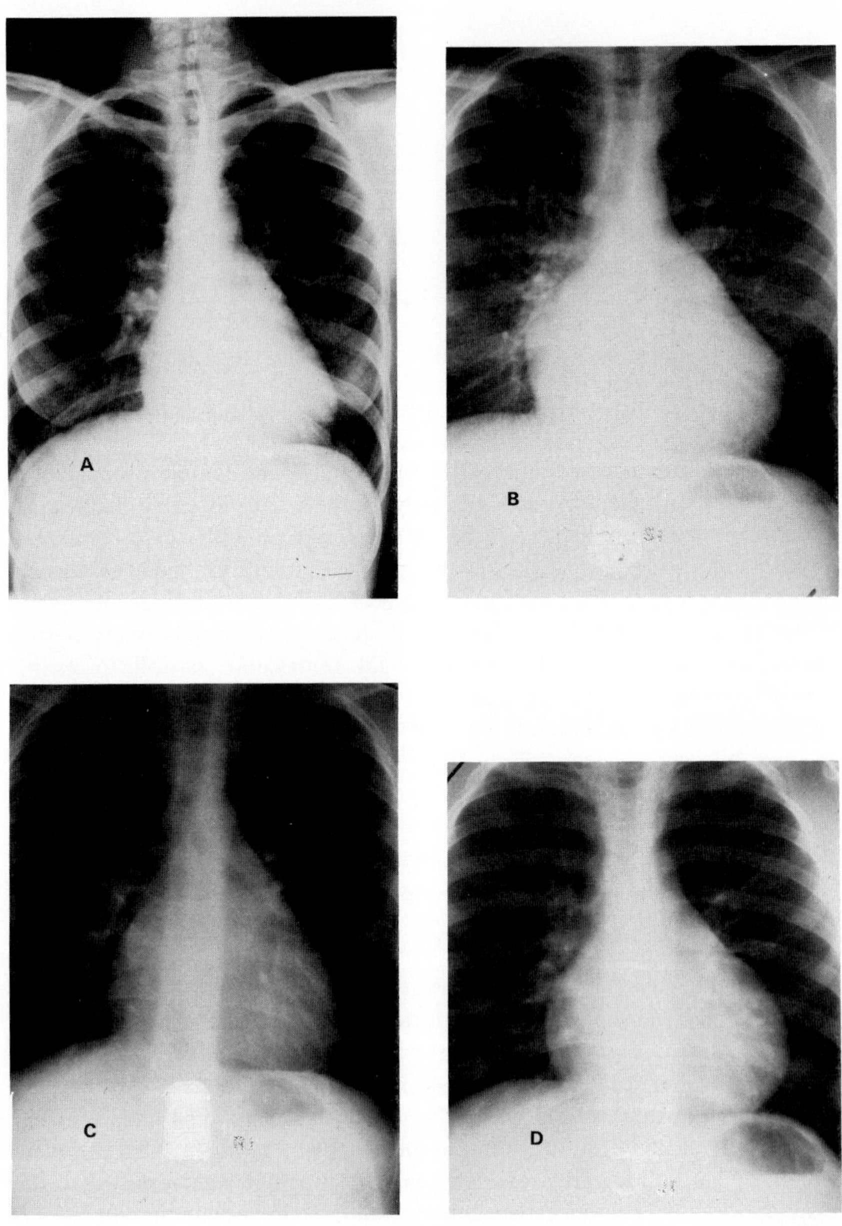

Figure 4. Cardiomyopathy. Chest radiographs of family with cardiomyopathy which simulated Ebstein's anomaly. A. Mother; B. Sixteen-year-old son; C and D. Younger siblings of B. Note the similarity of the shape of the cardiac silhouette in all the family. The children have more cardiac enlargement than the mother has.

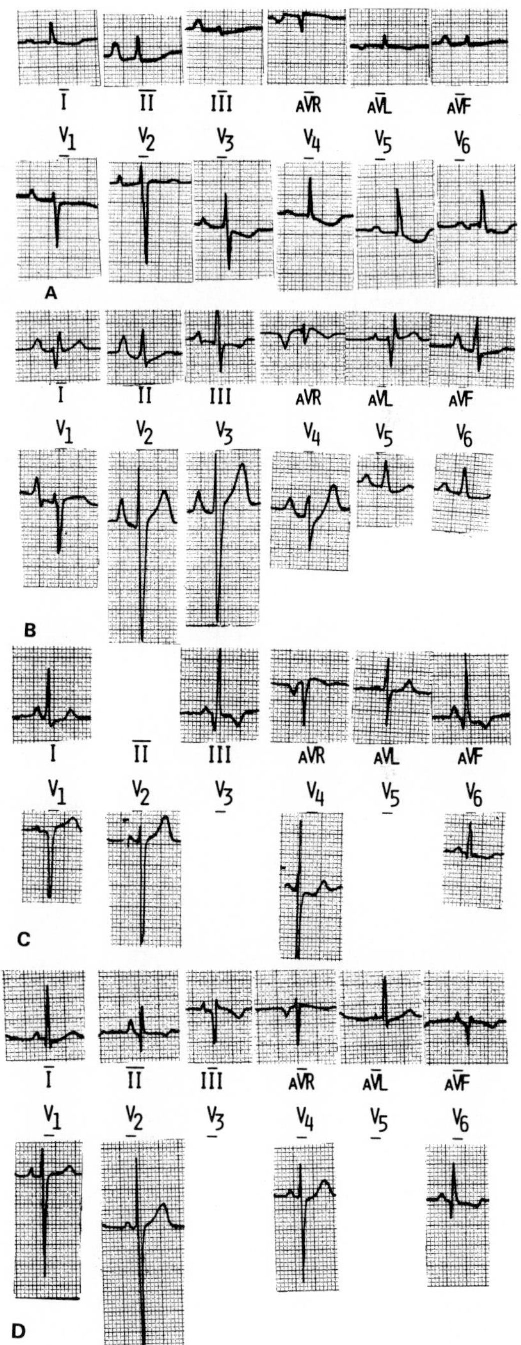

Figure 5. Cardiomyopathy. ECG's of the patients shown in Figure 4. A. Mother B. Sixteen-year-old son; C and D. Younger siblings of B. Note the large P wave in the mother's tracing and that of her elder son (SI); abnormal initial vectors in SI produce an rSR′ in leads 1 and aVL. The younger siblings RI and JI show Q waves in the diaphragmatic leads.

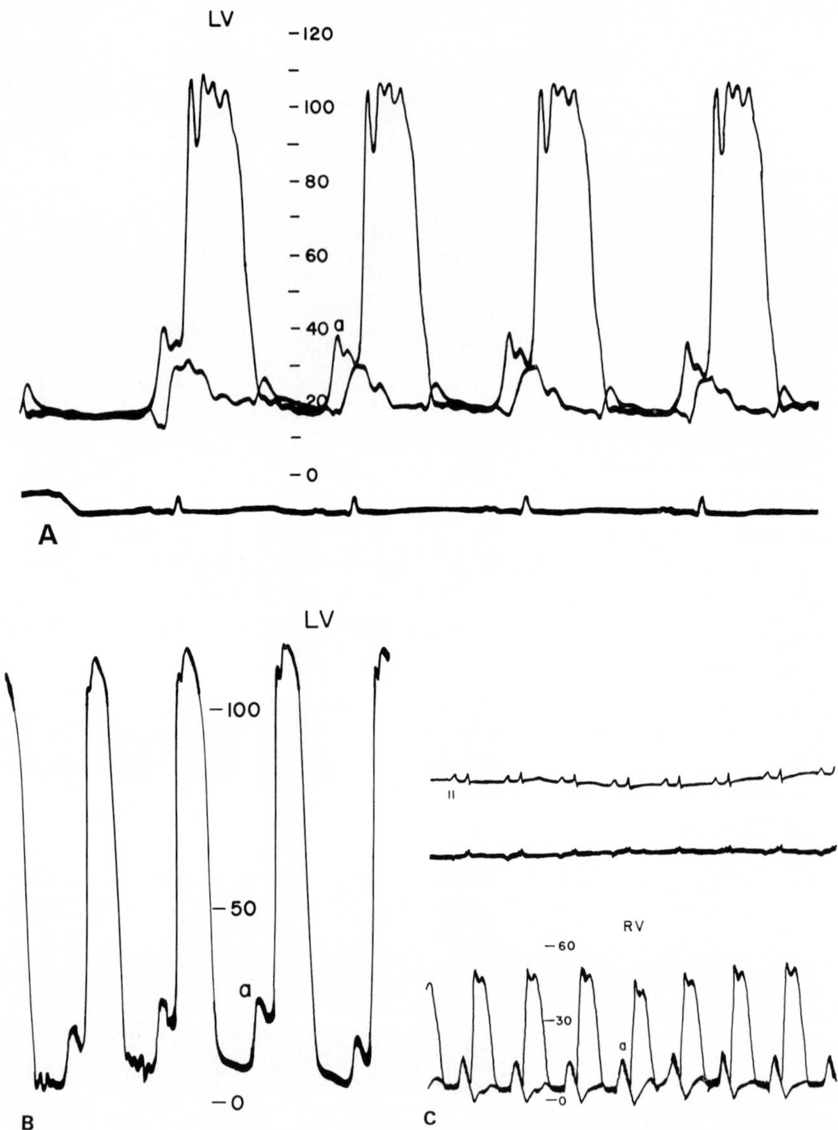

Figure 6. Cardiomyopathy. Ventricular pressure tracings of 2 of the patients in Figures 4 and 5. A. Note the large "a" wave in the mother's left ventricular diastolic pressure tracing. This wave is damped in the simultaneously recorded pulmonary wedge pressure record. The left ventricular end-diastolic pressure averaged 35 mm Hg. B. Sixteen-year-old-son. Note the striking similarity of her elder son's left ventricular pressure tracing. C. Elder son's right ventricular pressure tracing. From top down, ECG lead 2; intracardiac ECG, right ventricular pressure, and right atrial pressure. The "a" wave is prominent in the right ventricular and right atrial pressure tracings and the "x" descent is sharp in the right atrial pressure record. The "y" descent is flat.

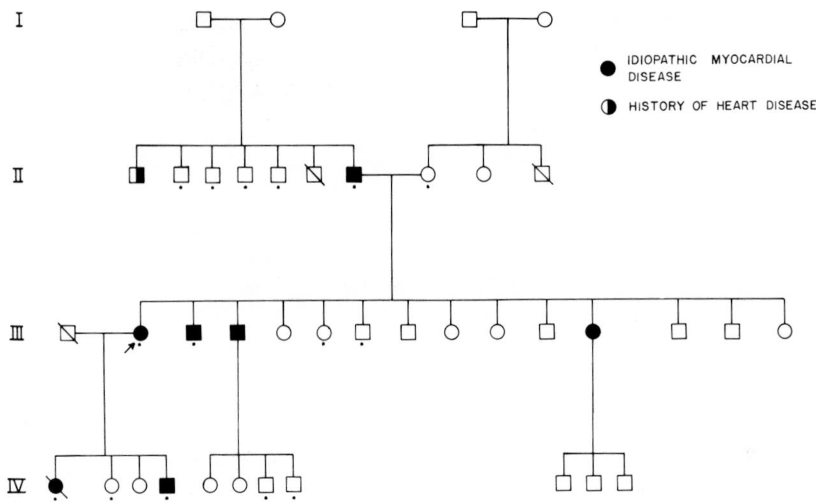

Figure 7. Congestive Cardiomyopathy. Pedigree showing autosomal dominant inheritance. A dot under a symbol indicates that the patient was examined by one of the authors.

was too late to carry out a simple therapeutic abortion. Her condition deteriorated and hysterotomy was advised. The patient died after this procedure. The autopsy confirmed the diagnosis of congestive cardiomyopathy.

A 16-year-old boy was treated without success for fulminating biventricular failure of abrupt onset. Autopsy showed massive dilatation of the heart and findings characteristic of congestive cardiomyopathy. The family history included a pair of monozygotic twins who had died in childhood of endocardial fibroelastosis. Both parents were of healthy Irish stock. Neither the mother, who was a nurse, nor the father, who was an internist, could find other cases in their families or family records in spite of an intensive search. We concluded that the children received the gene in an autosomal recessive manner which is the accepted mode of transmission of subendocardial fibroelastosis [41]. Subsequently, when he was in his sixties, the father developed a systolic murmur, a gallop rhythm, and slight cardiac enlargement. It seems unlikely, that this was the same lethal disease that caused his children's death. However, it is still possible that the father's illness represented expression of the heterozygote, that is the carrier state. Alternatively, the father's disease may have represented mild expression of an autosomal dominant gene. Finally, the father's illness may have been coincidental, for example, early ischemic heart disease. However, since

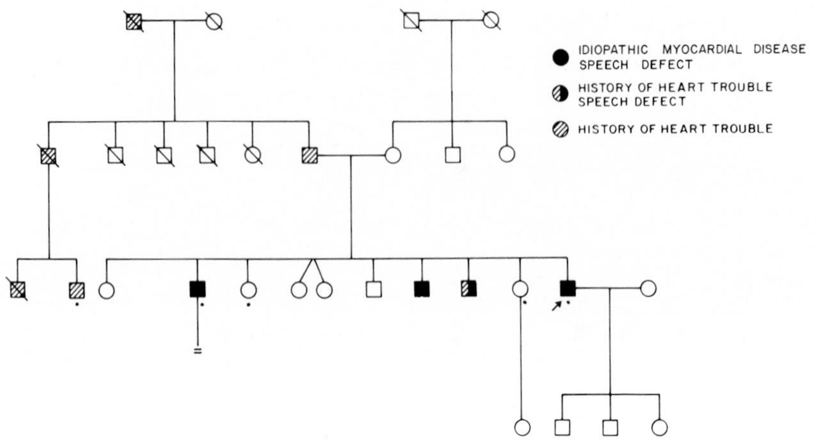

Figure 8. Cardiomyopathy. Pedigree showing 3 affected sons ($III_{4,9,10}$). This suggests X-linked recessive inheritance. In addition to cardiomyopathy, all had strikingly similar facial appearance and a speech defect (palatine weakness) as manifestations of generalized somatic myopathy. A dot under a symbol indicates that the patient was examined by one of the authors.

the symptoms were mild, hemodynamic studies and coronary arteriography were not carried out, and therefore the question remains unsettled.

Figure 8 depicts a family with congestive cardiomyopathy. The proband also had a congenital anomaly of the coronary arteries (all 3 vessels arose from a single ostium and common stem). The pedigree shows 3 affected sons, a finding consistent with X-linked recessive inheritance. The 3 men bore a striking facial resemblance to each other, and all of them had speech defects secondary to palatine weakness. The facial expression and unusual speech were manifestations of somatic myopathy.

These cases illustrate that when congestive cardiomyopathy is taken as a whole, no familial pattern emerges. However, when more specific syndromes are dissected from this whole, certain of them can be shown to be heritable.

To obtain the prevalence of idiopathic myocardial disease in eastern Kentucky, we listed all cases known to our clinic. We inquired about other cases from all internists and cardiologists registered to practice in the eastern half of the state. Using the ascertainment probability, estimated from the distribution of probands among sibships, the corrected estimate of prevalence in eastern Kentucky is 2.45 instances per 100,000 of the population.

Much remains to be learned about the heritable and familial aspects of idiopathic myocardial disease. At present, certain conclusions are warranted. Idiopathic hypertrophic obstructive cardiomyopathy is usually, perhaps always, inherited as an autosomal dominant. Phenotypic expression is variable as exemplified by our monozygotic twins and may conceal the hereditary basis in some cases. Other nonfamilial cases of hypertrophic obstructive cardiomyopathy are examples of the secondary type. Friedreich's ataxia may be inherited as a dominant or, rarely, as a recessive trait, and heart disease has been known to be associated with it since the earliest descriptions [42]. Recently, it has been shown for the first time that this cardiac involvement sometimes takes the form of hypertrophic obstructive cardiomyopathy [43].

Many cases of congestive cardiomyopathy are acquired, but within this heterogeneous general category are several distinctive syndromes, some of which are inherited as autosomal dominants such as the syndrome which simulates Ebstein's anomaly, some as autosomal recessives, and some as X-linked recessives.

Genetical counseling may be asked of the physician in charge of patients with idiopathic myocardial disease, and probably should be offered in all cases. The majority of the families that we encountered were unaware that the condition was genetic. The age of onset of idiopathic myocardial disease is variable, and in many cases symptoms and signs are delayed until the patient is well advanced into adult life. Thus, many patients will have long completed their families before the truth becomes self-evident. Risk estimates are based on Mendelian probabilities, appropriately weighted when estimates are available for failure of penetrance, gametic and zygotic selection, age of onset, and sporadicity.

For hypertrophic obstructive cardiomyopathy, which is inherited as an autosomal dominant, the prior probability that the child of an affected parent will be affected is 0.5, whereas with complete penetrance, the risk for a child of an unaffected parent is zero. Apparent gametic selection in the male, however, requires a considerable reduction in the prior probability if the affected parent is a male. Our data established that male transmission does occur, and hence the adjustment required may not be great. If the distribution of age of onset is accurately known, the risk for the latent carrier state can be calculated. For example, if the probability that the disease would be manifest by the age of 20 stands at 0.6, the risk for a 20-year-old offspring of an affected mother falls from 0.5 to 0.28. These risk estimates are unaffected by the sex of the child, although they are reduced if the affected parent is the father.

For diseases transmitted as autosomal dominants, an autosomal recessive variant will usually be found. Thus, there are autosomal recessive varieties of idiopathic myocardial disease of which subendocardial fibroelastosis is the best known. The family of a 16-year-old boy who died of idiopathic congestive cardiomyopathy and whose twin brothers had died of subendocardial fibroelastosis is in all probability an example of this mode of inheritance. In autosomal recessive transmission, the prior probability of the child of an affected parent being affected is given by the same gene frequency which is probably no greater than 0.01. However, close inbreeding could substantially increase the risk.

For cardiomyopathies associated with diseases such as Duchenne's muscular dystrophy [44, 45], which produce weakness of the somatic muscles inherited as X-linked recessives, the risk for the child of an affected male is zero: The risk for a male child of a carrier mother is 0.5, and the risk for the female child of a carrier mother approaches zero unless she has an XO karyotype, in which case the risk is the same as that for a male. For more distant relatives, the risk calculations are more complex and such cases should be referred to a genetic counselor. Inbreeding is not relevant to the risk since it has no effect on the incidence of autosomal dominant or X-linked recessive diseases.

Chromosomal analysis is not indicated except when an affected female has cardiomyopathy and somatic muscle disease. Similarly, buccal smears, chromatography of the urine, and enzyme assays are not generally considered useful. However, in a recent paper, Klajman et al. [46] described elevated serum enzyme levels in 11 of 38 members of 10 families with familial cardiomyopathy. In the same study, heart antibodies were discovered in 14 of 28 clinically affected cases and 2 of 10 unaffected relatives but in only 2 of 36 healthy controls. Heart antibodies have been found helpful in the diagnosis of idiopathic myocardial disease by some investigators [47], but less so by others [48]. The paper [46] by Klajman et al., however, is of special importance because it is the first to report heart antibodies in unaffected members of affected families.

In our studies, we found cases associated not only with the neuromuscular and muscular disorders but also with Hageman factor deficiency and acanthocytosis. Although these may be chance associations, remote inbreeding in a genetic isolate such as eastern Kentucky would be likely to yield multiple genetic abnormalities in single families. No evidence for linkage between idiopathic myocardial disease and other genetic markers is known, although we continue to search for this since close linkage would furnish a simple and convenient method of diagnosis in the preclinical stage, indeed, even in utero. The ECG has proved highly satisfactory as a means of screening families for myocardial disease. It is simple, inexpensive, readily obtained by unskilled personnel, and is frequently abnormal in affected family members. ECG abnormalities are particularly useful in the young, but in older subjects may be less specific and less striking since the pseudoinfarction pattern tends to decrease or disappear with increasing age [11, 49].

The risks to the mother who becomes pregnant are in a separate category. We advise that childbirth may be successfully undertaken if the patient has hypertrophic obstructive cardiomyopathy and does not have cardiac failure or atrial fibrillation. This advice is based on the report [50] by Turner and his colleagues on the obstetric management of hypertrophic obstructive cardiomyopathy. In congestive cardiomyopathy in a prospective father without evidence of familial involvement, we may advise that pregnancy may be undertaken provided that the prospective mother is healthy. We advise strongly against pregnancy if the prospective mother has congestive cardiomyopathy because of the high prevalence of heart failure and the relationship of congestive cardiomyopathy to peripartal (postpartum) cardiomyopathy.

REFERENCES

1. Muller, H.J. and Snyder, L.H.: Genetics Medicine and Man. Ithaca, New York, Cornell University Press, 1947.
2. Milhorat, A.T. and Wolff, H.G.: Studies in disease of muscle. Psychiat. 49:641, 1943.
3. Bell, J.: Pseudohypertrophic and allied types of progressive muscular dystrophy. Treas Hum Inherit 4:283, 1943.
4. Tyler, F.H. and Wintrobe, M.M.: Studies in disorders of muscle. Ann Intern Med 32:72, 1950.
5. Walton, J.N. and Nattrass, F.J.: On the classification, natural history and treatment of myopathies. Brain 77:168, 1954.
6. Bercu, B., Diettert, G.A., Danforth, W.A., Pund, E.E., Ahlvin, R.C., and Belliveau, R.R.: Pseudoaortic stenosis produced by ventricular hypertrophy. Am J Med 25:814, 1958.
7. Brent, L.B., Aburano, A., Fisher, D.L., Moran, T.L., Myers, J.D., and Taylor, J.W.: Familial muscular subaortic stenosis. Circulation 21: 167, 1960.
8. Garret, B., Hay, W.J., and Richards, A.G.: Familial cardiomegaly. J Clin Pathol 12:355, 1959.
9. Hollman, A., Goodwin, J.F., Teare, D., and Renwick, J.W.: A family with obstructive cardiomyopathy (asymmetrical hypertrophy). Br Heart J 22:449, 1960.
10. Paré, J.A.P., Fraser, R.G., Prozynski, W.J., Shanks, J.A., and Stubington, D.: Hereditary cardiovascular dysplasia. Am J Med. 31:37, 1961.
11. Kariv, I., Kreisler, B., Sherf, L., Feldman, S., and Rosenthall, T.: Familial cardiomyopathy: A review of 11 families. Am J Cardiol 28:693, 1971.
12. Braunwald, E., Lambrew, C.T., Rockoff, S.D., Ross, J., and Morrow, A.G.: Idiopathic hypertrophic subaortic stenosis. Circulation 28:958, 1964.
13. Weber, D.J., Gould, L., and Schaffer, A.I.: A family with idiopathic myocardial hypertrophy. Am J Cardiol 17:419, 1966.

14. Barold, S.S., Linhart, J.W., Hildner, F.J., Arkadi, R., and Samet, P.: Familial Cardiomyopathy. A clinical hemodynamic and angiographic study in one family. Chest 57:141, 1970.
15. Wood, R.S., Taylor, W.J., Wheat, M.W., and Schiebler, G.L.: Muscular subaortic stenosis in childhood. Pediatrics 30:849, 1962.
16. Schrader, W.H., Pankey, G.A., Davis, R.B., and Theologides, A. Familial idiopathic cardiomegaly. Circulation 24:599, 1961.
17. Tregar, A. and Blount, S.G.: Familial cardiomyopathy. Am Heart J 70:40, 1965.
18. Walther, R.J., Madoff, I.M., and Zinner, K.: Cardiomegaly of unknown cause occurring in a family. New Engl J Med 263:1104, 1966.
19. Battersby, E.J. and Glenner, G.G.: Familial cardiomyopathy. Am J Med 30: 382, 1962.
20. Bishop, J.M., Campbell, M. Wyn, and Jones, E.: Cardiomyopathy in four members of a family. Br Heart J 24:715, 1962.
21. Goodwin, J.: Congestive and hypertrophic cardiomyopathies. A decade of study. Lancet 1:731, 1970.
22. Bjork, G. and Orinius, E.: Familial cardiomyopathies. Acta Med Scand 176:407, 1964.
23. Nassar, W.L., Williams, J.F., Mishkin, M.E., Childress, R.H., Helemn, C., Merritt, A.D., and Genovese P.D.: Familial myocardial disease. Circulation 35:638, 1968.
24. Meerschwam, I.S.: Hypertrophic Obstructive Cardiomyopathy. Baltimore, Williams & Wilkins, 1969.
25. Teare, R.D.: Asymmetrical hypertrophy of the heart in young adults. Br Heart J 20:1, 1958.
26. Evans, W.: Familial cardiomegaly. Br Heart J 11:68, 1949.
27. Davies, L.G.: A familial heart disease. Br Heart J 14:206, 1952.
28. Campbell, M. and Turner-Warwick, M.: Two more families with cardiomegaly. Br Heart J 18:393, 1956.
29. Gaunt, R.T. and Lecutier, M.A. Familial Cardiomegaly. Brit Heart J 18:251, 1956.
30. Brock, R.: Functional obstruction of the left ventricle. Guy's Hosp Rept 108:221, 1957.
31. Brock, R.: Functional obstruction of the left ventricle. Guy's Hosp Rept 108:126, 1959.
32. Fowler, N.O.: Differential diagnosis of the cardiomyopathies. Prog Cardiovasc Dis 14:113, 1971.
33. Braunwald, E. and Aygen, M.M.: Idiopathic myocardial hypertrophy without congestive heart failure or obstruction to blood flow. Am J Med 35:7, 1963.
34. Shabetai, R. and McGuire, J.: Idiopathic cardiac hypertrophy simulating valvular heart disease. Am Heart J 65:124, 1963.
35. Brigden, W.: Uncommon myocardial disease. Lancet 11:1179, 1960.
36. Parker, D.P., Kaplan, M.A., and Connolly, J.E.: Coexistent aortic valvular and functional hypertrophic subaortic stenosis. Am J Cardiol 24:307, 1969.
37. Ellis, F.H. Jr., Ongley, P.A., and Kirklin, J.W.: Results of surgical treatment for congenital aortic stenosis. Circulation 25:29, 1962.
38. Hamby, R.I., Roberts, G.S., and Meron, J.M.: Hypertension and hypertrophic subaortic stenosis. Am J Med 51: 474, 1971.
39. Goodwin, J.F.: Obstructive cardiomyopathy. Cardiologia 52:69, 1968.
40. Shabetai, R.: A new syndrome in hypovolemic shock. Am J Cardiol 24:404, 1969.

41. Rosahn, P.D.: Endocardial fibroelastosis. Old and new concepts. Bull NY Acad Med 31:453, 1955.
42. Friedreich, N.: Ueber degenerative atrophic der spinalen hinterstrange. Arch Pathol Antatphysiol 26:391, 1863.
43. Gach, J.V., Andriange, M., and Franch, G.: Hypertrophic obstructive cardiomyopathy and Friedreich's ataxia. Am J Cardiol. 27:436, 1971.
44. Perloff, J.K., de Leon, A.C. Jr., and O'Doherty, D.: The cardiomyopathy of progressive muscular dystrophy. Circulation 33:625, 1966.
45. Pratt, R.T.C.: The genetics of neurological disorders. New York, Oxford Univ. Press, 1967.
46. Klajman, A., Nurit, K.B., Feldman, S., and Kariv, I.: Immunological studies in familial cardiomyopathy. Am J Cardiol 28:707, 1971.
47. Shaper, A.G., Kaplan, M.H., Foster, W.D., MacIntosh, D.M., and Wilks, N.E.: Immunohistological studies in endomyocardial fibrosis. Lancet 1:598, 1967.
48. Camp, T.F., Hess, E.V., Conway, G., and Fowler, N.O.: Immunologic findings in idiopathic cardiomyopathy. Am Heart J 77:610, 1969.
49. Kariv, I., Sherf, L., and Solomon, M.: Familial cardiomyopathy with special consideration of electrocardiographic findings. Am J Cardiol 13:734, 1964.
50. Turner, G.M., Oakley, C.M., and Dixon, H.G.: Management of pregnancy complicated by hypertrophic obstructive cardiomyopathy. Br Med J 4:281, 1968.

TIMOTHY J. REGAN, M.D.

Alcoholic Cardiomyopathy

Although the association of alcoholism with cardiomyopathy is generally recognized, the exact nature of this relationship has not been defined. A recent review has indicated the varied acceptance of the concept over the past 100 years [1]. During the latter part of the nineteenth century, there were repeated reports of diffuse involvement of the heart in chronic alcoholic individuals, but it was not until 1906 that Graham Steell first adverted to the possible relationship of alcoholic heart disease and beriberi [2]. During the period of economic depression in this country in the 1930s, the beriberi syndrome dominated the view of alcoholic cardiomyopathy. Cardiovascular manifestations often coexisted with peripheral neuritis; the hyperkinetic nature of this circulatory disorder was evidenced by rapid circulation time, wide pulse pressure, high cardiac output, and low peripheral resistance. The clinical spectrum of thiamine-deficiency heart disease was eventually broadened to include subjects with low-output heart failure, and the pathogenetic role of ethanol was either deemphasized or ignored [3].

It is evident that identification of the pathogenesis of the cardiac involvement in alcoholism is of more than theoretic interest. If ethanol, per se, is a predominant etiologic factor, then major emphasis on the nutritional aspects of therapy rather than alcoholism itself would be erroneous. During

From the Department of Medicine, College of Medicine and Dentistry of New Jersey at Newark.

This investigation was supported in part by U.S.P.H.S. NIH Research Grant No. MH 17007 and Graduate Training Grant No. HE 05510.

the latter 1950s, three separate reports drew attention to the many cardiac patients with long-standing alcoholism without evidence of significant nutritional deficiency in the majority. Eliaser related cardiac abnormalities seen in alcoholics to the severity and duration of the alcoholism and concluded that a significant number of alcoholics with heart failure had no detectable vitamin deficiency or important hepatic disease [4].

Brigden and Robertson, reporting observations in 50 patients, noted the difficulty in obtaining a history of alcoholism, often obtained only through persistent questioning of the patient or from relatives [5]. The diagnosis of alcoholic heart disease was made primarily by exclusion of other causes of heart disease, namely, hypertension and coronary artery disease, cor pulmonale, and congenital or valvular disease. Heart disease apparently developed earlier in those who drank spirits rather than beer, and only 10 percent presented with the high-output failure of beriberi, which usually responded to thiamine. In addition to pointing out the usual lack of specificity of the clinical signs and symptoms, these observers noted that high diastolic arterial blood pressure was sometimes found during periods of severe congestive heart failure, which may lead to the false diagnosis of hypertensive heart disease. The blood pressure returned to normal following response to therapy. No cases of hepatic cirrhosis were found, and clear evidence of peripheral neuritis was rare. Their experience with cardiac beriberi as a thiamine-responsive disease was similar to that of other groups; clinical evidence of thiamine deficiency was rare in alcoholic patients with myocardial disease.

The occupational background of patients with alcoholic cardiomyopathy was emphasized by Evans [6], in that the majority of his 20 patients held executive positions in contrast to the patient population at an urban hospital [7]. A male predominance has been observed repeatedly in these and subsequent series, presumably due to the greater prevalence of alcoholism in men. However, a lesser sensitivity of women to the myocardial effects of ethanol has not be excluded. An ethnic or racial predilection to alcoholism and alcoholic heart disease is more difficult to establish, but has been suggested on the basis of a relatively high prevalence in the urban areas of the northeast [8]. The duration of alcoholism reported by most authors is usually at least 10 years before cardiac symptoms appear. Consequently, if a population sample for disease prevalence consists predominantly of short-term addicts, a relatively small number of individuals would be expected to have clinically detectable heart disease.

It is now pertinent to consider the prevalence of alcoholism in the general population. In view of the difficulty in obtaining reliable histories, we can assume that alcoholism is likely to be underestimated. In a recent survey, Cahalan and his associates found that two-thirds of the population used alcohol, and he divided them into four categories: infrequent, light, moderate, and heavy users [8]. The group considered to be heavy users represented about 12 percent of the adult population. An important element in considering prevalence is the variation between different regions of the country and between hospitals of a given region. In addition, there is the problem of obtaining reliable information on quantity, frequency, and duration of alcohol intake in individuals addicted to alcohol.

With these reservations in mind, cardiac changes observed at postmortem examination in subjects who were chronic heavy users of alcohol are of interest. In a recent survey, 97 patients with a clinical history of excess alcohol intake were studied at necropsy [9]. Diffuse interstitial myocardial fibrosis of varying severity was present in 90 percent; this fibrosis did not appear to be the result of coronary artery disease. Almost half the subjects had myofiber vacuolization, and nearly a third had heart weights greater than 500 gm. Hypertension was unusual, but no information was provided on the prevalence of anemia, which might have an important bearing on cardiac hypertrophy. Hepatic changes, ranging from fatty infiltration to end-stage cirrhosis, did not correlate with the cardiac lesions. Death resulted from clinically obvious myocardial disease in 20 percent of this group, but the contribution of the cardiac alteration to death in the remainder was unknown. These studies suggest a high incidence of cardiac-muscle disease in alcoholics dying in hospitals, but, without rigorous exclusion of nutritional factors, the primary role of alcohol can only be presumed.

In a prior study of the failing heart in alcoholics, focal areas of myocardial fibrosis were found to be associated with histochemical evidence of diffuse lipid deposition within myocardial fibers [10]. Electron microscopic studies [11, 12] showed abnormalities of mitochondria with swelling and disappearance of cristae, swelling of the sarcoplasmic reticulum, and varying degrees of myofibril degeneration. The structural changes in the myocardium appeared to differ from those of obstructive cardiomyopathy in that the latter demonstrates abnormal myofiber size and orientation. In the hearts of patients with hypokalemic myocardial disease, isolated sarcomere units undergo degeneration in the early stages in contrast to the changes in the heart of the alcoholic. Unfortunately, once cardiac symptoms have appeared in the alcoholic, the myocardial morphologic alterations may be diffuse and similar in appearance to those of idiopathic myocardopathy so that the clinical value of myocardial biopsy is limited.

Despite the emphasis on associated nutritional deficiencies in the alcoholic cardiac patient during the first half of this century, relatively little attention was paid to their nutritional problems prior to this period. Clinicians attributed the heart failure of chronic alcoholics to the effects of alcohol [1]. On the other hand, the nutritional status of alcoholics today appears to be improved over that of the 1930s when approximately 100 cases of thiamine deficiency were recognized in one hospital during a single year. In contrast, during the past 2 decades, there have been few published cases fulfilling the criteria for beriberi heart disease.

A recent nutritional survey of alcoholics who were generally considered not to be indigent revealed a relatively low incidence of nutritional deficiency, although 36 percent of their calories were derived from alcohol [13]. Only 15 percent of these patients had thiamine deficiency as determined by diet history and excretion of vitamin metabolites. Riboflavin, niacin, and protein deficiency occurred in less than 10 percent of this group, and low levels of serum albumin were observed in an even smaller segment of the group. Whether the myocardial response to chronic alcoholism differs in the minority of patients with nutritional deficiency, when compared to the better-nourished alcoholic, remains to be evaluated. It should be noted that blood vitamin levels assayed in hospitalized patients frequently reveal no clear distinction between alcoholics with and those without evidence of liver disease [14]. Blood vitamin concentrations may also be low as a nonspecific effect of chronic illness in the absence of alcoholism.

Inasmuch as nutritional problems were not evidenced in the majority of the patients in recent reports of cardiomyopathy [7, 15, 16, 17, 18], a study was undertaken of alcoholic subjects with no symptoms or clinical evidence of heart disease, in order to exclude the possible secondary role of malnutrition as a complication of heart failure [19]. To minimize the potential contribution of malnutrition, a group of alcoholic subjects with normal cardiovascular clinical examinations and no clinical evidence of vitamin deficiency and malnutrition were chosen for hemodynamic study. They were within 5 percent of normal weight for their age, and there was no hypoalbuminemia, edema, peripheral neuropathy, nor anemia of significance. These subjects were normotensive, had no electrocardiographic evidence of coronary disease, and were in an age group in which clinically important coronary artery disease would be expected to have a relatively low prevalence. Documentation of duration of alcoholism and the type of ethanol used by these subjects was obtained from the patients' histories and information derived from close relatives. The subjects had used ethanol habitually for 10 to 15 years. Whiskey was the predominant alcoholic beverage; as a rule, it was consumed several times a week in amounts ranging from 0.5 to 2 pints/day. The alcoholic group was further defined by the presence of fatty liver without fibrosis. Arterial blood concentrations of pyruvate and lactate were normal, and the uptake of these substrates by

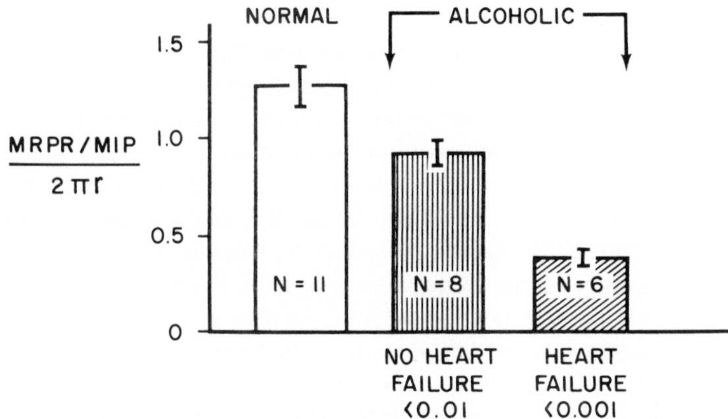

Figure 1. MRPR = maximum rate of pressure rise in the left ventricle; MIP = maximum isometric pressure $2\pi r$ = circumferential fiber lengths. (Reprinted from J Clin Invest 48:397-407, 1969, by permission.)

the myocardium was also within normal limits, diminishing the likelihood of thiamine deficiency.

Left ventricular performance was studied by increasing afterload with angiotensin to the same extent in control and alcoholic subjects. The noncardiac alcoholic exhibited a significantly greater rise of ventricular end-diastolic pressure with minimal increment of stroke volume compared to nonalcoholic controls, so that by this standard ventricular performance was diminished. Similar observations have been made during exercise in cirrhotic patients without clear evidence of cardiac disease [20] as well as in beer-drinking subjects with cardiomyopathy who were restored to an apparently normal state clinically after removal of trace metal excess [21]. To test the contractile state of the ventricle at rest in the same group of noncardiac alcoholics, the investigators used a contractility index, expressing the maximum rate of left ventricular rise with a normalized preload and afterload. The noncardiac alcoholics showed significantly lower left ventricular contractility than the normal subjects did, but their values were significantly higher than those of alcoholic patients who had progressed to heart failure (Fig. 1).

To explore the possible relationship of ethanol to abnormalities of left ventricular function, we studied a similar group of noncardiac alcoholics during acute ingestion of ethanol over a 2-hour period [19]. One group received 6 oz and the other 12 oz of Scotch during 2 hours. With the 6-oz dose there was no significant change of left ventricular filling pressure or stroke output. With the 12-oz dose, there was a substantial rise of left ventricular end-diastolic pressure associated with a modest decline of cardiac stroke output. These values returned to control after alcohol feeding was interrupted. It is apparent from this and other studies that the acute hemodynamic response to ingested ethanol may vary depending on dose, duration of administration, and time of measurement, as well as the previous hemodynamic state of the patient.

In contrast to these findings in noncardiac alcoholics, the alcoholic patient with heart failure may have a greater sensitivity to the 6-oz dose of ethanol. Figure 2 illustrates a patient with alcoholic cardiomyopathy and persistent elevation of left ventricular end-diastolic pressure and volume. The stroke volume and cardiac output rose only moderately despite a 50 to 60 percent increment of left ventricular end-diastolic pressure and end-diastolic volume. Thus, low doses of alcohol which may be innocuous to normal subjects can adversely affect cardiac function when myocardial disease is present. The observations outlined below show that the cardiac subject with advanced disease of the left ventricle, who is not habituated to ethanol, may well have a greater than normal myocardial depression in response to an equivalent dose.

A recent study of normal subjects who were not habituated to ethanol suggested that prior experience is an important determinant of the cardiovascular response [22]. While the subjects drank 6 oz of Scotch over a 2-hour period, left ventricular systolic time intervals were measured intermittently. After 1 hour, when blood ethanol concentration averaged 75 mg percent, there was a significant increase of the preejection period and isovolumic contraction time as well as an increased ratio of the preejection period to ventricular ejection time (Fig. 3). Feeding isocaloric solutions of sucrose did not prolong the ejection times. It was concluded that ethanol doses which produce only mild intoxication can elicit depression of cardiac function in nonalcoholics in contrast to the response in the individual habituated to ethanol [19]. Although part of the difference in response may be due to enhanced oxidation of ethanol by the liver after habituation, it would appear that the myocardium itself may participate in the adaptation to chronic alcohol ingestion. In studies of the isolated rat heart, animals that had ingested ethanol over an 18-month period, exhibited significantly less depression of ventricular function on exposure to ethanol than control animals did [23]. Thus, the acute effects of modest doses of ethanol taken with moderate frequency may have significance only for the patient with severe cardiac disease. However, when alcohol is combined with pentobarbital or other myocardial depressants [24], serious consequences may result.

Altered ionic permeability appears to be an important factor in the direct influence of ethanol on cardiac cells. After 12-oz of whiskey, losses of potassium and phosphate from the left ventricle, reflected by rises in

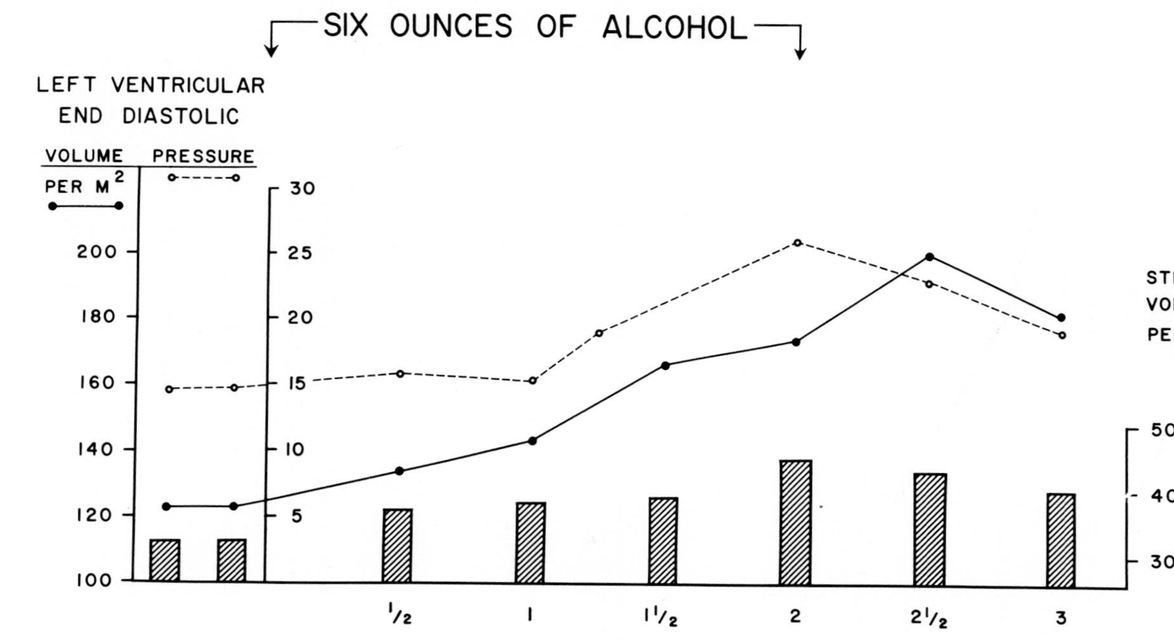

Figure 2. These observations during the ingestion of 6 oz Scotch in an alcoholic patient with cardiac decompensation reveal a depressant effect on the left ventricle at a dose that had no effect in the noncardiac alcoholic. (Reprinted from Circulation 44:957-963, 1971, by permission.)

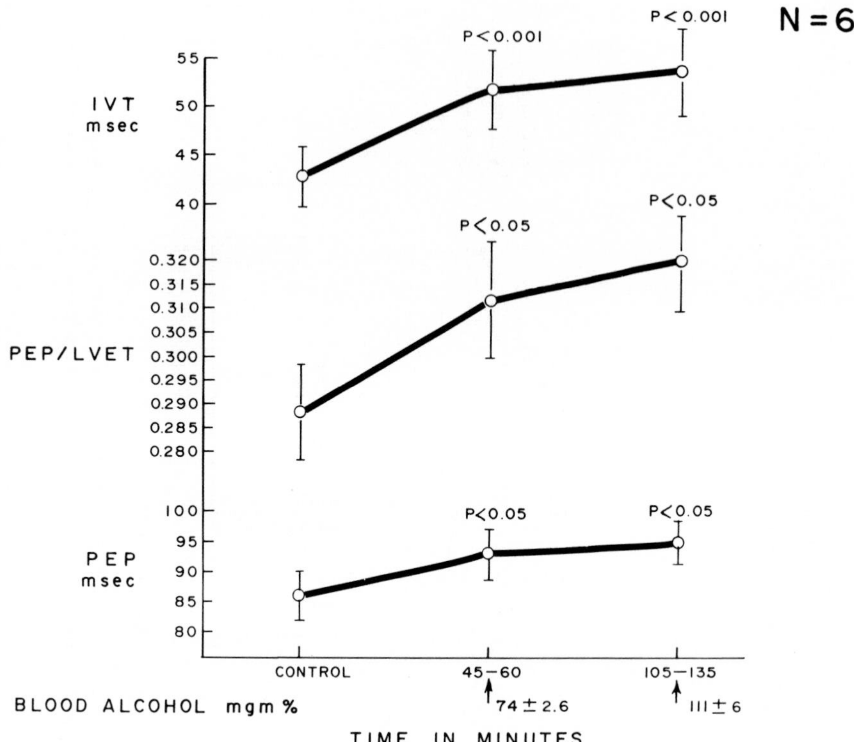

Figure 3. Six normal subjects were fed 6 oz of Scotch whiskey over a 2-hour period. Prolongation of left ventricular ejection times (LVET) was evident after 60 minutes. PEP = pre-ejection period; IVT = isovolumic time. (Courtesy of Dr. S. S. Ahmed.)

coronary venous concentrations, have been observed in noncardiac alcoholics [19]. The leakage was transient, with recovery to control about 2 hours after interrupting alcohol ingestion. There was no reduction of coronary blood flow. Lipid transport in the myocardium was altered by acute alcoholism in these studies. Free fatty acid uptake by the left ventricle was reduced, and triglyceride uptake was enhanced. This response may contribute to pathologic changes observed at postmortem examination, at which substantial increases in lipid, presumably triglyceride, have been observed in the myocardium of alcoholics [10]. However, the duration of chronic ethanol intake required to produce persistent abnormality of heart-muscle composition is unknown. As in the liver, the acute response to ethanol is characteristically associated with lipid accumulation [25], but the mechanism by which this evolves into a chronic process is unknown.

That ethanol can diminish ventricular function acutely does not signify that chronic disease will necessarily result from habitual use. To

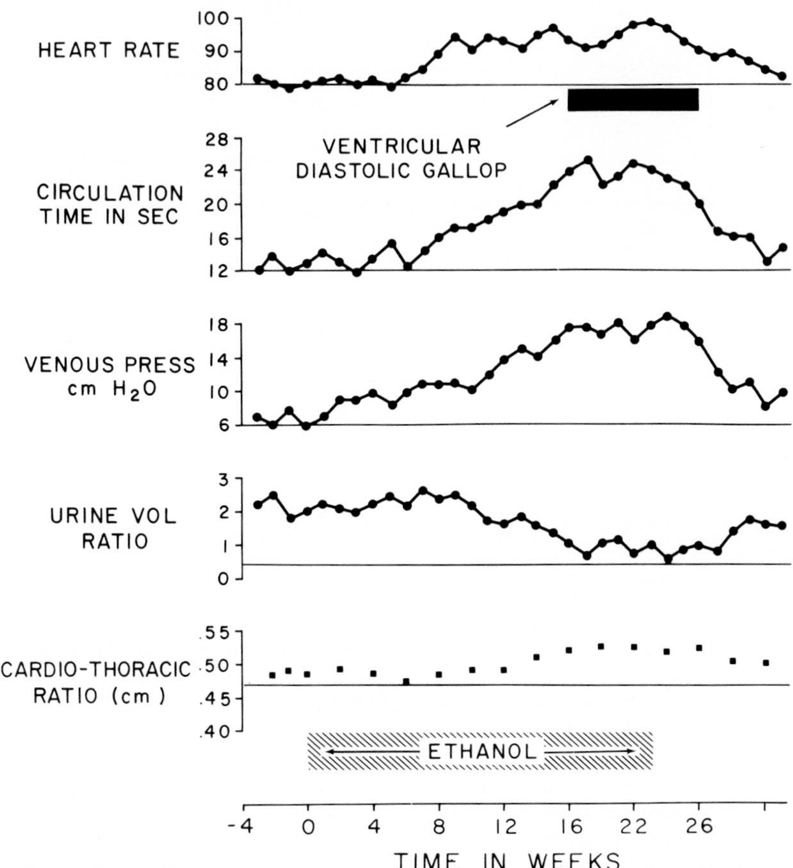

Figure 4. These are observations in a single, well-nourished patient receiving daily Scotch, which resulted in evidence of heart failure. The heart failure regressed without medical treatment after interrupting alcohol intake. (Reprinted from J Clin Invest 48:397-407, 1969, by permission.)

test the thesis that cumulative effects of ethanol over a period of time may result in cardiac abnormality despite adequate nutrition, a well-compensated patient was given 12 to 16 oz of Scotch per day for a period of 5.5 months. After 6 weeks (Fig. 4), his resting heart rate rose, and there was prolongation of circulation time and elevation of venous pressure without evidence of malnutrition. Serum albumin, blood glucose, lactate, pyruvate, and electrolytes remained normal over the observation period. After 4 months, a

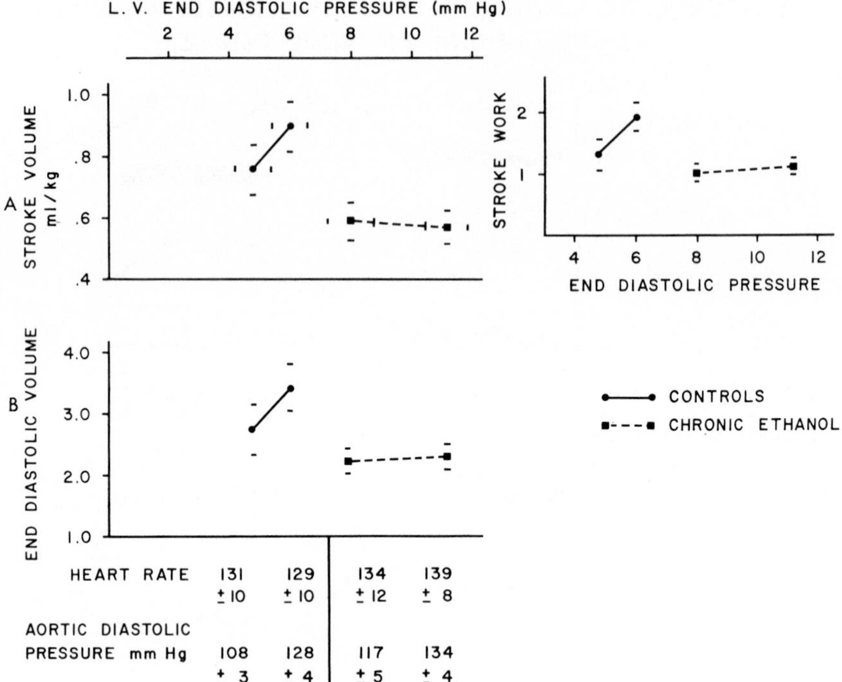

Figure 5. A study of left ventricular function in control dogs and in dogs with chronic exposure to ethanol. A. Plot of left ventricular end-diastolic pressure versus stroke volume (left side) and stroke work (right side). Angiotensin was infused intravenously to raise aortic diastolic pressure by about 20 mm Hg. B. The chronic alcoholic animals did not increase stroke output and work. This was presumably related to failure to raise end-diastolic volume. The isolated vertical and horizontal bars refer to standard errors.

ventricular gallop rhythm appeared and persisted until ethanol was interrupted. After the Scotch whiskey was stopped, there was spontaneous restoration to normal cardiovascular function without specific cardiac therapy. A major role of ethanol in the production of left heart failure in this subject was substantiated by the gradual reversion of the cardiocirculatory abnormality after alcohol ingestion was interrupted. This observation supports the thesis that the myocardial disease is reversible at certain stages if intake of ethanol is discontinued as demonstrated in several studies of ambulatory patients [17, 26].

In view of the variables that can obscure the pathogenesis of human disease, a study has been undertaken in young full-grown, male mongrel dogs receiving 36 percent of their calories from ethanol for an average period of 18 months [27]. These animals were maintained on normal

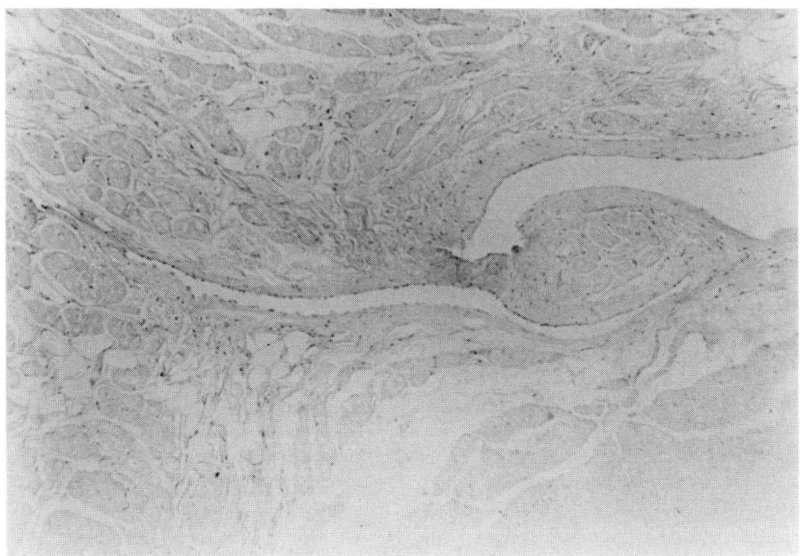

Figure 6. Section of apical myocardium from chronic ethanolic animal. Alcian blue positive staining material in the interstitium is presumably mucopolysaccaride. Left ventricle from control animals did not stain. (Courtesy of Dr. M. M. Lyons.)

protein intake and received supplementary vitamins. Microbiological assay for the vitamin B series as well as vitamins A, C, D, and E, revealed no difference in serum vitamin levels from controls. Their original weight was maintained and their hematocrit and serum albumin were normal. During an angiotensin test, the animals receiving ethanol exhibited a larger rise of ventricular end-diastolic pressure and reduced level of stroke output and stroke work when compared to controls (Fig. 5). Ventricular diastolic filling appeared to be impeded, resulting in a diminished stroke volume and ejection fraction. Histochemical analysis, demonstrated an increase in Alcian-blue-stained material in the interstitium of the myocardium without any notable change in collagen (Fig. 6). This may be considered the predominant early morphologic lesion of the myocardium since the myofibers appeared normal on electron microscopy and the mitochondria and sarcoplasmic reticulum showed only occasional swelling or dilatation. The requirements for progression of alcoholic cardiomyopathy from this lesion to heart failure with or without cardiac hypertrophy are not known. However, a longer ingestion period is presumably the major requirement as judged by the experience in man in whom 10 to 15 years of alcoholism is common before heart failure is seen.

The importance of duration of exposure to alcohol is illustrated by studies of left ventricular conduction times in dogs receiving ethanol for 2 years [28]. In animals receiving alcohol for less than a year, the His-Q time measured by the electrode catheter technique was in the normal range, whereas animals observed over 2 years had a greater than 30 percent prolongation of the His-Q interval. The QRS duration was prolonged by nearly 50 percent in the longer term animals and was less abnormal in the short-term experiments. Accumulation of myocardial triglycerides, reminiscent of that seen in alcoholic patients [10], was observed on chemical analysis. A similar observation was previously made in the myocardium of dogs that had received ethanol for 10 weeks [29]. During the initial months of observation, plasma triglyceride and plasma cholesterol rose. Such changes have been reported in dogs fed alcohol for 12 weeks [30]. However, in our study, after approximately 6 months, the plasma levels fell to control levels with the exception of free fatty acid which progressively rose during the subsequent year. To assess the metabolism of free fatty acid, the investigators infused ^{14}C oleic acid systemically. Extraction, myocardial uptake, and $^{14}CO_2$ production judged by the product of arterial-coronary venous differences and coronary blood flow were not significantly different from control. However, the incorporation of fatty acid was shifted from phospholipid to predominantly triglyceride. The lack of abnormality in oxidation of fatty acids suggested that the carnitine system was not involved in the lipid accumulation. Other possible mechanisms, including an inhibition of the triglyceride lipase or enhanced activity of phospholipases are under scrutiny. It is of interest that the distribution of lipid on electron microscopy did not appear to be related to particular subcellular organelles.

Most cardiac diseases have clinical manifestations that include not only heart failure but also arrhythmias and conduction abnormalities. Thus, it is noteworthy that during infusion of ethanol in animals, isolated ventricular ectopic beats may appear with moderate blood levels of ethanol [25]. In these studies of dogs with chronic disease, there were changes in electrolyte composition in the myocardium suggesting a possible mechanism of ventricular arrhythmias. Maines' investigation of chronic alcohol ingestion in the rat indicated a distinct tendency to ventricular arrhythmias [31]. Hence, it is important to be aware that sudden unexpected death has been observed in a relatively high incidence in a group of young adult alcoholics [32]. These subjects had fatty livers as the principal pathologic finding. In this respect they were similar to alcoholics previously found to have physiologic evidence of cardiac malfunction [19]. Ventricular fibrillation may have occurred in these subjects. Additional information in this regard is derived from a study of outpatient alcoholics in Oslo, in whom an increased incidence of sudden cardiac death was observed [33].

Burch et al. [34] and others [27, 31] recently reported that feeding ethyl alcohol daily to mice for as little as 7 to 10 weeks resulted in ultrastructural abnormalities in the myocardium despite adequate nutrition [34]. Animals with reduced food intake had no greater abnormality than the well fed. Despite the large quantities of ethyl alcohol relative to human intake that were used, this study and the others involving 3 different species reveal that chronic ethanol ingestion can produce deleterious effects on cardiac conduction, rhythm, function, and structure, apparently independent of nutritional deficit. Although a great deal of variability was not observed in these animals, it is likely that in man, there is a variable cardiac response to ethanol. Whether this is related to exogenous or endogenous factors or both remains a large area for study. The form in which ethanol is ingested may be an important factor. In most clinical studies the use of whiskey in large amounts appears to be a common factor. The production of myocardial disease may be related to high concentrations of ethanol in blood achieved in a relatively short time. In patients with cardiomyopathy who are exclusively or predominantly drinkers of beer in large quantities, the production of cardiac disease may be attributed in many instances to an associated excess intake of trace metals. That the clinical manifestations of cardiac disease disappeared in patients after the cobalt [21] or arsenic was removed from the beer, despite continued use of this alcoholic beverage, supports this interpretation.

The pathogenesis of alcoholic cardiomyopathy is of more than academic interest since if a critical mechanism involved in alcohol-induced injury can be modified, the long-term effects on the myocardium may be obviated. During acute administration of ethanol, a significant rise in plasma osmolality occurs associated with an increase in plasma volume, which presumably indicates a transfer of fluid from the extravascular space [25]. Thus, the osmotic gradient that exists during the early period after alcohol administration may account for the initial depression of cardiac function, as observed when hyperosmolar solutions are administered intravenously [25]. Whether or not oral administration of alcohol is also associated with a significant hyperosmotic effect on myocardium has not been established. A direct action of ethanol on the cardiac cell and its membranes, possibly by affecting the intracellular transfers of calcium ion or myosin ATPase activity, may contribute to the late stage of myocardial depression. It has recently been reported that the first metabolite of ethanol, acetaldehyde, when infused at rates to simulate blood levels associated with moderate ethanol ingestion, can significantly depress left ventricular function [35] (Fig. 7). This suggests that acetaldehyde may have a role in the pathogenesis of the cardiomyopathy. Although there is no evidence that alcoholic dehydrogenase is induced in the myocardium

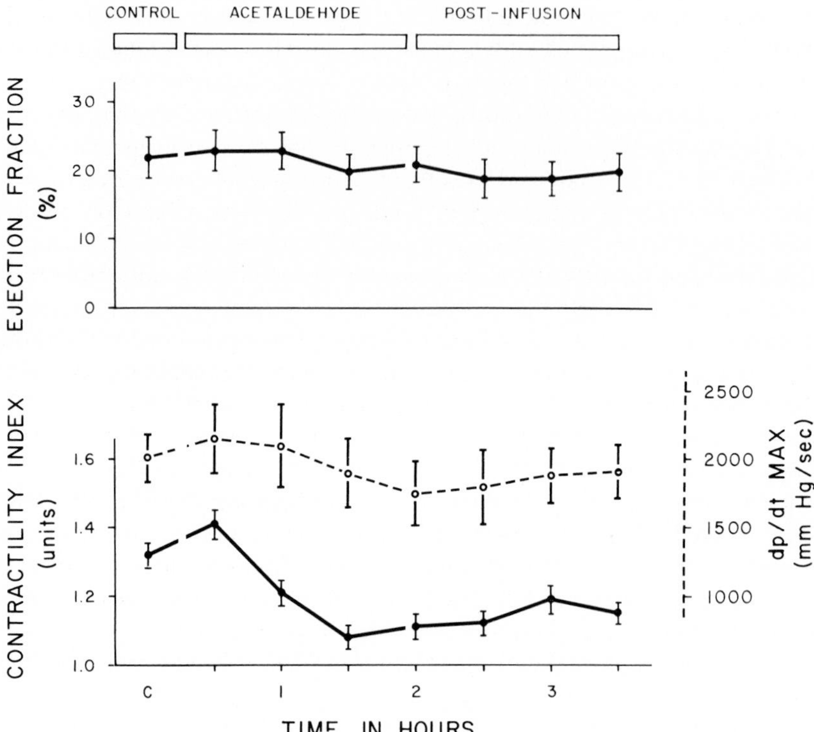

Figure 7. Acetaldehyde was infused at 50 μg/kg/minute for 2 hours in the intact anesthetized dog. Left ventricular *dp/dt* max and contractility index were depressed between 1 to 2 hours of infusion with moderate recovery postinfusion. Left ventricular ejection fraction was affected less substantially, whereas heart rate and aortic pressure did not significantly change. (Courtesy of Dr. M. U. Jesrani.)

during chronic alcohol experiments [23], such an event would presumably increase the concentration of acetaldehyde in the cardiac cells.

The altered lipid metabolism produced by ethanol may be dependent in part on plasma lipid concentrations, and thus composition of the diet. Alterations in lipid composition and function of myocardial cellular membranes may be responsible for the early changes in sarcoplasmic reticulum and mitochondria in which swelling and distortion of these organelles was observed. An additional consideration involves the role of magnesium ion. Primary magnesium deficiency does produce cardiac lesions in immature experimental animals. Unequivocal disease in adults is difficult to demonstrate, however, although secondary potassium loss could have important consequences. In patients with chronic alcoholism, magnesium deficiency may be present and is readily corrected [36]. How early in the disease hypomagnesemia appears and its possible interaction with ethanol to produce cardiac malfunction or arrhythmias in adults remain to be examined.

Involvement of other organs in chronic alcoholism has already been mentioned, in that patients with cardiomyopathy usually have minimal evidence of hepatic disease. Chronic studies of alcohol in the dog revealed relatively modest increments in tryglyceride in liver without cirrhotic change [27]. Although alcoholic cardiac disease has been reported in conjunction with skeletal myopathy [37], the two seem to occur more often separately than together. A critical examination of the skeletal and cardiac muscle on a morphologic, functional, and biochemical basis has not yet been reported. Careful examination of autopsy material from patients with alcoholism not known to have myopathy has indicated skeletal muscle involvement in 22 percent of the subjects, with abnormalities of myofilaments and mitochondria [38]. One may expect some difference in the incidence of abnormalities in cardiac and skeletal muscle on the basis of the lower rate of blood flow and ethanol delivery to the skeletal muscle. If the mitochondria are a critical organelle in the pathogenesis of the disease, the lower number of these particles in skeletal muscle may account for some discrepancies in the incidence of abnormalities in these two organs.

Detection of preclinical cardiomyopathy in the noncardiac alcoholic would be desirable, but at present most subjects are seen after the onset of cardiac symptoms. As a group, these patients are younger than the average coronary patient and exhibit nonspecific findings. As exemplified by the patient in Figure 4, sinus tachycardia and a third heart sound gallop rhythm are frequent findings and may exist with only mild restriction of exercise capacity. Commonly, however, some degree of orthopnea and effort dyspnea are present. Often there are physical findings consistent with low-output heart failure, including a narrow arterial pulse pressure and a prolonged circulation time, as well as an increased systemic venous pressure, pulmonary rales, and cardiac enlargement. These abnormalities usually become intensified after the first episode of heart failure; precordial pain is common.

In cardiomyopathic patients between 40 and 60 years of age, the differential diagnosis of coronary artery disease may present a difficulty. In alcoholics without liver cirrhosis, atherosclerotic disease of coronary arteries has been observed to be similar to that of the nonalcoholic population of the same age group [39]. Ventriculographic studies may be helpful; generalized hypokinesis of the left ventricle favors a primary myopathy. However, localized areas of asynergy have been observed in over a quarter of patients with primary myocardial disease of multiple etiology [40], and ethanol administration may intensify this abnormality [41]. The failure to demonstrate significant obstructive lesions by coronary angiography would also favor the diagnosis of cardiomyopathy.

Occasionally, palpitation is a major complaint in alcoholic cardiomyopathy and is presumably due to cardiac arrhythmias. Atrial fibrillation has been observed during alcoholic episodes, and may regress after abstinence [42]. Sinus tachycardia associated with ventricular premature beats has been suggested as an important clue to the diagnosis of alcoholic cardiomyopathy, but this combination is common in other forms of heart disease. On the electrocardiogram abnormalities of repolarization are the rule, but the spinous or cloven-shaped T waves originally described by Evans [6] are found infrequently. Further, these changes appear to be related to cardiac muscle damage rather than to a specific cause. Whether or not there are early electrocardiographic abnormalities which antedate clinical disease is obviously of interest. Levine and his coworkers concluded that the sharpness of T waves was the only possible electrocardiographic clue to alcoholism [43]. Our own experience suggested that a sizable proportion of alcoholics without clinical heart disease have in midprecordial leads prominent T waves which usually exceed in sharpness and size those in the normal population. The absence of septal Q waves in the alcoholic has been suggested as grounds for considering the diagnosis of cardiomyopathy [44], and the localized absence or reduced amplitude of R waves may simulate the changes of old myocardial infarction. Conduction changes have been observed in about one-third of patients and have included varying degrees of AV block and left or right bundle branch block [44].

Treatment

The treatment of alcoholic cardiomyopathy depends on the stage of the disease. If noninvasive measurements prove sufficiently sensitive, the feasibility of early diagnosis and therapy will be improved. In addition to the evidence cited above [19], 2 other studies of alcoholics without evident heart disease have detected reduced ventricular function during stress testing [20, 21]. If an abnormality of ventricular function is demonstrable prior to clinical evidence of heart disease, then therapeutic intervention should begin at once. The key to treatment at all stages involves complete abstinence.

The alcoholic with cardiac abnormality may be approached effectively on an individual physician-patient relation rather than exclusively relying on group therapy, since several reports of individual treatment have described regression of disease after prolonged abstinence [17, 26]. Thus, in a study in which 22 patients stopped or substantially curtailed their drinking, there was a 9 percent mortality in a follow-up as long as 10 years, as opposed to 57 percent in those who continued to drink heavily. Patients with the shortest duration of symptoms were more likely to show a return of heart size to normal, indicating the importance of prompt intervention as well as the feasibility of adequate treatment without prolonged bed rest.

After the onset of clinical manifestations, traditional antiarrhythmic agents, D.C. electric shock treatments, digitalis and diuretics may be used as needed. Electrolyte abnormalities may either exist during the acute stage or may develop readily in patients with moderate to advanced disease. Since thromboembolism from endocardial thrombi is a prominent feature, occurring in as many as 80 percent of individuals in one series [21], anticoagulants are important. Finally, where facilities are available, prolonged bed rest can reduce the size of excessively dilated hearts and, more importantly, may contribute to control of alcohol intake [42].

SUMMARY

Since a significant fraction of the population are heavy consumers of ethanol, and recent postmortem studies suggest that most alcoholics have some degree of cardiac abnormality, eludication of the mechanism of alcoholic cardiomyopathy is of importance. Intoxicating amounts of ethanol depress ventricular function acutely and effect leakage of myocardial cell components.

Studies in 3 animal species and in man show that the cumulative effects of chronic ethanol intake can, without evident malnutrition, depress ventricular function and produce metabolic and morphologic abnormalities of the myocardium which precede the clinical manifestations. Progression of the disease to heart failure, cardiac arrhythmias, or thromboembolism, separately or in combination, occurs under multiple circumstances that are not clearly defined. These appear to include the cumulative effects of ethanol alone or an intensified drinking episode, simultaneous exposure to trace metals in excess, and occasional specific nutritional deficiency or superimposed infection. The low prevalence of clear-cut manifestations of nutritional deficiency in patients with alcoholic cardiomyopathy supports the view that the cardiac abnormality is commonly not dependent on malnutrition.

Finally, clinical data indicate that cessation of alcohol intake may reverse the disease or interrupt its progression in many patients. Anticoagulant therapy is recommended at least during the early recovery stage.

REFERENCES

1. Ferrans, V.J.: Alcoholic cardiomyopathy. Am J Med Sci 252:123, 1966.
2. Steell, G.: The three cardinal symptoms of heart disease. In, Textbook on Diseases of the Heart. Philadalphia, Blakiston, 1906, p 19.
3. Blakenhorn, M.A., Vilter, C., Scheinker, I.M., and Austin, R.S.: Occidental beriberi heart disease. J Am Med Assoc 131:717, 1946.
4. Eliaser, M. and Giansiracusa, F.: Heart and alcohol. Calif Med 84:234, 1956.
5. Brigden, W. and Robinson, J.: Alcoholic heart disease. Br Med J 2:1283, 1964.
6. Evans, W.: The electrocardiogram of alcoholic cardiomyopathy. Br Heart J 21:445, 1959.
7. Burch, G.E. and Walsh, J.J.: Cardiac insufficiency in chronic alcoholism. Am J Cardiol. 6:864, 1960.
8. Cahalan, D., Cisin, I.H., and Crossley, H.M.: American drinking practices: A national survey of drinking behavior and attitudes. New Brunswick, N. J., Rutgers Univ. Center of Alcohol Studies, Monograph 6, 1969.
9. Schenk, E.A. and Cohen, J.: The heart in chronic alcoholism. Pathol Microbiol (Basel) 35:96, 1970.
10. Ferrans, V.J., Hibbs, R.G., Weilbaecher, D.G., Black, W.C., Walsh, J.J., and Burch, G.E.: Alcoholic cardiomyopathy: A histochemical study. Am Heart J 69:748, 1965.
11. Hibbs, R.G., Ferrans, V.J., Black, W.C., Walsh, J.J., and Burch, G.E.: Virus-like particles in heart of the patient with cardiomyopathy. Am Heart J 69:327, 1965.
12. Alexander, C.S.: Idiopathic heart disease II. Electron microscopic examination of myocardial biopsy specimens in alcoholic heart disease. Am J Med 41:229, 1966.
13. Neville, J.N., Eagles, J.A., Sampson, G., and Olson, R.E.: The nutritional status of alcoholics. Am J Clin. Nutr 21: 1329, 1968.
14. Leevy, C.M., Baker, H., Ten-Hove, O., Frank, O., and Cherrick, G.R.: B-complex vitamins in liver disease of the alcoholic. Am J Clin Nutr 16:339, 1965.
15. Fowler, N.O., Gueron, M., and Rowlands, D.T.: Primary myocardial disease. Circulation 23:498, 1961.
16. Massumi, R.A., Rios, J.C., Gooch, A.S., Nutter, D., Vita, V.T., and Datlow, D.W.: Primary myocardial disease. Circulation 31:19, 1965.
17. Tobin, J.R., Jr., Driscoll, Lim, M.T., Sutton, G.C., Szanto, P.B., and Gunnar, R. M.: Primary myocardial disease and alcoholism. Circulation 35: 4, 1967.
18. Wendt, V.E., Wu, C. Balcon, R., Doty, G., and Bing, R.J.: The hemodynamic and metabolic effects of chronic alcoholism in man. Am J Cardiol 15:175, 1965.
19. Regan, T.J., Levinson, G.E., Oldewurtel, H.A., Frank, M.J., Weisse, A.B. and Moschos, C.B.: Ventricular function in noncardiacs with alcoholic fatty liver: Role of ethanol in the production of cardiomyopathy. J Clin Invest. 48:407, 1969.
20. Gould, L.: Cardiac hemodynamics in alcoholic patients with chronic liver disease and presystolic gallop. J Clin Invest. 48:860, 1969.
21. Morin, Y.Q.: Beer-drinkers' cardiomyopathy: Hemodynamic alterations. Can Med Assoc J 97:901, 1967.
22. Ahmed, S.S., Levinson, G.E., and Regan, T.J.: Altered systolic time intervals with low doses of ethanol in man. Circulation 44:II-35, 1971.

23. Lochner, A., Cowley, R., and Brink, A.J.: Effect of ethanol on metabolism and function of perfused rat heart. Am Heart J 78:770, 1969.
24. Newman, W.H. and Valicenti, J.F., Jr.: Ventricular function following acute alcohol administration: A strain-gauge analysis of depressed ventricular dynamics. Am Heart J 81:61, 1971.
25. Regan, T.J., Koroxenidis, G., Moschos, C.B., Oldewurtel, H.A., Lehan, P.H., and Hellems, H.K.: The acute metabolic and hemodynamic responses of the left ventricle to ethanol. J Clin Invest 45:270, 1966.
26. Demakis, J.G., Rahimtoola, S.H., Sutton, G.C., Jamil, M., Proskey, A. Rosen, K.M., and Gunnar, R.M.: The clinical course of cardiomyopathy associated with alcoholism. Circulation 44:II-157, 1971.
27. Regan, T.J., Khan, M.I., Ettinger, P.O., Jesrani, M.U., Lyons, M., and Oldewurtel, H.A.: Myocardial function and metabolism in the well-nourished chronic alcoholic animal. Circulation 44: II-49, 1971.
28. Ettinger, P. O., Khan, M. I., Oldewurtel, H. A., and Regan, T. J.: left ventricular conduction abnormalities in chronic diabetes and alcoholism. Circulation 42: III-98, 1970.
29. Marciniak, M., Gudbjarnason, S., and Bruce, T.A.: The effect of chronic alcohol administration on enzyme profile and glyceride content of heart muscle, brain and liver. Proc Soc Exper Biol Med 128:1021, 1968.
30. Beard, J.D. and Barboriak, J.J.: Plasma lipids of dogs during and after chronic ethanol administration. Proc Soc Exper Biol Med 118:1151, 1965.
31. Maines, J.E. and Aldinger, E.E.: Myocardial depression accompanying chronic consumption of alcohol. Am Heart J 73:55, 1967.
32. Kramer, K., Kuller, L., and Fisher, R.: The increasing mortality attributed to cirrhosis and fatty liver, in Baltimore (1957-1966). Ann Intern Med 69:273, 1968.
33. Sundby, P.: Alcoholism and mortality. Oslow, Norway. Universitetsfordaget, 1967 (Alcohol Research in the Northern Countries), publ 6, Stockholm, National Institute for Alcohol Research and New Brunswick, N. J., Rutgers Univ Center of Alcohol Studies, 1969.
34. Burch, G.E., Colcolough, H.L., Harb, J.M., and Tsui, C.Y.: The effects of ingestion of ethyl alcohol, wine and beer on the myocardium of mice. Am J Cardiol 27:522, 1971.
35. Jesrani, M.U., Gopinathan, K., Khan, M.I., Oldewurtel, H.A., and Regan, T.J.: Acetaldehyde and the myocardial depressant effects of ethanol. Circulation 44: II-127, 1971.
36. Jones, J.E., Shane, S.R., Jacobs, W.H., and Flink, E.B.: Magnesium balance in chronic alcoholism. Ann NY Acad Sci 162 (Suppl 2):934, 1969.
37. Erlenborn, J.W. and Pilz, C.G.: Paroxysmal myoglobinuria associated with cardiomegaly and electrocardiographic abnormalities. J Am Med Assoc 181: 1111, 1962.
38. Kahn, L.B. and Meyer, J.S.: Acute myopathy in chronic alcoholism: A study of 22 autopsied cases with ultrastructural observations. Am J Clin Pathol 53:516, 1970.
39. Hirst, A.E., Hadley, G.G., and Gore, I.: The effect of chronic alcoholism and cirrhosis of the liver on atherosclerosis. Am J Med Sci 249:143, 1965.
40. Kreulen, T.H., Herman, M.V., and Gorlin, R.: Ventriculographic patterns and hemodynamics in primary myocardial disease (PMD). Circulation 43 and 44: II-40, 1971.

41. Herman, M.V., Heinle, R.A., Klein, M.D., and Gorlin, R.: Localized disorders in myocardial contraction. N Engl J Med 277:222, 1967.
42 Burch, G.E. and DePasquale, N.P.: Alcoholic cardiomyopathy. Am J Cardiol 23:723, 1969.
43. Levine, H.D., Piemme, T.E., and Monroe, K.E.: A brisk electrocardiogram observed in chronic alcoholics. Am Heart J 69:140, 1965.
44. Horan, L.G., Flowers, N.C., Thomas, J.R., and Tolleson, W.J.: The spatial vectorcardiogram in idiopathic cardiomyopathy. Prog Cardiovasc Dis 7:115, 1964.

WALTER H. ABELMANN, M.D.

Clinical Aspects of Viral Cardiomyopathy

This chapter will include a summary of what is known about involvement of the myocardium in specific viral infections, a description of the clinical manifestations of viral myocarditis in general, a discussion on differential diagnosis, consideration of therapeutic approaches, and finally brief comments on the question of late sequelae.

Almost any viral infection may be accompanied by clinical evidence of altered cardiac function [1], but most frequently by abnormal formation or conduction of cardiac impulses or abnormal repolarization. Morphologic alterations of the heart muscle have been associated with most viral infections [2, 3]. In cases of proven fatal viral infection, however, they are usually demonstrated only after prolonged, severe illness, associated with hypoxia, acid-base imbalance, secondary infections, administration of multiple drugs, or hypotension. The only pathogenic viruses which have regularly been recovered from human cardiac tissues are poliomyelitis, Coxsackie and echoviruses. Furthermore, at least in experimental animals, virus has been shown to replicate in cardiac tissue without clinical or light microscopic abnormalities [4]. Thus, it is not always easy to decide when a viral infection actually involves the heart [1].

For the purposes of this chapter, morphologic, physiologic or clinical abnormalities observed in association with proved or at least clinically presumptive viral infections will be accepted as presumptive viral myocarditis. It is understood that this is likely to include toxic, metabolic, and possibly

From the Thorndike Memorial Laboratory and the Harvard Medical Unit, Boston City Hospital, Boston, Massachusetts.

immunologic effects of viral infection in addition to effects of replication of virus in the heart. On the other hand, it is also recognized that multiple blocks of cardiac tissue subjected to serial sections indicate a considerably higher prevalence of inflammatory lesions in the myocardium of patients with viral infections than clinically suspected [2].

THE LESION

Classically, myocarditis is an inflammatory lesion, characterized in its mildest interstitial form by cellular infiltrate, usually predominantly mononuclear [2, 3]. Lesions often, but not necessarily, are perivascular. They may be focal or diffuse; they may show predilection for the subendocardial or subepicardial regions. There may be varying degrees of myocytolysis and necrosis. Anitschkow cells, giant cells, eosinophils may be seen but are not diagnostic. Subepicardial lesions are often associated with pericarditis. Lesions are not limited to the interstitium and muscle, but may also involve specialized tissues such as nodes and conduction system. The specific location as well as the extent of lesions may determine what, if any, functional impairment or clinical manifestations may ensue. Focal lesions of small size, if strategically placed, may give rise to life-threatening arrhythmias or conduction disturbances. Remarkably diffuse interstitial infiltrates may be found incidentally in patients dying of extracardiac causes without clinical heart disease having been evident. When diffuse myocarditis is associated with diffuse loss of muscle tissue, however, heart failure may ensue.

The spectrum of acute viral myocarditis ranges from subclinical myocarditis to arrhythmias, conduction defects, electrocardiographic changes, to heart failure, collapse and sudden death. Myocarditis may be truly asymptomatic, or its symptoms may be overshadowed by systemic effects of the viral infection.

INCIDENCE OF MYOCARDITIS

A thorough review of 40,000 autopsies drawn from a predominantly young and male population by Gore and Saphir [5] revealed 1,402 cases of myocarditis. Seventy of these were associated with viral illness, and an additional 84 cases of isolated myocarditis could have been of viral etiology. Thus, the maximal autopsy incidence of viral myocarditis was 0.38 percent. According to official United States statistics [6], which probably represent underestimates, 860 deaths or 0.4 per 100,000 population were attributed to acute nonrheumatic myocarditis in 1967.

Reliable data on morbidity of viral myocarditis are lacking. In most viral infections, involvement of the heart appears to be rare, and overt clinical myocarditis is the exception. Reliable clinical criteria of cardiac involvement, however, have not been established. Many surveys rely on electrocardiographic abnormalities which are nonspecific and of dubious value in the diagnosis of myocarditis. Scott and collaborators [7] found electrocardiographic abnormalities not only in 1.5 percent of 737 children with acute respiratory infections but also in 1.8 percent of a control group of 108 children. Laboratory evidence of recent viral infection was obtained in 42.6 percent of 13 patients with abnormal electrocardiograms and in 49.5 percent of the 832 patients with normal tracings. Other evidence, however, suggests that asymptomatic myocarditis may be rather frequent. Among 323 healthy persons killed accidently, Stevens and Underwood-Ground [8] found 9 cases of isolated focal myocarditis, a prevalence of 2.8 percent.

MYOCARDITIS ASSOCIATED WITH SPECIFIC VIRUSES OR VIRAL SYNDROMES

Myocarditis may occur in the usual childhood diseases. In these diseases, clinical myocarditis is quite rare and usually benign. Fatal myocarditis is so unusual that cases tend to be reported in the literature. Inasmuch as bacterial superinfections are frequently also present, the etiology of myocardial lesions is sometimes in doubt. It may be pertinent to recall how common these diseases really are. For the year 1964-1965, when the reference population of the United States was 188,430,000, 10,020,000 cases of measles were reported, 6,810,000 cases of German measles, 4,110,000 cases of chicken pox, and 3,026,000 cases of mumps [9].

Rubeola

A review of the cardiac findings in 91 fatal cases of rubeola by Degen [10] revealed myocarditis in 4 hearts, in association with pericarditis. The interstitial infiltrates were mainly lymphocytic. It is not clear, however, to what extent secondary bacterial infection may have played a role. Transient electrocardiographic abnormalities were demonstrated by Ross [11] in more than half of 71 children with measles. Prolongation of the P-R interval was the most common abnormality. Complete heart block as well as ventricular tachycardia have been described but are rare. An example is shown in Figure 1.

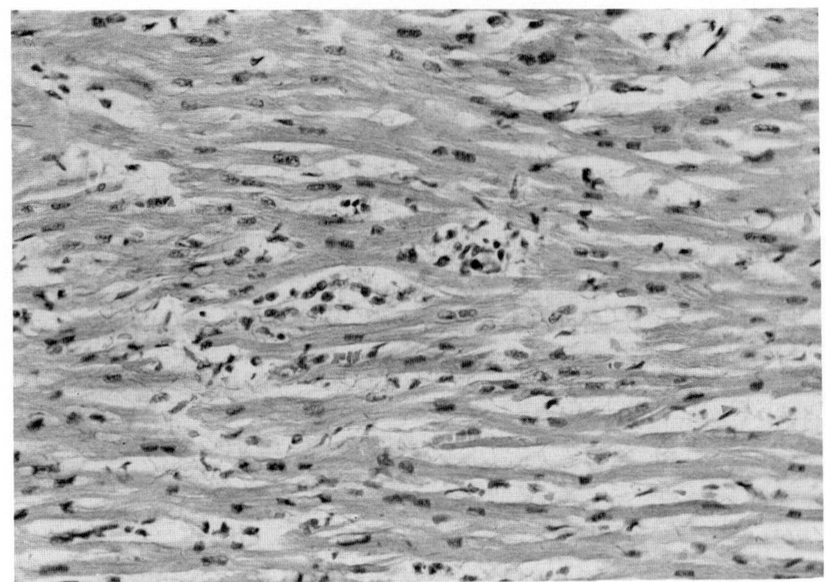

Figure 1. Myocarditis. Myocardium with interstitial myocarditis from a 2-year-old girl who died of measles and pneumonia on the first hospital day. Typical rash had developed 5 days prior to admission, accompanied by fever, anorexia, emesis, cough, and dyspnea. Physical findings included a temperature of 103.6, sinus tachycardia 140 to 200/minute, tachypnea 40-80/minute, rales, cyanosis, rash, and dehydration (×400; H + E).

Rubella

Special mention should be made of maternal rubella during the first trimester of pregnancy. In addition to the well known congenital cardiac defects, focal-to-diffuse myocardial necrosis may result [12]. These lesions may heal *in utero* or persist into neonatal life. Conduction disturbances have been observed, including partial [13] and complete heart block [14].

Variola, Varicella, and Vaccinia

Among 9 cases of fatal smallpox, Gore and Saphir [5] found 1 case of myocarditis.

Frank myocarditis with congestive heart failure has been reported to accompany chicken pox, followed by full clinical recovery [15]. The histological changes in the heart in cases of subclinical myocarditis have been described [16]. The usual picture is that of focal perivascular mononuclear infiltrates with occasional interstitial involvement and rare myocytolysis.

One case of fatal varicella myocarditis presented with paroxysmal atrial tachycardia [17]. Sudden and unexpected death of a 10-month-old boy, 4 weeks after onset of varicella, was associated with myocarditis affecting preferentially the bundle of His and its branches [18]. Sudden death from myocarditis has also been reported following vaccinia [19].

Mumps

Gore and Saphir [5] found 1 case of myocarditis among 8 cases of fatal mumps. In an epidemic of mumps studied by Rosenberg [20], abnormal electrocardiograms were encountered in 16 of 104 cases, but only in 4 of these was there clinical evidence of cardiac involvement. Among the electrocardiographic abnormalities were diphasic or inverted P waves, changes in ST or T waves, and first-degree heart block. Bengtsson and Orndahl [21] studied 564 cases of mumps and found electrocardiographic abnormalities in 4.4 percent, mainly depression of ST segments and flattening or inversion of T waves. However, heart block was observed in 2 patients and extrasystoles in 1. Congestive heart failure has been described by Roberts and Fox [22].

Infectious Mononucleosis

In 6 of 9 fatal cases of infectious mononucleosis [5], myocarditis was observed. Electrocardiographic abnormalities were found in 5 of 100 patients surveyed by Hoagland [23], including persistent complete heart block in 1. Bengtsson [24] reported a 20-year-old man who presented with acute myocarditis simulating an acute myocardial infarction and subsequently developed infectious mononucleosis. Pericarditis has been reported [25] and may also be the first clinical manifestation of disease. One patient with pericardial effusion and tamponade later developed constrictive pericarditis [26].

Viral Hepatitis

In fatal epidemic hepatitis, myocarditis has been observed [27]; interstitial and perivascular infiltrates may be associated with focal necrosis and subendocardial hemorrhages. Whereas clinical heart failure has not been reported, Loeffler [28] reported cardiac dilatation, especially of the right atrium and ventricle, in 6 of 14 fatal cases. Sanghvi and Misra [29] observed electrocardiographic abnormalities in 44 percent of 140 cases. The largest series is that of Maretic and Kuze-Capar [30], who found electrocardiographic abnormalities in 283 cases or 17.3 percent of 1634 patients with hepatitis, observed between 1964 and 1970. Except for children, who usually manifested tachycardia, bradycardia was frequent, the heart rate being less than 50/minute in 10 cases. Several paroxysms of atrial fibrillation were encountered in an 11-year-old girl. Nodal rhythm was seen in 4 patients and wandering pacemaker in 5. P waves were of low amplitude or negative in 11 cases. Abnormalities of the ST segment or T wave were seen in 262 patients, and the Q-T interval was prolonged in 33. Abnormalities were usually transient, but persisted for several months in 5 instances. It is not known to what extent the changes are a function of inflammatory lesions in the myocardium, changes in myocardial metabolism secondary to altered hepatic function, alterations in electrolytes, or elevations in serum bilirubin or bile salts [31]. The bradycardia has been explained on the basis of increased vagal tone inasmuch as it can be abolished by changes in position and exercise [32].

Pneumonia Due to Adenovirus

Among 222 cases of fatal pneumonia attributed to viral infection, there were 32 cases of myocarditis [5]. Transient electrocardiographic abnormalities have been reported in this syndrome [33]. It remains unknown which virus was responsible for these early cases. However, adenovirus, a cause of pneumonitis in infants and children, has been isolated from children with acute myocarditis [35].

Mycoplasma Pneumoniae

In a recent preliminary communication, Lewes and Rainford [34] report myocarditis associated with proved infection with *Mycoplasma pneumoniae*. Electrocardiographic abnormalities, however, were the only clinical manifestations.

Influenza

In 1945, Finland and associates [36] reported the isolation of influenza-A virus from the heart of a 34-year-old woman who died of acute myocarditis after a 6-day illness. Clinical influenza 4 months earlier was followed by persistent cough and fatigue. The final illness was characterized by prostration, fever, chills, progressive dyspnea, bradycardia, complete heart block, substernal distress, and finally circulatory collapse. The heart weighed 490 grams, and its chambers were slightly dilated. There was diffuse necrosis of myofibers and extensive interstitial infiltration with mononuclear cells. In the lungs, congestion dominated over inflammatory changes. A second patient with proved influenza who died of pneumonia also had myocarditis.

Circulatory collapse, sudden death, congestive heart failure, all degrees of heart block, and other electrocardiographic abnormalities had previously been reported to be associated with clinical influenza, especially during the pandemic of 1918 [31]. Gross and light microscopic changes in the heart of patients dying of influenza are quite rare. Cardiovascular symptoms and signs accompanying influenza are often attributable to extracardiac circulatory changes or to secondary bacterial infections. Most documented cardiac complications of influenza have occurred during convalescence from the initial illness.

Psittacosis and Ornithosis

Myocarditis has been repeatedly observed in well-documented fatal cases of psittacosis [37-40]. Heart failure is a prominent manifestation. Sutton and associates [41] serologically studied 599 patients with suspected acute myopericarditis and found 9 patients with acute myocarditis, pericarditis, or both, whose complement antibody to psittacosis agent antigen was present at least twice in dilutions of 1:16 or greater or displayed either a fourfold rise or fall. Precordial pain was present in 4 cases, a pericardial friction rub in 2, pericardial effusion in 2; the heart was enlarged in 7, an S_3 gallop was heard in 2, and an S_4 gallop in 2. Atrial tachycardia was observed in 1, acute ST-T changes in 8. Intraventricular conduction defects were also seen. In 4 of the 9 patients, however, there was preexistent heart disease. The other 5 patients recovered fully.

Cytomegalovirus Disease

Focal myocarditis has been described in association with cytomegalovirus infection, especially in infants. Ahvenainen [42] reported a 3-month-old infant with chronic diarrhea who died of pneumonia and meningitis; there was diffuse myocarditis, and inclusion bodies were seen in the heart. Myocardial involvement has also been described in cytomegalovirus infection associated with leukemia [43]. The severe general illness and involvement of other organ systems appear to overshadow cardiovascular manifestations of the disease, at least in the fatal cases reported.

Poliomyelitis

A wide variety of clinical cardiovascular abnormalities and pathologic lesions have been described in patients with poliomyelitis. The etiology of such changes has not always been clear, especially in view of coexisting hypoxia, electrolyte and acid-base imbalance, and superinfection. However, poliomyelitis virus has been isolated from the heart [44]. Histologic lesions include focal necrosis, edema, and mononuclear infiltrates, often perivascular. Fibrosis has also been described. The most comprehensive clinical study is that of Weinstein and Shelokov [45], who analyzed cardiovascular manifestations in 428 cases of poliomyelitis, about half of them adults. Acute systemic hypertension was observed in 7 percent of the patients, usually in association with severe illness and cyanosis; it was attributed to hypoxia. Acute pulmonary edema was observed in a number of bulbar cases. Abnormal electrocardiograms were recorded in 25 percent of the cases, comprising mainly abnormal ST segments or T waves, first-degree AV block, or prolongation of Q-T inteval. Of 16 fatal cases examined, 12 showed histologic evidence of myocarditis; right-sided dilatation was common. In another series [46], interstitial myocarditis was found in three-fourths of 22 cases who died in cardiovascular collapse, usually with terminal pulmonary edema.

Coxsackie Virus Infection

Coxsackie group B viruses are considered the most frequent cause of viral myocarditis in the newborn, in the child, and in the adult [47-49]. Infants are very susceptable to the virus. Several outbreaks in nurseries have included cases of myocarditis, often fatal [47, 50]. Kibrick and Benirschke [51] reported fatal myocarditis associated with meningoencephalitis in a 6-day-old infant. Coxsackie virus B type 3 was recovered from the thoracic spinal cord, and the authors present evidence for intrauterine acquisition of the infection from the mother, who had an upper respiratory tract infection 2 days prior to delivery and subsequently developed neutralizing antibodies to the recovered virus. Such a history of minor febrile illness is often obtained from the mother of infants who develop myocarditis. The initial nonspecific symptoms of the illness in infants—difficulty in feeding, fever, lethargy—are followed by tachycardia, tachypnea, pallor, cyanosis, and abnormal ST and T changes of the electrocardiogram. There may be cardiac enlargement and florid heart failure with hepatomegaly; arrhythmias have been observed. Cardiovascular manifestations may be overshadowed by evidence of meningoencephalitis. Myocarditis has also been encountered in children in association with both sporadic and epidemic Coxsackie B infections, generally more benign in course [47].

Cardiac involvement by Coxsackie B virus in adults is now well accepted [47, 49, 52, 53], and may account for many cases of "idiopathic nonspecific benign myopericarditis." The disease generally being benign, the true incidence is not known. It is the more severe case which tends to be recognized clinically and reported. Some data collected during the 1965 outbreak of Coxsackie B 5 virus infection in Europe yield valuable estimates of incidence of myopericarditis. According to a report from the Public Health Laboratory Service in the United Kingdom [54], 41 percent of infections reported occurred in children less than 10 years old, and 19 percent in patients aged 10 to 19. Of 900 cases with proved Coxsackie B 5 virus infection, 31 percent had infections of the central nervous system, 23 percent myalgia and pleurodynia, 15 percent upper respiratory symptoms, 9 percent gastrointestinal symptoms. Forty-eight patients were reported to have cardiac symptoms, attributed to pericarditis in 41 and to myocarditis in 5. Two of the latter were fatal: one in an infant of 11 days and the other in an adult. Analyzing reports from Finland and Scotland, Grist and Bell [47] conclude that cardiac syndromes comprised 12 and 5 percent of proved Coxsackie B 5 cases, respectively. They also suggest that the true contribution of Coxsackie viruses to cardiac disease may be considerably greater because relatively few patients with acute heart disease are recognized early and investigated virologically.

A similar analysis of sporadic cases of heart disease studied virologically outside epidemic periods yielded evidence of Coxsackie B virus infection in from 3 to 39 percent [47]. In a subsequent report, Grist and Bell [55] analyzed 234 patients with evidence of acute and chronic heart disease who were studied virologically. Isolation of any Coxsackie B virus, a fourfold rise in antibody titer or a neutralizing antibody titer of 256 or greater were accepted as indicating Coxsackie B infection. In this manner, 55 percent of 46 cases of acute myocarditis and 22 percent of 51 cases of acute pericarditis could be attributed to Coxsackie B virus.

The clinical manifestations of Coxsackie B virus myocarditis in the adult are usually, but not invariably, preceded or accompanied by systemic manifestations of viral disease. Frequent among these are fever, symptoms of an upper respiratory tract infection, and abdominal symptoms, including nausea and emesis. Myalgia, pleurodynia, and arthralgia are common. Cutaneous eruptions may be rubelliform or, on occasion, vesicular, or purpuric. Other manifestations may include pneumonitis, meningoencephalitis, encephalomyelitis, orchitis, ovaritis, hepatitis, pancreatitis, or nephritis. Chest pain is the symptom most frequently encountered in Coxsackie B virus myopericarditis, usually but not always pleuropericardial in nature, aggravated by respiration and relieved by sitting up and leaning forward. Pain resembling angina pectoris has been described in some patients [49, 55]. Others complain of palpitation, usually associated with ventricular premature beats. A pericardial or pleuropericardial friction rub, at times transient, is heard in at least one-third of adult cases. Cough and dyspnea usually indicate congestive heart failure, which is present in about one-fourth of most adult series and, in contradistinction to infants and children, is only rarely associated with edema and hepatomegaly, but usually with cardiomegaly and pulmonary congestion and often with pleural effusions.

The electrocardiographic changes observed most frequently are elevations of ST segments, and flattening to inversion of T waves. The characteristic picture of pericarditis may evolve, or serial changes may suggest localized ischemia. Transient Q waves [49, 53] and even the pattern of myocardial infarction have been described [49]. Ventricular premature beats are not infrequent. Ventricular tachycardia and fibrillation have on rare occasions been documented [49, 53]. Atrial premature beats appear to be less frequent than ventricular premature beats; single cases of atrial fibrillation have been observed [49]. Transient second- or third-degree heart block as well as bundle branch block have been described [49, 53].

The chest radiograph may reveal generalized cardiomegaly with or without pulmonary congestion, and on rare occasions florid pulmonary edema. Pleural effusion tends to be either left-sided or bilateral. Patchy pulmonary infiltration may be seen.

A mild-to-moderate leukocytosis with predominance of neutrophils is the rule, even in the absence of superinfection. The erythrocyte sedimentation rate tends to be elevated. A mild-to-moderate rise in serum enzymes is often seen. Thus, Sainani and collaborators [53] found that in their group of 22 adults with Coxsackie B myocarditis the lactic dehydrogenase was elevated in all, aldolase was elevated in 11, and serum glutamic oxalacetic transaminase was increased in 7.

Recent evidence suggests that Coxsackie A viruses, albeit more difficult to isolate, may be responsible for myocarditis in infants and, occasionally, in adults [47]. Clinical manifestations include congestive heart failure and sudden death.

Echovirus Disease

More recently it has been established that the echovirus group of enteroviruses may, like the Coxsackie viruses, cause acute myopericarditis in man [56]. Single cases of paroxysmal atrial tachycardia [47, 57] and of isolated fulminant myocarditis with complete heart block [58] were associated with proved echovirus type 9 virus infection; in the latter case, the virus was isolated from the myocardium. Russell and Bell [59] report a 6-week-old infant with refusal to eat, vomiting, choking attacks, cyanosis, and dyspnea. The respiratory rate was 72 per minute and the heart rate was 240 per minute. The electrocardiogram showed inverted T waves in all three standard leads. Echovirus type 22 was isolated from the feces, and convalescent serum showed a delayed rise in antibody titer to this virus. The infant was treated with digoxin and steroids and made an uneventful recovery. Like Coxsackie viruses, echoviruses have regularly been associated with outbreaks of pleurodynia [56]. Figure 2 was obtained from a sporadic case.

GENERAL CLINICAL MANIFESTATIONS

The preceding section might suggest that different viruses have specific or characteristic cardiac effects or manifestations. This is probably not so. When virologic methods become more widely available, it is likely that the above-cited cardiac manifestations for specific viruses will be found to be associated with all. Although as a group, patients infected with a specific virus may show characteristic cardiovascular manifestations, the clinician faced with a single patient will not be able to differentiate the various viruses on the basis of cardiovascular manifestations. If this can be done at all clinically, it will be done on the basis of associated systemic manifestations.

Thus, almost all clinical manifestations of viral myocarditis have already been discussed. By way of recapitulation, myocarditis may be clinically silent and may be detected only by abnormalities on a screening electrocardiogram or chest radiograph, although even these may be normal. Myocarditis may give rise to arrhythmias or conduction disturbances; it may lead to acute myocardial failure with weakness, pallor, cyanosis, hypotension with narrow pulse pressure, and ultimately, circulatory collapse, or it may result in congestive heart failure. The latter is probably always biventricular, but in infancy and childhood the manifestations of right ventricular failure tend to predominate, whereas in the adult, symptoms and signs of left ventricular failure may gain the upper hand. Electrocardiographic abnormalities are often transient or display evolution. Heart failure tends to respond well to digitalis glycosides and diuretic agents. By the time myocarditis is recognized, it has usually reached its most severe stage: the patient either succumbs to it or to associated involvement of other organ systems, or he responds to therapy and shows steady improvement.

One manifestation of viral myocarditis deserves mention: sudden unexpected death. Gormsen [60] reported 17 cases of myocarditis among

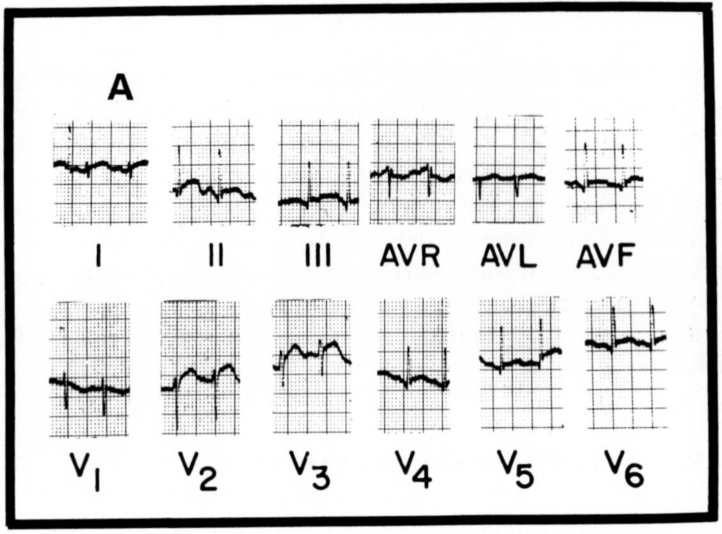

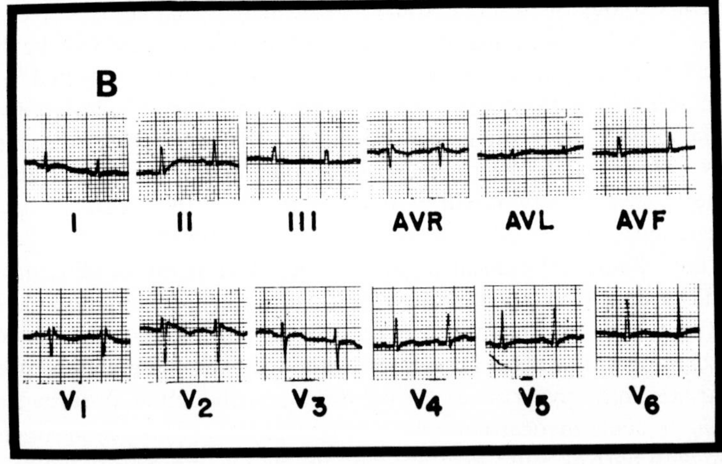

Figure 2. Acute Myopericarditis. Electrocardiograms taken on the third and ninth day of illness of a 20-year-old housewife in the first trimester of pregnancy with acute myopericarditis, attributed to echovirus type 9, which was isolated from the nasopharynx. Serial convalescent sera, unfortunately, were lost. The illness started with pleuropericardial pain and nausea. Cough, increasingly severe dyspnea, and tachycardia followed. Pain became severe, a pericardial friction rub was heard, and bilateral pleural effusions developed. On nonspecific therapy, she made a gradual but complete recovery. A. Sinus tachycardia at 145/minute with widespread borderline elevations of ST segments and low T waves. B. Sinus tachycardia at 115/minute with decrease in voltage and further lowering of T waves. (Courtesy of Dr. J.V. Varnum and Dr. D.E. Bragdon, Chelmsford, Mass.)

1,378 cases of sudden, unexpected death. Histological examination, however, had been carried out only in 117 cases. Corby [61] attributed 32 cases of sudden, obscure death to focal myocarditis, representing 0.35 percent of medicolegal autopsies surveyed. In his series, 9 individuals had "dropped dead," 7 had been found dead at home, and 4 collapsed with chest pain and died in a few hours. On the other hand, a review of 72 autopsied cases of sudden, unexpected death [62] yielded only 1 case of myocarditis: a 20-year-old woman who died suddenly at work. In a review of 275 sudden deaths in 20- to 45-year-old adults, Luke and Helpern [63] attributed only 1 death to myocarditis, presumed to be viral. In this series, however, the extent of histological examination was not commented on, and alcoholic patients and patients hospitalized for more than 24 hours had been excluded. Stevens and Underwood-Ground [8] cite the case of a pilot in which the cause of an accident was attributed to myocarditis.

DIAGNOSIS OF VIRAL MYOCARDITIS

The prerequisite to the diagnosis of myocarditis is the awareness of its existence and alertness to its manifestations. Unfortunately, the clinical diagnosis of myocarditis, even in fatal cases, is often not made. Some physicians are satisfied with a diagnosis of manifestations (e.g., arrhythmia, congestive heart failure) and treat without an etiological diagnosis. Admission of some patients to cardiac care units with the implied diagnosis of coronary disease may also be prejudicial to further diagnostic considerations. Another cause of erroneous diagnosis is the dominance of extracardiac problems which may obscure the cardiac lesion. The viral infection may have cutaneous, cerebral, hepatic, or other systemic involvement of a severity that all symptoms are accounted for and a thorough cardiovascular evaluation does not appear to be indicated. Preexisting heart disease—congenital, rheumatic, or arteriosclerotic—may fully account for cardiac manifestations if myocarditis is not suspected.

Being aware of the possibility of myocarditis complicating any acute viral infection, the alert clinician will pay attention to persistent undue tachycardia, irregularities of the heart beat, right or left ventricular S_3 or S_4 gallops, cough, dyspnea, and—especially in children—an enlarging liver and venous distention. Involvement of the pericardium, which is especially frequent in the myopericarditis associated with Coxsackie and echoviruses, may facilitate early detection by giving rise to pleuropericardial pain with or without a friction rub, which may be transient. Any of these findings should prompt electrocardiographic and radiographic assessment and follow-up. Leukocytosis, elevation of erythrocyte sedimentation rate and abnormal level of serum enzymes are frequent but nonspecific. The clinical approach to the diagnosis of subclinical myocarditis and its possible value have been discussed previously [64]. Electrocardiographic abnormalities during and after exercise may be especially valuable [65].

The viral etiology of myocarditis in a given patient is not easy to establish with certainty [1]. Early in the course of illness, virus may be isolated from throat washings, feces, blood, pericardial fluid, or myocardium. To this end, myocardial biopsy may, on occasion, be of value [66]. Isolation of a virus, however, does not necessarily establish its etiological role in the myocardial disease [1].

Presence of antibody to a specific virus in the serum in rising titer during convalescence represents evidence of a recent infection. A fourfold increase in virus neutralizing antibody, complement fixation, or hemagglutination inhibition titers is generally accepted as indicating a current infection. Both identification of antigen in body fluids or tissue by means of immunofluorescence [67] and demonstration of virus in tissue by electron microscopy [68] are now possible and may come into clinical use.

DIFFERENTIAL DIAGNOSIS

Nonviral myocarditis. The circulatory manifestations of nonviral myocarditis may be and generally are not distinguishable from those of viral myocarditis. The important exception is rheumatic myocarditis (v.i.). Nonviral myocarditides are usually associated with acute or subacute systemic infections which give rise to general symptoms as well as symptoms pointing to other affected organ systems. It must be recognized that almost any infectious agent may give rise to myocarditis [64]. The etiologic agent may be recognized by characteristic symptoms or regional prevalence. Thus, periorbital edema, myalgia, and a history of ingestion of raw pork suggest trichinosis, which may be confirmed by skin test, precipitin test, or muscle biopsy. Cardiac irritability and T-wave abnormalities in association with lobar pneumonia suggest pneumococcal myocarditis; in such cases sputum and blood cultures are usually positive. Right heart failure associated with malaise, fever, and splenomegaly in a child in the interior of Brazil is most likely due to infection with *Trypanosoma cruzi* or Chagas' disease, which may be confirmed by blood smear, xenodiagnosis, or rising antibody titer. Severe tachycardia or partial heart block in association with a tonsillar and occasionally cutaneous ulcer and membrane may indicate toxic myocarditis secondary to *Corynebacterium Diphtheriae.* Prompt examination of smear and culture are most helpful.

Toxic myocarditis, seen after ingestion of phosphorus or in association with emetine therapy, may be indistinguishable clinically from viral myocarditis.

Myocarditis of unknown etiology may also be difficult to differentiate from viral myocarditis. Furthermore, it is likely that many cases of this entity may be of viral etiology.

Rheumatic myocarditis is almost always associated with pericarditis and endocarditis; that is, it is a true pancarditis. Although a pericarditis may not develop or be so evanescent as not to be detected, a heart murmur is likely to be heard sooner or later. Extracardiac manifestations, so valuable diagnostically, may on occasion be fleeting or absent, especially in adulthood. Throat culture and serial antistreptolysin titers may be most helpful.

Tuberculous myocarditis is much rarer than tuberculous pericarditis, with which it is usually associated. It is of clinical importance inasmuch as specific and effective therapy is available. Associated pulmonary disease, mediastinal nodes, change in tuberculin reactivity, recovery of tubercle bacilli from sputum, gastric aspirate, pericardial fluid, or pericardial biopsy are of diagnostic value.

Viral Myocarditis Presenting as Congestive Heart Failure

When myocarditis presents as acute congestive heart failure, it may be difficult to differentiate from biventricular failure due to a *recent silent myocardial infarction* in an individual with coronary atherosclerosis and previous infarct and fibrosis, in whom the electrocardiogram may suggest localized damage. The latter may be revealed by a vectorcardiogram. A meticulous history and a search for prior electrocardiograms may also be helpful.

Acute pericardial effusion and early tamponade must be differentiated from diffuse myocarditis and failure. When there is no associated myocardial disease, gallop sounds are absent, but may be mimicked by pericardial sounds. In the absence of pulmonary disease, pulsus paradoxus points to a pericardial problem. Radiographic visualization of the right atrium by means of either carbon dioxide or contrast material injected intravenously or selectively will aid in the determination of pericardial fluid, which may also be demonstrated by means of echocardiography. Routine radiography and fluoroscopy have been disappointing in this regard.

Acute cor pulmonale, usually secondary to multiple pulmonary emboli, may be difficult to distinguish from myocarditis, especially if the emboli are silent or associated with minor pulmonary symptoms or radiographic densities suggesting infiltration compatible with viral pneumonitis. In both entities, right ventricular failure dominates, clinically. The presence of left ventricular failure points to myocarditis, especially in the absence of coronary disease. Evidence of right heart strain on electrocardiograms favors cor pulmonale. Pulmonary emboli should be especially suspected in association with recent surgical procedures, immobilization, pregnancy, and thrombogenic medications. A lung scan may be helpful. A pulmonary angiogram is the definitive diagnostic procedure. Pulmonary arterial pressure and vascular resistance should be determined at the same time; occasionally, elevated values in the absence of emboli establish the presence of sufficient pulmonary vascular or parenchymatous disease to account for right heart failure.

Beriberi heart disease characteristically has a rapid clinical evolution, although the deficiency of thiamine is usually chronic. As in myocarditis, there is biventricular failure with clinical dominance of right ventricular failure. Initial bradycardia yields to tachycardia. Electrocardiographic manifestations are nonspecific, but arrhythmias are rare. History of poor nutrition and increased demand for thiamine (e.g., growth, pregnancy, or hyperthyroidism) is helpful. Beriberi heart disease is not seen in the absence of neuropathy, but the latter may be mild and easily missed on routine examination. Untreated thiamine deficiency can be proved by means of the red blood cell transketolase assay. Except for the terminal stage, cardiac beriberi is characterized by high cardiac output and a narrow arterio-venous oxygen difference, whereas viral myocarditis is presumably associated with low-output failure.

Noninflammatory cardiomyopathies often remain clinically silent for a long time and present as heart failure. Unless a previous abnormal radiograph or electrocardiogram can be located, it is not possible to be certain whether one is dealing with an acute disease such as myocarditis or an acute manifestation of a chronic disease. Occasionally, a family history of cardiomyopathy is helpful. In general, in chronic cardiomyopathies patients the first attack of heart failure responds well to nonspecific therapy for congestive heart failure. Therefore, when the response is poor, one should favor myocarditis. However, especially in children, the latter usually also responds well [69]. A secondary cardiomyopathy may be recognized by characteristic extracardiac features [70]. For example, *hemochromatosis*, which presents most frequently as biventricular failure, is characterized by the association of pigmentary cirrhosis with diabetes mellitus and bronzing of the skin; determination of serum iron and liver biopsy establish the diagnosis. Congestive heart failure, supraventricular arrhythmias, and the abnormalities of conduction are frequent, whereas ventricular arrhythmias are rare.

Amyloidosis which most commonly presents as insidious and intractable congestive heart failure, is rare under the age of 40. It is a multisystem disease, often associated with chronic inflammatory or neoplastic diseases. A true restrictive cardiomyopathy, it may be characterized by a small, stiff heart with manifestations identical to those seen in constrictive pericarditis. Arrhythmias are frequent, especially atrial fibrillation. Heart block of all degrees may occur.

The differential diagnosis in children must include glycogen-storage disease [69] or *cardiac glycogenosis* (Cori's type II or Pompe's disease), a rare familial disorder. This disease which usually becomes manifest before the child's sixth month results in marked cardiac enlargement and ultimately leads to heart failure unless a fatal arrhythmia supervenes. Survival past the first year it rare. There is usually electrocardiographic evidence of left ventricular hypertrophy. The definitive diagnosis is made by demonstration of increased glycogen in skeletal muscle.

Endocardial fibroelastosis is a much more common disorder of childhood [69]. Only the primary form, that is, the form not associated with other congenital heart diseases, will be considered here. This is characterized by diffuse thickening of the endocardium, primarily in the left atrium and the left ventricle. Although it is usually considered a congenital lesion and results in death before age 5, similar lesions have been observed in older children and occasionally in adults. Clinically, the patient presents with biventricular heart failure. Although the process may involve both the mitral valve and aortic valve, heart murmurs and gallop sounds are rare. Electrocardiographic evidence of left ventricular hypertrophy may be helpful in the differentiation from myocarditis, but is not regularly seen. The clinical differentiation of acute myocarditis is most difficult.

Viral Myocarditis Presenting as Arrhythmia or Conduction Disturbance

Cardiac arrhythmia or conduction disturbance is probably the most frequent manner of presentation of viral myocarditis. This statement, however, holds true for most all myocarditides, regardless of etiology. In the usual setting of an acute febrile illness, or a routine screening examination, when as a rule a history of recent upper respiratory tract infection or gastrointestinal upset is obtainable, the most frequent and perhaps also the most difficult differential diagnosis is the so-called functional arrhythmia. Occasional atrial and even ventricular premature beats, bradycardia, shifting auricular pacemaker, and first-degree heart block are observed so frequently in association with febrile illness or with the stress of a screening medical examination that alone they can, at best, justify a raised sense of suspicion, leading to further investigation. Yet, it is unknown in what proportion of patients with such isolated phenomena foci of myocarditis actually exist. Functional irritability is often associated with increased vagal tone; if heart rate is increased by exercise, the irritability may subside. In contrast, exercise in myocarditis may bring out irritability [65, 71]. Whereas atrial and ventricular premature beats and first-degree heart block may be seen in healthy individuals, newly occurring atrial tachycardia, fibrillation or flutter, as well as ventricular tachycardia, and second- or third-degree heart block must always be considered associated with organic heart disease. In the United States, in adult patients, *ischemic heart disease* must again be given first consideration. It is not at all unusual for a coronary occlusion or myocardial infarction to have cardiac arrhythmia or block as its dominant manifestation. The possibility of a *coronary embolus* must be kept in mind, especially in cases of acute or chronic valvulitis with possible valvar verrucae or mural thrombi. Mural thrombi are also common in primary cardiomyopathy. Even in the absence of any inflammatory component, cardiomyopathy may be associated with fibrosis, which may result in arrhythmias or heart block when strategically located. Among the *secondary cardiomyopathies*, sarcoidosis is commonly associated with conduction disturbances, whereas arrhythmias are common in sarcoidosis, amyloidosis, carcinoid, and tumors metastatic to the heart, and may also occur in collagen diseases—here again, often in association with inflammatory lesions [70].

Viral Myocarditis Presenting as Valvar Insufficiency

When a patient with acute myocarditis is first seen in flagrant congestive heart failure, murmurs and other manifestations of mitral and tricuspid insufficiency, or both, may dominate the picture. Acute rheumatic carditis may thus be mimicked, and the picture may be difficult to differentiate from rheumatic or congenital heart disease. Even a good response to anticongestive therapy in insufficiency of the atrioventricular valves does not necessarily favor the diagnosis of myocarditis inasmuch as it is also characteristic of functional tricuspid and mitral regurgitation seen in association with some congenital and rheumatic lesions.

Viral Myocarditis Presenting as Circulatory Collapse

When myocarditis develops either rapidly or in association with depletion of circulatory blood volume, vascular collapse rather than congestive heart failure may result. The clinical picture may resemble that of acute myocardial infarction, or it may suggest hemorrhage or a surgical emergency. In the presence of epigastric pain due to an associated pericarditis, exploratory laparotomy may be resorted to, an unfortunate decision.

The response to expansion of plasma volume may be gratifying, and the primacy of the myocardial lesion may become evident when the ventricular filling pressures rise progressively as fluid is being replaced.

THERAPY

Specific Therapy

As yet, there is no specific therapy for true viral diseases. For clinical reasons, infections due to *Mycoplasma pneumoniae** and psittacosis* have been included in this chapter; these respond to tetracycline although it has not been established that the course of myocarditis per se is altered by antibiotics.

Control of Bodily Activity and Cardiac Overload

Inasmuch as myocardial function or at least cardiac reserve may be impaired, limitation of cardiac work load is advisable. Clinical experience suggests that myocarditis may be more severe in working or exercising individuals [29, 66]. The enhancing effect of exercise on experimental Coxsackie A and B myocarditis has been well established [4, 48]. It would thus seem wise to prescribe rest for the patient with acute myocarditis. Inasmuch as control of cardiac output is the goal, symptomatic therapy of pain, pruritis, anxiety, and fever may also be protective of the heart. Caution must be observed in the administration of parenteral fluids, both with regard to quantity and rate of delivery, lest the heart be overloaded and congestive heart failure be induced or aggravated.

* *Editorial Note:* These organisms are now usually considered to be intermediate between viruses and true bacteria.

Oxygen

Studies by Pearce with experimental vaccinia and pseudorabies infections suggest that hypoxia increases both incidence and severity of myocarditis [72]. Clinically, hypoxia plays a major pathogenic role in myocarditis seen in patients with influenza and poliomyelitis. A good case can thus be made for assuring adequate ventilation and oxygenation, especially in the presence of pulmonary infiltration, congestion or hypoventilation, or an irritable myocardium. Hyperbaric conditions, on the other hand, have been shown to enhance replication of Coxsackie B-1 virus in mouse hearts and to double mortality rate [73].

Surveillance and Resuscitation

In view of the unpredictability of cardiac arrhythmias, heart block, and sudden death [60-63], it is recommended that patients with acute myocarditis be placed under cardiac surveillance just as patients with acute myocardial infarction. Electrical cardioversion, defibrillation, and cardiac resuscitation [49, 53] have been used successfully in the management of acute myocarditis.

Artificial Pacemaker

In the presence of either second- or third-degree heart block [74] or Stokes-Adams attacks [75, 76] with ventricular escape, the insertion of a temporary artificial pacemaker may be indicated.

Antiarrhythmic Drugs

Atrial flutter or fibrillation with rapid ventricular response, rarely persistent in the absence of other heart disease, may require digitalization, which should be done cautiously. A lowered threshold for digitalis toxicity in patients with myocarditis has been postulated but not proved. Ventricular irritability may be treated with quinidine, procaine amide, or lidocaine. These antiarrhythmic agents, however, depress myocardial contractility and should be used with caution.

Digitalis Glycosides

Patients in congestive heart failure tend to respond well to digitalis glycosides, especially in childhood [69]. As mentioned, one must remain alert for digitalis toxicity. Other agents with positive inotropic action have been used, but their effect is less well documented. Isoproterenol may be useful if low cardiac output is associated with hypotension.

Diuretics

When there is fluid retention, hypervolemia, pulmonary congestion, or peripheral edema, limitation of sodium intake and judicious use of diuretics is generally effective. One must guard against loss of potassium and magnesium, which may enhance myocardial necrosis and lower the threshold of digitalis toxicity. Except in life-threatening situations or when there is evidence of considerable fluid retention, thiazide and mercurial diuretics should be given preference over more potent agents such as ethacrynic acid or furosemide which potentially may lead to depletion of plasma volume and hypotension [77].

Pericardiocentesis

Early detection of cardiac tamponade and pericardial paracentesis may be life saving.

Corticosteroids

Steroids have been used widely in the therapy of viral myocarditis and, by some, have been considered of clinical value [78]. However, controlled observations are lacking. It must be remembered that there is good evidence that in experimental viral infections steroids render the myocardial lesions more severe and increase mortality. Thus, Kilbourne and collaborators [79] reported evidence of synergistic action of cortisone and Coxsackie B-3 virus. This strain by itself produced only minimal focal lesions in the myocardium of healthy mice. Cortisone-treated mice, however, developed disseminated myocardial necrosis. Cortisone may well act by impairing the production of interferon [80].

It may thus be wise to reserve steroid therapy for the patient who does not respond to therapy and whose life appears threatened [49, 53] and then to withdraw steroids as soon as feasible. Finally, steroid therapy may facilitate secondary bacterial infections, which should be prevented when possible, or detected early and treated when not preventable.

Prevention

Considering the effectiveness of vaccination against smallpox, rubella, poliomyelitis, and influenza, it is evident that the ultimate approach to the more common and life-threatening viral infections will be prevention.

IMMEDIATE AND LONG-TERM PROGNOSIS

Whereas clinically evident acute viral myocarditis in infancy tends to be severe and carries a guarded prognosis [47, 50, 51], viral myocarditis in adulthood is generally benign, and fatal cases are rare [47, 49, 53, 56]. Recovery, however, may be delayed, symptoms and electrocardiographic abnormalities may be present for weeks to months, and clinical symptoms are known to recur. Bengtsson and Lamberger [81] report that of 90 patients presumed to have acute myocarditis who were observed for 5 years, 20 percent still had cardiac symptoms, most frequently precordial pain, oppression, or arrhythmia; 19 showed electrocardiographic abnormalities, and the exercise electrocardiogram was abnormal in 30 percent. The physical working capacity was reduced in 40 percent, and the heart volume was increased in 20 percent. Without control series, it is difficult to know to what extent some of these residual symptoms reflect residual heart disease or postinfectious asthenia [82, 83]. Of 22 patients with acute myocarditis associated with evidence of Coxsackie B virus infection, Sainani and associates [53] reported that 5 developed chronic heart failure, the time interval not being specified. Smith [49] reports that of 42 adult patients with myopericarditis attributed to Coxsackie B virus, recovery was complete in 82 percent, although in 12 patients it was prolonged to 3 months or more. In 17 percent of the cases there were 1 or more recurrences, over as long as 2 years. Two patients died during attacks of recurrent heart failure, but autopsy was not performed.

Kline and Saphir [84] reported 6 cases of chronic, pernicious myocarditis drawn from 225 cases of myocarditis examined pathologically. An enlarged heart with chronic interstitial myocarditis and replacement fibrosis was associated with a protracted, relentless downhill course and progressive heart failure. They culled 23 additional cases from the literature. The duration of the disease ranged from 1 month to 8 years. In none of Kline's cases was a viral illness identified, and only one of the cases cited from the literature followed a viral illness, namely measles. There is no evidence linking the clinical syndromes observed after viral myocarditis with chronic pernicious myocarditis.

That the majority of chronic cardiomyopathies appear primary or idiopathic has given rise to speculation that they might represent end-stages of an earlier acute myocarditis. Such a relationship now accepted for rheumatic myocarditis, Chagas' disease, and toxoplasmosis has been postulated for psittacosis [41, 85]. Perhaps insufficient time has elapsed for follow-up observations on cases with proved viral myocarditis to be available to confirm this point.

By means of fluorescent antibody techniques, however, viral antigens have occasionally been detected in a case of cardiomyopathy [86]. Only recently has it been shown that experimental murine infection with Coxsackie B-3 virus may be associated with persistent inflammation progressing to chronic myocardial fibrosis [87].

Immunofluorescent studies have also identified Coxsackie virus antigens in the mitral [67] and aortic [88] valves of patients dying with cardiomyopathy and myocarditis, respectively, suggesting that viral endocarditis may possibly be a precursor of chronic valvular heart disease.

REFERENCES

1. Abelmann, W. H.: Virus and the heart. Circulation 44:950, 1971.
2. Saphir, O.: Nonrheumatic inflammatory diseases of the heart. C. Myocarditis. In, Gould, S.E. (Ed.): Pathology of the Heart, 2nd ed. Springfield, Ill., Charles C Thomas, 1960, pp. 779-823.
3. Hudson, R. E. B.: Cardiovascular Pathology. Baltimore, Williams & Wilkins, 1965, Vol. 1, pp. 782-803; 1970; Vol. 3, pp. 483-498.
4. Tilles, J. G., Elson, S. H., Shaka, J. A., Abelmann, W. H., Lerner, A. M., and Finland, M.: Effects of exercise on Coxsackie A9 myocarditis in adult mice. Proc Soc Exp Biol Med 117:777, 1964.
5. Gore, I. and Saphir, O.: Myocarditis. A classification of 1402 cases. Am Heart J 34:827, 1947.
6. Vital Statistics of the United States 1967. Vol. II, Mortality, Part A. U.S. Department of Health, Education and Welfare, Public Health Service, Washington, D.C., 1969.
7. Scott, L. P., III, Gutelius, M. F., and Parrott, R. H.: Children with acute respiratory tract infections. An electrocardiographic survey. Am. J Dis Child 119: 111, 1970.
8. Stevens, P. J. and Underwood-Ground, K. E.: Occurrence and significance of myocarditis in trauma. Aerospace Med 41:776, 1970.
9. Acute Conditions, Incidence, and Associated Disability. United States, July 1964-1965. National Center for Health Statistics. Series 10, No. 26 (December) 1965.
10. Degen, J.A., Jr.: Visceral pathology in measles. A clinicopathologic study of 100 fatal cases. Am J Med Sci 194:104, 1937.
11. Ross, L. J.: Electrocardiographic findings in measles. Am J Dis Child 83:282, 1952.
12. Korones, S.B., Ainger, L.E., Monif, G.R.C., Roane, J., Sever, J.L., and Fuste, F.: Congenital rubella syndrome: Study of 22 infants. Myocardial damage and other new clinical aspects. Am J Dis Child 110:434, 1965.
13. Goldfinger, D., Schreiber, W., and Wosika, P.H.: Permanent heart block following German measles. Am J Med 2:320, 1947.
14. Logue, B.L. and Hanson, J.L.: Complete heart block in German measles. Am Heart J 30:205, 1945.
15. Moore, C.M., Henry, J., Benzing, G., III, and Kaplan, S.: Varicella myocarditis. Am J Dis Child 118:899, 1969.

16. Hackel, D.B.: Myocarditis in association with varicella. Am J Pathol 29:369, 1953.
17. Tatter, D., Gerard, P.W., Silverman, A.H., Wang, C., and Pearson, H.E.: Fatal varicella pancarditis in a child. Am J Dis Child 108:88, 1964.
18. Morales, A.R., Adelman, S., and Fine, G.: Varicella myocarditis. A case of sudden death. Arch Pathol 91:29, 1971.
19. Mant, K.: Mort subite due à une myocardite focale suivant une vaccination contre la variole. Ann Med Leg 43:1, 1963.
20. Rosenberg, E.H.: Acute myocarditis in mumps (epidemic parotitis). Arch Intern Med 76:257, 1945.
21. Bengtsson, E. and Orndahl, G.: Complications of mumps with special reference to the incidence of myocarditis. Acta Med Scand 149:381, 1954.
22. Roberts, W.C. and Fox, S.M., III: Mumps of the heart. Clinical and pathologic features. Circulation 32:342, 1965.
23. Hoagland, R.J.: Cardiac involvement in infectious mononucleosis. Am J Med Sci 232:252, 1956.
24. Bengtsson, C.: Infektiös mononukleos debuterande med cardit-symptom. Nord Med 22:1265, 1964.
25. Roseman, D.M. and Barry, R.M.: Acute pericarditis as the first manifestation of infectious mononucleosis. Ann Intern Med 47:351, 1957.
26. Wilson, D.R., Lenkei, S.C., and Paterson, J.F.: Acute constrictive epicarditis following infectious mononucleosis. Circulation 23:257, 1961.
27. Saphir, O., Amromin, G.D., and Yokoo, H.: Myocarditis in viral (epidemic) hepatitis. Am J Med Sci 231:168, 1956.
28. Loeffler, H.: Ueber 14 todesfaelle an hepatitis epidemica. Gastroenterologia 69:258, 1944.
29. Sanghvi, L.M., and Misra, S.N.: Electrocardiographic abnormalities in epidemic hepatitis, Circulation 16:88, 1957.
30. Maretic, Z. and Kuze-Capar, Z.: Das elektrokardiogramm bei infektioeser hepatitis. Z. Kreislaufforsch 59: 1116, 1970.
31. Lyon, E.: Virus Diseases and the Cardiovascular System. A Survey. New York, Grune & Stratton, 1956, p. 215.
32. Abelmann, W.H., Kowalski, H.J., and McNeely, W.F.: Cardiovascular studies during acute infectious hepatitis. Gastroenterology 27:61, 1954.
33. Painton, J.F., Hicks, A.M., and Hartman, S.: Clinical analysis of primary atypical pneumonia. Ann Intern Med 24:775, 1946.
34. Lewes, D. and Rainford, D.J.: Symptomless myocarditis and myalgia in viral and mycoplasma pneumoniae infections. Br Heart J 33:613, 1971.
35. Henson, D. and Mufson, M.A.: Myocarditis and pneumonitis with type 21 adenovirus infection. Association with fatal myocarditis and pneumonitis. Am J Dis Child 121:334, 1971.
36. Finland, M., Parker, F., Barnes, M.W., and Joliffe, L.S.: Acute myocarditis in influenza A infections—two cases of nonbacterial myocarditis, with isolation of virus from the lungs. Am J Med Sci 209:455, 1945.
37. Adamy, G.: Klinische studie ueber psittakose. Dtsch. Arch Klin Med 169:301, 1930.
38. Grist, N.R. and McLean, C.: Infections by organisms of psittacosis/lymphogranuloma venereum group in the west of Scotland. Br Med J 2:21, 1964.
39. Jannach, J.R.: Myocarditis in infancy with inclusions characteristic of psittacosis. Am J Dis Child 96:734, 1958.

40. MacLennan, W.J., Dymock, I.W., and Ross, C.A.C.: Cardiac involvement in psittacosis. Br Med J 4:620, 1967.
41. Sutton, G.C., Morrissey, R.A., Tobin, J.R., Jr., and Anderson, T.O.: Pericardial and myocardial disease associated with serological evidence of infection by agents of the psittacosislymphogranuloma venereum group (Chlamydiaceae). Circulation 36:830, 1967.
42. Ahvenainen, E.K.: Inclusion disease or generalized salivary gland virus infection. Report of five cases. Acta Pathol Microbiol Scand Suppl 93:159, 1952.
43. Bodey, G.P., Wertlake, P.T., Douglas, G., and Levin, R.H.: Cytomegalic inclusion disease in patients with acute leukemia. Ann Intern Med 62:899, 1965.
44. Jungeblut, C.W. and Edwards, D.E.: Isolation of poliomyelitis virus from the heart in fatal cases. Am J Clin Pathol 21:601, 1951.
45. Weinstein, L. and Shelokov, A.: Cardiovascular manifestations in acute poliomyelitis. New Engl J Med 244:281, 1951.
46. Hildes, J.A., Schaberg, A., and Alcock, A.J.W.: Cardiovascular collapse in acute poliomyelitis. Circulation 12:986, 1955.
47. Grist, N.R. and Bell, E.J.: Coxsackie viruses and the heart. Editorial. Am. Heart J 77:295, 1969.
48. Lerner, A.M.: Coxsackie virus myocardiopathy. Editorial. J Infect Dis 120:496, 1969.
49. Smith, W.G.: Coxsackie B. myopericarditis in adults. Am Heart J 80:34, 1970.
50. Javett, S.N., Heymann, S., Mundel, B., Pepler, W.J., Lurie, H.I., Gear, J., Measroch, V., and Kirsch, Z.: Myocarditis in the newborn infant. A study of an outbreak associated with Coxsackie group B virus infection in a maternity home in Johannesburg. J Pediat 48:1, 1956.
51. Kibrick, S. and Benirschke, K.: Acute aseptic myocarditis and meningoencephalitis in the newborn child infected with Coxsackie virus group B, type 3. New Engl J Med 255:883, 1956.
52. Helin, M., Savola, J., and Lapinleimu, K.: Cardiac manifestations during a Coxsackie B5 epidemic. Br Med J 3:97, 1968.
53. Sainani, G., Krompotic, E., and Slodki, S.J.: Adult heart disease due to the Coxsackie virus B infection. Medicine 47:133, 1968.
54. Report to the Director of Public Health Laboratory Service from various laboratories in the United Kingdom: Coxsackie B5 virus infections during 1965. Br Med J 4:575, 1967.
55. Grist, N.R. and Bell, E.J.: Enteroviruses and cardiac disease. Lancet 2:1188, 1970.
56. Bell, E.J. and Grist, N.R.: Echo viruses, carditis, and acute pleurodynia. Am Heart J 82:133, 1971.
57. Cherry, J.D., Jahn, C.L., and Meyer, T.C.: Paroxysmal atrial tachycardia associated with ECHO 9 virus infection. Am Heart J 73:681, 1967.
58. Monif, G.R.G., Lee, C.W., and Hsiung, G.D.: Isolated myocarditis with recovery of ECHO type 9 virus from the myocardium. New Engl J Med 277:1353, 1967.
59. Russell, S.J.M. and Bell, E.J.: Echoviruses and carditis. Lancet 1:784, 1970.
60. Gormsen, H.: Sudden unexplained death due to myocarditis. Acta Pathol Microbiol Scand Suppl 105:30, 1955.
61. Corby, C.: Isolated myocarditis as a cause of sudden obscure death. Med Sci Law 1:23, 1960.
62. Kuller, L., Lilienfeld, A., and Fisher, R.: Sudden and unexpected deaths in young adults. An epidemiological study. JAMA 198:158, 1966.

63. Luke, J.L. and Helpern, M.: Sudden unexpected death from natural causes in young adults. A review of 275 consecutive autopsied cases. Arch Pathol 85:10, 1968.
64. Abelmann, W.H.: Current Concepts: Myocarditis. New Engl J Med 275:832, 944, 1966.
65. Levander-Lindgren, M.: Studies in myocarditis. II. Electrocardiographic changes. Cardiologia 47:73, 1965.
66. Sutton, G.C., Harding, H.B., Trueheart, R.P., and Clark, H.P.: Coxsackie B4 myocarditis in an adult: Successful isolation of virus from ventricular myocardium. Aerospace Med 38:66, 1967.
67. Burch, G.E., Sun, S.C., Colcolough, H.L., Sohal, R.S., and DePasquale, N.P.: Coxsackie B viral myocarditis and valvulitis identified on routine autopsy specimens by immunofluorescent techniques. Am Heart J 74:13, 1967.
68. Haas, J.E. and Yunis, E.J.: Viral crystalline arrays in human Coxsackie myocarditis. Lab Invest 23:442, 1970.
69. Rosenbaum, H.D., Nadas, A.S., and Neuhauser, E.B.D.: Primary myocardial disease in infancy and childhood. Am J Dis Child 86:28, 1953.
70. Wheeler, R.C. and Abelmann, W.H.: Cardiomyopathy associated with systemic diseases. Cardiovasc Clin 4:283-303, 1972.
71. Bengtsson, E.: Working capacity and heart volume in patients with electrocardiographic abnormalities suggestive of acute myocarditis during various acute infectious diseases. Acta Med Scand 159:499, 1957.
72. Pearce, J.H.: Heart disease and filtrable viruses. Circulation 21:448, 1960.
73. Orsi, E.V., Mancini, R., and Barriso, J.: Hyperbaric enhancement of Coxsackievirus infection in mice. Aerospace Med 41:1169, 1970.
74. Johnson, J.L.: Complete atrioventricular heart block secondary to acute myocarditis requiring intracardiac pacing. J Pediat 78:312, 1971.
75. Pansini, R., Fersini, C., Farinelli, A., Sbrighi, V., Ripa, R., and Grandi, L.: Miocardite primitiva dell'adulto da virus Coxsackie (gruppo B, tipo 5) ad espressivita sincopale pluriricorrente da iperattivita ventricolare parossistica. Primo contributo anatomoclinico. Minerva Med 55:1641, 1964.
76. Harris, R., Siew, S., and Lev, M.: Smoldering myocarditis with intermittent complete AV block and Stokes-Adams syndrome. A histopathologic and electrocardiographic study of "trifascicular" bundle branch block. Am J Cardiol 24:880, 1969.
77. Ramirez, A. and Abelmann, W.H.: Hemodynamic effects of diuresis by ethacrynic acid. Arch Intern Med 121:320, 1968.
78. Ainger, L.E.: Acute aseptic myocarditis: Corticosteroid therapy. J Pediat 64:716, 1964.
79. Kilbourne, E.D., Wilson, C.B., and Perrier, D.: The induction of gross myocardial lesions by a Coxsackie (pleurodynic) virus and cortisone. J Clin Invest 35:362, 1956.
80. Rytel, M.W.: Interferon response during Coxsackie B-3 infection in mice: I. The effect of cortisone. J Infect Dis 120:379, 1969.
81. Bengtssen, E. and Lamberger, B.: Five-year follow-up study of cases suggestive of acute myocarditis. Am Heart J 72:751, 1966.
82. Pruitt, R.D.: Acute myocarditis in the adult. Progr Cardiovasc Dis 7:73, 1964.
83. Levander-Lindgren, M.: Studies in myocarditis. IV. Late prognosis. Cardiologia 47:209, 1965.

84. Kline, I.K. and Saphir, O.: Chronic pernicious myocarditis. Am Heart J 59:681, 1960.
85. Sutton, G.C., Demakis, J.A., Anderson, T.O., and Morrissey, R.A.: Serologic evidence of a sporadic outbreak in Illinois of infection by Chlamydia (psittacosis-LGV agent) in patients with primary myocardial disease and respiratory disease. Am Heart J 81:597, 1971.
86. Kawai, C.: Idiopathic cardiomyopathy. A study on the infectious immune theory as a cause of the disease. Jap Circ J 35:765, 1971.
87. Wilson, F.M., Miranda, Q.R., Chason, J.L., and Lerner, A.M.: Residual pathologic changes following murine Coxsackie A and B myocarditis. Am J Pathol 55:253, 1969.
88. Burch, G.E. and Colcolough, H.L.: Progressive Coxsackie viral pancarditis and nephritis. Ann Intern Med 71:963, 1969.

EVELYN V. HESS, B.CH., B.A.O., M.D.
and ALAN KIRSNER, M.D.

Immunologic Studies in Myocardial Diseases

INTRODUCTION

The etiology and pathogenic mechanisms of many types of myocardial disease are not known. Research on these aspects of myocardial disease has involved many disciplines. With the advent of modern immunology, it was logical that this new discipline with all its new techniques be applied to the problems of idiopathic myocardial disease. An association between immunological abnormalities and some forms of heart disease has been known since the early 1930s. With the introduction of immunofluorescent techniques, heart-reactive antibody [1], and antibody cross reactive with Group A streptococci [2] were demonstrated in the sera of rheumatic fever patients. Subsequent work showed that immune mechanisms played a major role in the pathogenesis of the carditis of acute rheumatic fever [3]. Heart-reactive antibody (HRA) has also been found in patients with chronic rheumatic heart disease, endomyocardial fibrosis, "idiopathic" cardiomyopathy, postcardiotomy and postmyocardial infarction syndrome, bacterial endocarditis, and idiopathic hypertrophic subaortic stenosis. Gamma globulin bound to heart tissue has been demonstrated by the direct immunofluorescent technique in acute rheumatic fever, rheumatic heart disease, idiopathic cardiomyopathy, and endomyocardial fibrosis. Finally, cardiac transplant has added the problem of cardiac rejection and has shown the physical relationship between the immune system and the myocardium.

The myocardium is antigenically complex [4]. Myocardial antigens can be classed as organ specific (present in cardiac myofibers), tissue specific (present in both cardiac and skeletal muscle), and antigens common to

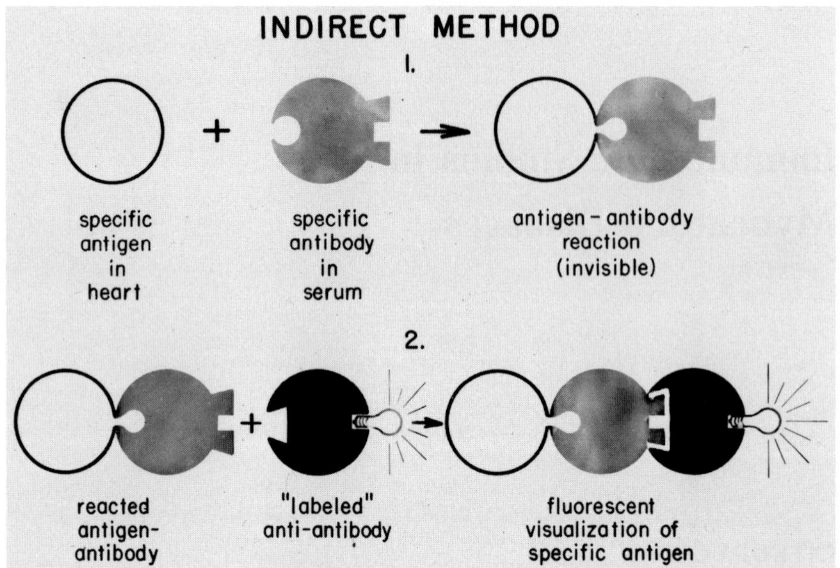

Figure 1. Indirect immunofluorescence technique to demonstrate serum heart reactive antibody (sandwich technique). If the serum to be tested contains antibody to various sites in heart muscle, they will be visualized as bright green fluorescence with ultraviolet light.

myocardium and other organs and tissues. Both soluble and insoluble antigens have been described. There are also myocardial antigens cross reactive with group A streptococcal cell walls, cell wall extracts, and cell membranes.

The antibodies reactive with myocardium have been demonstrated by immunofluorescence (Fig. 1) complement fixation, tanned cell hemagglutination, antiglobulin consumption, precipitation, and collodion particle agglutination testing [5]. Kaplan and coworkers, using immunofluorescence, demonstrated 3 patterns of staining: sarcolemmal-subsarcolemmal (SS), intermyofibrillar (IMF), and diffuse (D) sarcoplasmic [6]. The sarcolemmal-subsarcolemmal staining is observed most frequently in rheumatic fever. Intermyofibrillar staining is less commonly noted. The diffuse sarcoplasmic staining has been seen in inflammatory conditions and infection. These observations have been confirmed by other groups [7, 8].

It is the purpose of this chapter to summarize the recent literature with emphasis on the role of immune mechanisms in myocardial disease. Several comprehensive reviews covering the whole subject of autoimmunity and the heart have recently appeared [5, 9, 10].

RHEUMATIC FEVER AND RHEUMATIC CARDITIS

Evidence supporting the concept of an immune mechanism in the pathogenesis of heart disease is most convincing in the carditis of rheumatic fever, and the Group A streptococcus is now accepted as the etiologic agent of this disease. The evidence for this includes: (1) The lag period between a streptococcal infection and the onset of carditis provides time for antibody formation; (2) Elevated antibody titers are found to multiple streptococcal extracellular antigens; (3) Recurrent attacks of acute rheumatic fever are more commonly seen with a high titer response; (4) Heart-reactive antibody is found in rheumatic fever, and the titers are higher and percent positivity greater in acute rheumatic fever than in chronic rheumatic heart disease; (5) Autopsy studies have demonstrated gamma globulin and complement in cardiac tissue of rheumatic carditis patients; (6) An immunological cross reaction has been demonstrated between Group A streptococcal cell wall and cell membrane antigens and human heart tissue, and these cross-reactive antibodies have been detected in the sera of patients with rheumatic fever; (7) An immunological cross reaction between Group A streptococcus polysaccharide and the structural glycoproteins of the heart valves has been demonstrated.

With a variety of immunologic techniques, heart-reactive antibody has been demonstrated in 25 to 63 percent of patients with acute rheumatic fever. The percentage of positive tests is lower in rheumatic heart disease without carditis [11]. Using indirect immunofluorescence, Hess and coworkers have demonstrated heart reactive antibodies in 41.5 percent of 171 patients with acute rheumatic fever, 16.4 percent of 201 patients with inactive rheumatic disease, and 3 percent of 66 normal individuals. Sixty-three percent of 71 patients with carditis but only 26 percent of 74 patients with rheumatic fever without carditis had positive reactions [7]. Kaplan and coworkers reported that 77 percent of 40 patients with acute rheumatic fever and 63 percent of 79 patients with inactive rheumatic heart disease exhibited heart-reactive antibody using indirect immunofluorescence [6]. Studies using antiglobulin consumption and passive hemagglutination tests have yielded similar results [3].

Gamma globulin deposits in auricular appendage biopsy [12, 13] and immunoglobulins in postmortem rheumatic heart tissues [14] have been demonstrated by immunofluorescence and electron microscopy. These were present in 18 percent of 100 auricular appendages from rheumatic hearts. One of 33 nonrheumatic hearts showed bound gamma globulin. Deposits were observed in myofibers, sarcolemma, interstitial connective tissues, and vessel walls. The tissue sites demonstrating fixation of gamma globulin

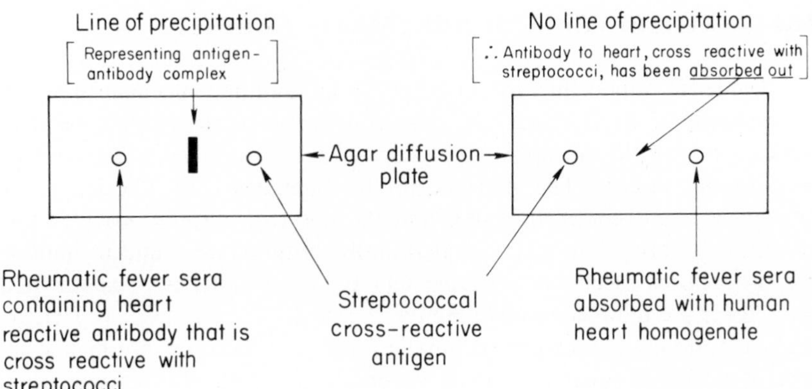

Figure 2. Demonstration of a positive reaction in precipitation-absorption test. In the left agar diffusion plate, serum from a patient with rheumatic fever is shown to have heart-reactive antibody cross reactive with streptococcal antigen. On the right, absorption of the same rheumatic fever sera with human heart homogenate, "absorbs out" the antibody to heart, cross reactive to streptococcal antigen, and precipitation does not occur.

frequently exhibited alteration as indicated by affinity for eosin and by strongly positive reactions with the periodic acid-Schiff stain (PAS) [12]. Immunofluorescence showed widespread deposition of immunoglobulin and C3 (third component of complement) in the hearts of 5 children who died of acute rheumatic fever with carditis. Deposits were localized primarily in sarcolemma of cardiac myofibers and also in smooth muscle of vessel walls, in the endocardium, and in interstitial connective tissue [14].

Evidence of an immunologic cross reaction between the cell walls of Group A streptococci and human heart tissue was first reported in 1962 [2]. Kaplan and Meyeserian demonstrated that rabbit antisera to the cell walls of a type 5 strain, cross reacted with human heart by both immunofluorescent and complement fixation tests [Fig. 2]. The streptococcal cross-reactive antigen was shown to be a protein constituent of streptococcal cell walls and was consistently found associated with M protein, the virulence factor of the Group A streptococcus [3, 15]. Subsequent work showed that type 12, type 19 streptococcal cells, and acid-extract preparations, including highly purified M protein preparations, were cross reactive [3].

However, the more recent studies of Zabriskie and coworkers suggest that all Group A strain streptococci possess this antigen which is present regardless of the type-specific M protein [16]. They pointed to the cell (protoplast) membrane of the Group A streptococcus as the locus of the antigenic determinant of a cross-reactive antibody system [17]. Recent data from these investigations suggest that the cell membrane is the antigen responsible for the cross reaction with the cardiac myofibers.

An immunological cross reaction between the polysaccharide specific to the Group A streptococcus and the structural glycoproteins isolated from human heart valves has been demonstrated [18].

Various techniques have been used to demonstrate antibodies to myocardium in the sera of patients with streptococcal disease [3, 19], cross reactive with Group A streptococci. Kaplan and Svec demonstrated that sera from patients with streptococcal infections may contain antibody to heart. This antibody also reacted with streptococcal antigen in gel diffusion plates and could be completely absorbed from serum with heart but not other organ tissue [19].

Zabriskie and associates have recently shown that the heart-reactive antibody in rheumatic fever sera can be absorbed out with streptococcal cell membranes, but that the heart-reactive antibody in sera from patients with the postcardiotomy syndrome is not absorbed. Absorption with human heart tissue (mostly muscle) absorbs out both antibodies [20]. Investigators have recently begun to study the role of cellular immune mechanisms in heart disease. Lymphocytes from rheumatic fever patients have been shown to be cytotoxic to human cardiac cells [21], and other work has shown that lymphocytes play a role in the rat experimental myocarditis model [22]

There is now ample evidence to support the hypothesis that immune mechanisms are related to the pathogenesis of the carditis of rheumatic fever. Patients with Group A streptococcal infections who develop rheumatic carditis produce heart-reactive antibodies that cross react with the Group A streptococcus. The titer of these heart-reactive antibodies correlates well with the presence of acute rheumatic processes. Thus in Zabriskie's work, strong immunofluorescent staining of cardiac tissue by circulating antiheart antibody in serologic titers over 1:10 was not seen except in rheumatic fever. Immunoglobulins have been demonstrated in the myocardium of patients with rheumatic carditis. To date, studies to demonstrate either antiheart or antistreptococcal antibody activity in these deposits have not been reported. These would require either study of the specific antibody activity of the immunoglobulin eluted from rheumatic fever hearts or direct immunofluorescent staining of such hearts with labeled antistreptococcal and antiheart antibodies.

There is a good temporal relationship also between the active process and the heart-reactive antibodies as shown by a number of investigators. It is of interest to note that patients with rheumatic fever lack the secondary phenomena such as rheumatoid factors, antinuclear antibody and associated connective tissue disorders that are so common in the presence of autoimmune reactions [7]. Humoral factors do not explain the other manifestations of acute rheumatic fever. It is possible that cellular mechanisms are important in their causation.

IDIOPATHIC CARDIOMYOPATHY

Idiopathic cardiomyopathy (IC) is a disease of unknown etiology in which immunologic mechanisms have been considered. There are several reports of heart-reactive antibody in patients with IC, and two groups have reported gamma and immunoglobulins bound to heart tissue. Using a direct immunofluorescence technique, Sanders and Ritts found gamma globulin in the ventricular musculature of 5 of 9 patients. Two of 16 control subjects hearts showed weak immunofluorescent staining [23]. Das and coworkers demonstrated immunoglobulin by direct immunofluorescence in heart tissue from 3 patients with severe congestive cardiomyopathy. Complement (C3) was found in 2 of the hearts. Heart-reactive antibody was not present in any of these sera [24].

Several groups have searched for circulating heart-reactive antibody. Robinson and coworkers noted an 11 percent incidence of heart-reactive antibody [25], and Fletcher and Wenger found that the frequency was not significantly different from that of a mixed control group [26]. Using an indirect immunoflourescent method, Das and coworkers found heart reactive antibody in 6 of 35 patients (17 percent) with idiopathic cardiomegaly, 7 of 8 patients (88 percent) with idiopathic hypertrophic subaortic stenosis, and in 1 of 43 control subjects [27].

Studies at the University of Cincinnati Medical Center were carried out in two groups of patients. The first group, composed of 33 patients (studied on 1 occasion), had a 12 percent incidence of heart-reactive antibody. This was greater than found in controls (4 percent) but less than in patients with other cardiac diseases (33.33 percent) [8]. The second group of patients was studied serially over a period of 2 years. The presence of heart-reactive antibody was correlated with exacerbation and remission of disease and serum complement (C3) level. Twenty-eight percent were found to have heart-reactive antibody at some time during their course, but it did not correlate with exacerbation or remission of disease. The titers were low; the staining pattern was predominantly subsarcolemmal. The C3 levels were normal during both remission and exacerbation of disease. It does not appear that humoral immunologic factors play a role in the etiology or pathogenesis of idiopathic cardiomyopathy. It is more likely that heart-reactive antibody represents an as yet undetermined secondary immunologic phenomenon [28].

ENDOMYOCARDIAL FIBROSIS, INFECTIVE ENDOCARDITIS, AND SEPSIS

Endomyocardial fibrosis (EF) is a disease mainly of the tropics, characterized by progressive fibrous thickening of the endocardium and inner aspect of myocardium of either or both ventricles [10]. The cause is unknown, but immunologic mechanisms have been suggested. Immunofluorescent studies of the organs of 8 patients who died of endomyocardial fibrosis revealed the presence of fibrin deposits in heart, kidney, spleen, liver, pancreas, thyroid, and lungs. In addition, immunoglobulin (IgG) was demonstrated, confined mainly to sacrolemmal and subsarcolemmal sites. Heart-reactive antibodies (IgG) were demonstrated by immunofluorescence in the sera of 9 of 25 female patients and 14 of 18 male patients with endomyocardial fibrosis. Cryoglobulins were detected in the sera of 38 of 43 patients with endomyocardial fibrosis, and there was an increased incidence of gastric parietal cell and thyroid antibodies [29]. Using immunofluorescence, Shaper et al. reported heart-reactive antibody in 71 percent of patients with endomyocardial fibrosis, 47 percent with mixed cardiac diseases, 46 percent with rheumatic heart disease, 43 percent with pulmonary tuberculosis, and 27 percent with hypertension. They also showed a positive correlation between the presence of malarial antibody titers and heart-reactive antibody [30]. Subsequently, they described an immunological syndrome consisting of high titers of malarial antibody, high levels of IgM and circulating autoantibodies to heart, thyroid and gastric parietal cells in immigrant and indigenous peoples of Uganda [31]. These patients had a variety of diseases, mostly of infectious nature. It is suggested that such an abnormal immunologic diathesis, presumably related to malarial infection, might have pathogenetic significance for endomyocardial fibrosis [11]. Thus, although ample evidence has been presented for an increased incidence of heart-reactive antibody and heart-bound antibody in endomyocardial fibrosis and other diseases present in African patients, there is currently no direct evidence for an immunologic role in the etiology or pathogenesis of the disease.

Das and coworkers recently reported heart-reactive antibody in 7 of 9 patients with infective endocarditis. Follow-up study of sera obtained 3 to 6 weeks following institution of antimicrobial treatment showed negative reactions [32]. With an indirect immunofluorescent technique, 10 patients with subacute bacterial endocarditis and positive latex tests for rheumatoid factors were studied for heart-reactive antibody at the University of Cincinnati Medical Center. Serial samples of serum were available on each patient, and heart-reactive antibody was present in the serum of 9 of the 10 cases. The appearance of heart-reactive antibody tended to parallel the appearance and disappearance of rheumatoid factor and positive blood cultures. Myocardial immunofluorescent staining was sarcolemmal-subsarcolemmal or intermyofibrillar with occasional diffuse staining. Two patients with septicemia unrelated to infective endocarditis also showed weak sarcolemmal-subsarcolemmal and diffuse staining [33].

Patients with chronic infections (leprosy, pulmonary tuberculosis, syphilis, and subacute bacterial endocarditis) often produce large amounts of rheumatoid factors [34, 35]. Shaper and associates reported 2 cases with syphilitic aortitis and 6 of 14 patients with pulmonary tuberculosis with heart antibody [30].

These data suggest that antibody to heart tissue may be found in diseases in which there is no direct involvement of the myocardium but in which antibody production may be stimulated by chronic infection. Syphilis, tuberculosis, and subacute bacterial endocarditis would fall in this category. Rheumatoid factor has also been demonstrated in these diseases [34]. Antigen-antibody complex with *P. Malaria* antigen has been shown to be present in the kidneys of Nigerian children with nephrotic syndrome and suggests the possibility that a similar mechanism may be operative in EF to account for the in vitro and in vivo findings in this disease, especially if the condition is related to chronic infection or malaria [36].

THE POST-THORACIC-CARDIAC INJURY SYNDROMES

The post-thoracic cardiac injury syndromes which have been shown to have heart-reactive antibody include: (1) the post-thoracic injury syndrome which may follow either blunt or penetrating trauma; (2) The post-thoracotomy or post-pericardiotomy syndrome; (3) The postmyocardial infarction syndrome (Dressler's); and (4) The syndrome of idiopathic nonspecific pericarditis.

Using an immunofluorescent test for heart-reactive antibody (HRA), Kaplan and associates reported a 78 percent incidence in patients with rheumatic heart disease tested 1 to 3 weeks after mitral valve surgery [6], but did not relate the presence of these antibodies to the postcardiotomy syndrome in these patients. Using a tanned red cell test, Robinson and Brigden reported positive tests for heart-reactive antibody in 6 of 30 patients following cardiotomy of whom 5 developed clinical features of the postcardiotomy syndrome. Tests were negative in 30 patients whose postcardiotomy course was uneventful. In some patients, HRA were detected prior to the evolution of clinical features and all became negative with spontaneous or steroid-induced remission [37].

In an earlier study, a striking increase in the incidence of HRA after cardiac surgery for rheumatic heart disease was noted [7]. Using indirect immunofluorescence and an antiglobulin consumption test, Van der Geld reported HRA in the sera of 13 of 15 cases with the post-pericardiotomy syndrome and in 8 of 14 cases with the postmyocardial infarction syndrome. In 3 cases of myocardial infarction, HRA were observed in the serum although the patient had no symptoms of the postmyocardial infarction syndrome. HRA were also found after cardiac surgery in sera of patients without concomitant signs of the postpericardiotomy syndrome [38].

Diffuse staining heart-reactive antibody was noted in 6 of 22 patients with myocardial infarction and SS-IMF staining was found in an additional patient [7]. Dodson and coworkers reported heart hemagglutinins in 29 percent of myocardial infarction patients compared to 6 percent of normal control subjects [39]. In an early report, using a tanned cell hemagglutination test Ehrenfeld et al. reported obtaining positive reactions in 12 of 53 patients with a history of acute myocardial infarction and 3 of 33 patients with chronic coronary artery disease of whom several patients were found a number of years following the infarction [40]. In a recent study, Ebringer et al. reported that serum immunoglobulin G (IgG) levels fell over a period of 5 to 7 days after myocardial infarction and subsequently became elevated considerably above control levels. Patients with chest pain without myocardial infarction failed to show this biphasic response [41].

Using a tanned red cell hemagglutination test for heart-reactive antibody, Robinson and Brigden reported positive tests in 6 of 15 patients with idiopathic pericardit There were no differences in the clinical features, past history, or n. .ber of recurrences in patients with positive and negative reactions. Three of 4 patients with postmyocardial infarction syndrome had positive tests for HRA. Twelve of 14 patients with postcardiotomy syndrome had positive tests for HRA, and in all except 1, the reactions became negative with clinical resolution of the disease. In some cases, antibody returned and heralded the onset of clinical exacerbation [42].

Although there is ample evidence that there is a higher incidence of heart-reactive antibody in patients with the postthoracic-cardiac injury syndrome than in normal controls, at present it is uncertain whether or not immune mechanisms play a role in their pathogenesis. Certain features which suggest such mechanisms include fever, arthralgias and at times arthritis, serositis (pericarditis and pleuritis), a latent period following injury, the temporal correlation of serum antibody to diathesis of disease, and the decreasing titer of serum antibody with clinical remission. However, this is all indirect evidence, and the nature of these interrelationships remains obscure. Zabriskie has shown that the sera of postsurgery patients contains HRA which is not related to streptococcal-induced antigen [20].

Much further study is required before deciding if the immune mechanisms noted above are all secondary to cardiac injury and unrelated to etiology or pathogenesis.

THE IMMUNOLOGY OF CARDIAC TRANSPLANTATION

The fate of the acute untreated cardiac homograft is similar to that of other organs. It presents the characteristic gross appearance of congestion, edema, and extensive subendocardial hemorrhage. There is early infiltration with mononuclear cells, associated with injury to vascular endothelium which results in interstitial hemorrhage and edema and anoxic injury to the muscle fibers. The major pathologic process associated with chronic rejection is one of continuous or repeated subclinical damage to the intima of the arterial vessels, which results in proliferation and fibrosis with progressive luminal narrowing. The process proceeds insidiously until late in the course of rejection. This coronary arterial narrowing is presumably the result of immunologic damage to the endothelium [43].

As currently used, tissue typing usually means the typing of leukocyte antigens. These have been identified principally by leukoagglutination and lymphocyte cytotoxicity reactions using allogenic antisera. All of these antigens are determined by a single genetic locus called HL-A. Several groups have now reported HL-A histocompatibility and survival data in patients with heart transplantation. Terasaki and coworkers in a preliminary report correlating HL-A histocompatibility and survival in 48 patients with heart transplantation felt that there was some relation between survival and compatibility for HL-A antigens [44]. Botha reviewed the HL-A histocompatibility data of 5 patients receiving cardiac transplants in South Africa. He also felt that there was evidence to suggest that the degree of mismatching in heart transplantation may be correlated with rejection and suggested that grade D mismatches (mismatches for 4 or more antigens) be avoided [45].

Fernback, Nora, and Cooley observed that of 7 patients who died of rejection, 4 were D matches. Their longest surviving recipient had the best tissue match (C+) and had shown no evidence of rejection. They felt their data indicated a high risk of rejection in poorly matched cases and suggested that it would seem imperative that adequate prospective histocompatibility typing be used in each situation [46].

However, data recently reported by the Stanford University transplantation team did not support the above conclusions. The HL-A typing in 30 cases of cardiac transplantation revealed no significant relationship between the number of mismatches and postoperative survival, rejection history, or clinical status. Their most striking finding was that HL-A mismatching does not preclude long-term survival with satisfactory graft function. Three of their 4 recipients living more than 2 years after transplantation were mismatched for 4 antigens [47].

Rosen and coworkers examined cardiac tissue from transplanted hearts and found bound immunoglobulins in all 15 hearts. Most patients had HRA in the serum prior to transplantation. Very little bound globulin was found in the original hearts. Thirteen of 19 had positive lymphocytoxicity testing post-transplant [48].

At the present time, therefore, the data assessing the usefulness of HL-A histocompatibility antigens are conflicting and point to the need for more experience with this system in long-term follow-up of cardiac transplantation patients.

CONNECTIVE TISSUE DISEASE

Systemic lupus erythematosus (SLE) and rheumatoid arthritis (RA) are systemic diseases that involve the heart as well as other organ systems. The etiology is unknown, but there is ample evidence of altered immune mechanisms in the pathogenesis of both diseases. In recent years, these relationships have been clarified in regard to the kidney in systemic lupus erythematosus and to the joints in rheumatoid arthritis, but the mechanism of cardiac involvement in both conditions remains obscure.

Systemic Lupus Erythematosus

Immune complexes have been shown to play an important role in the pathogenesis of the renal lesions [49] and, perhaps, of cutaneous lesions [50] in systemic lupus erythematosus. Numerous investigators have demonstrated gamma globulin [51] and various complement components [52] in the renal glomeruli of patients with lupus nephritis. Schur and Sandson [49] correlated the immunologic factors and clinical activity in patients with SLE. They found that reduced serum complement levels and high titers of complement-fixing antibodies to DNA were associated with active disease, whereas the absence of these abnormalities usually indicated inactive disease. These serologic findings may reflect the in vivo formation of immune complexes associated with nephritis and possibly with the skin lesions as well as the autoimmune hemolytic anemia of SLE.

Although carditis frequently occurs in SLE, similar immunologic correlations have not been made. In our experience, serum complement is not reduced with the carditis of SLE, unless there is active "complex" disease elsewhere. Results of heart-reactive antibody studies in SLE are conflicting. Das et al. found such antibodies in 20 of 32 consecutive patients with SLE [53]. Hess et al. [7] and Zabriskie [16] failed to find HRA in 28 patients with systemic lupus erythematosus. Kaplan et al. [6] reported HRA in 5 of 11 patients. All these patients had antinuclear factor that reacted with heart muscle nuclei.

Rheumatoid Arthritis

Although myocarditis and arteritis occur in patients with rheumatoid arthritis, the mechanism is not understood [54]. The arthritis of rheumatoid arthritis is thought to be due in part to the release of hydrolytic and proteolytic enzymes into the joint space secondary to immune processes [55, 56].

Hess et al reported that 4 of 25 patients with rheumatoid arthritis had HRA [7]. Kaplan et al. [6] found HRA in 6 of 27 cases of rheumatoid arthritis, and Zabriskie [16] in none of 15 patients. As in SLE, the incidence of HRA appears low, but the reported studies were not directed primarily at patients with heart involvement.

Although various antibodies are found in dermatomyositis and systemic sclerosis, their relationship to the cardiac involvement of these diseases is unknown. Thus, although there is ample evidence in the inflammatory connective tissue diseases for the role of humoral factors in the pathogenesis of disease of selected organ systems, the mechanisms of the cardiac lesions remains obscure. It would appear unlikely that heart-reactive antibody is important in the pathogenesis of RA or SLE heart disease. The role of delayed hypersensitivity and other cellular immune mechanisms in the carditis of connective tissue disease therefore warrants investigation.

SUMMARY

In this chapter the evidence for immune mechanisms has been reviewed in the following: (1) Rheumatic fever and rheumatic carditis with particular emphasis on the cross reactivity between streptococcal and myocardial antigens; (2) Idiopathic cardiomyopathy; (3) Endomyocardial fibrosis and infective endocarditis; (4) the post-thoracic cardiac injury syndromes; as well as the data on immune mechanisms in cardiac transplantation and the evidence for immune mechanisms in the cardiac involvement of connective tissue disease.

The evidence for the existence of immune mechanisms in myocardial disease to date is inconclusive, and much further work remains to be done.

The presence of the various antiheart antibodies whether circulating or bound to the myocardium does not necessarily provide a mechanism for an immune disorder of the heart. However, the evidence to date, particularly in relation to cardiac transplantation data, suggests that this is a most worthwhile area for continuing investigation into the problem of myocardial disease.

REFERENCES

1. Kaplan, M.H.: The concept of autoantibodies in rheumatic fever and in the post-commissurotomy state. Ann NY Acad Sci 86:1960.
2. Kaplan, M.H. and Meyeserian, M.: An immunological cross-reaction between Group-A streptococcal cells and human heart tissue. Lancet 1:706, 1962.
3. Kaplan, M.H.: The cross-reaction of Group-A streptococci with heart tissue and its relation to induced autoimmunity in rheumatic fever. Bull Rheumatic Dis 19:560, 1969.
4. Espinosa, E., Kushner, I., and Kaplan, M.H.: Antigenic composition of heart tissue. Am J Cardiol 24:508, 1969.
5. Kaplan, M.H.: Autoimmunity to heart. In, Miescher P.A. and Muller-Eberhard H.J. (Eds.): *Textbook of Immunopathology*. New York and London, Grune & Stratton, 1969.
6. Kaplan, M.H., Meyeserian, M., and Kushner, I.: Immunologic studies of heart tissue IV. Serologic reactions with human heart tissue as revealed by immunofluorescent methods: Isoimmune, Wassermann, and autoimmune reactions. J Exp Med 113:17, 1961.
7. Hess, E.V., Fink, C.W., Taranta, A., and Ziff, M.: Heart muscle antibodies in rheumatic fever and other diseases. J Clin Invest 43:886, 1964.
8. Camp, T.F., Hess, E.V., Conway, G., and Fowler, N.O.: Immunologic findings in idiopathic cardiomyopathy. Am Heart J 77:610, 1969.
9. Kaplan, M.H.: Symposium on immunity and the heart. Am J Cardiol 24:458, 1969.
10. Kaplan, M.H. and Rakita, L.: Myocardial disease. In, Samter, M. (Ed.): *Immunological Diseases*. Boston, Little, Brown, 1971.
11. Kaplan, M.H. and Frengley, J.D.: Autoimmunity to the heart in cardiac disease. Am J Cardiol 24:459, 1969.
12. Kaplan, M.H. and Dallenbach, F.D.: Immunologic studies of heart tissue. III. Occurrence of bound gamma globulin in auricular appendages from rheumatic hearts. Relationship to certain histopathologic features of rheumatic heart disease. J Exp Med 113:1, 1961.
13. Lannigan, R. and Zaki, S.: Location of gamma globulin in the endocardium in rheumatic heart disease by the ferritin-labelled antibody technique. Nature 217:173, 1968.
14. Kaplan, M., Bolande, R., Rakita, L., and Blair, J.: Presence of bound immunoglobulins and complement in the myocardium in acute rheumatic fever. New Engl J Med 271:637, 1964.
15. Kaplan, M.H.: Immunologic relation of streptococcal and tissue antigens. J Immunol 90:595-606, 1963.

16. Zabriskie, J.B., Read, S.E., and Ellis, R.J.: Cellular and humoral studies in diseases with heart-reactive antibodies. In, Amos, B. (Ed.): Progress in Immunology. New York and London, Academic, 1971.
17. Zabriskie, J.B. and Freimer, E.H.: An immunological relationship between the Group-A streptococcus and mammalian muscle. J Exp Med 124:661-678, 1966.
18. Goldstein, I., Halpern, B., and Robert, L.: Immunological relationship between Streptococcus A polysaccharide and the structural glycoproteins of heart valve. Nature 213:44-47, 1967.
19. Kaplan, M.H. and Svec, K.H.: Immunologic relation of Streptococcal and tissue antigens III Presence in human sera of Streptococcal antibody cross-reactive with heart tissue. Association with Streptococcal infection, rheumatic fever, and glomerulonephritis. J Exp Med 119: 651-665, 1964.
20. Zabriskie, J.B., Hsu, K.C., and Seegal, B.C.: Heart-reactive antibody associated with rheumatic fever: Characterization and diagnostic significance. Clin Exp Immunol 7:147, 1970.
21. Read, S.E., Falk, R.E., and Zabriskie, J.D.: Cellular reactivity to streptococcal antigens in rheumatic heart disease. Clin Res 19:786, 1971 (Abstr).
22. Friedman, I., Lauter, A., Ron, N., and Davies, A.M.: Experimental myocarditis: *in vitro* and *in vivo* studies of lymphocytes sensitized to heart extracts and Group-A streptococci. Immunol 20:255, 1971.
23. Sanders, V. and Ritts, R.E.: Ventricular localization of bound gamma globulin in idiopathic disease of the myocardium. JAMA, 194:171, 1965.
24. Das, S.K., Callen, J.P., Dodson, V.N., and Cassidy, J.T.: Immunoglobulin binding in cardiomyopathic hearts. Circulation 44:612, 1971.
25. Robinson, J., Anderson, T., and Grieble, H.: Serologic anomalies in idiopathic myocardial disease. Clin Res 14:335, 1966 (Abstr).
26. Fletcher, G.F. and Wenger, N.K.: Autoimmune studies in patients with primary myocardial disease. Circulation 37:1032, 1968.
27. Das, S.K., Cassidy, J.T., and Petty, R.E.: Antibodies against heart muscle and nuclear constituents in cardiomyopathy. Am J Cardiol 25:91, 1970 (Abstr).
28. Kirsner, A.B., Hess, E.V., and Fowler, N.O.: Immunologic findings in idiopathic cardiomyopathy: a prospective serial study. Am Heart J. To be published.
29. van der Geld, H., Peetoom, F., Somers, K., and Kanyerezi, B.R.: Immunohistological and serological studies in endomyocardial fibrosis. Lancet 2:1210-1214, 1966.
30. Shaper, A.G., Kaplan, M.H., Foster, W.D., Macintosh, D.M., and Wilks, N.E.: Immunological studies in endomyocardial fibrosis and other forms of heart disease in the tropics. Lancet 1:598-600, 1967.
31. Shaper, A.G., Kaplan, M.H., Mody, N.J., and McIntyre, P.A.: Malarial antibodies and autoantibodies to heart and tissues in the immigrant and indigenous peoples of Uganda. Lancet 1:1342-1347, 1968.
32. Das, S.K., Cassidy, J.T., and Willis, P.W.: The significance of heart antibody in infective endocarditis. Circulation 46:II-107, 1971. (Abstr).
33. Kirsner, A.B., Phair, J., and Hess, E.V.: Unpublished data.
34. Williams, R.C.: Subacute bacterial endocarditis as an immune disease. Hosp Pract 6:111-122, 1971.
35. Bartfeld, H.: Distribution of rheumatoid factor activity in nonrheumatoid states. Ann NY Acad Sci 168:30-40, 1969.
36. Houba, V., Allison, A.C., Adenixi, A., and Houba, J.E.: Immunoglobulin classes

and complement in the biopsies of Nigerian children with the nephrotic syndrome. Clin Exp Immunol 8:761, 1971.
37. Robinson, J. and Brigden, W.: Immunological studies in the post-cardiotomy syndrome. Br Med J 2:706-709, 1963.
38. van der Geld, H.: Antiheart antibodies in the postpericardiotomy and the postmyocardial-infarction syndrome. Lancet 2:617-621, 1964.
39. Dodson, V.N., Willis, P.W., de Vries, L., and Clifford, M.E.: Certain immunologic substances in the serum of patients with myocardial infarction and other cardiovascular diseases. Am Heart J 73:221-226, 1967.
40. Ehrenfeld, E.W., Gery, I., and Davis, A.M.: Specific antibodies in heart disease. Lancet 1:1138, 1961.
41. Ebringer, A., Rosenbaum, M., Pincus, N., and Doyle, A.E.: Changes in serum immunoglobulin after myocardial infarction. Am J Med 50:297-301, 1971.
42. Robinson, J. and Brigden, W.: Recurrent pericarditis. Br Med J 2:272-275, 1968.
43. Lower, R.R., Kosek, J.C., Kemp, E., Grahm, W.H., Sewell, D.H., and Lim F.: Rejection of the cardiac transplant. Am J Cardiol 24:492-499, 1969.
44. Terasaki, P.I., von Dipeow, M., Davidson, C.J., and Mickey, M.R.: Serotyping for homotransplantation. XXIV Heart transplantation. Am J Cardiol 24:500-507, 1969.
45. Botha, M.C.: Leucocyte-antigen matching in donor selection for heart transplantation. Lancet 2:508-512, 1969.
46. Fernbach, D.J., Nora, J.J., and Cooley, D.A.: Prospective tissue-typing for heart transplants. Lancet 1:425-426, 1969.
47. Stinson, E.B., Payne, R., Griepp, R.B., Dong, E., and Shumway, N.E.: Correlation of histocompatibility matching with graft rejection and survival after cardiac transplantation in man. Lancet 2:459-462, 1971.
48. Rosen, R.D., Butler, W.T., Johnson, A.H., and Mittal, K.K.: Immunofluorescent and serologic studies of the humoral antibody response to cardiac allotransplantation. Transplant Proc 3:445-448, 1971.
49. Schur, P.H. and Sandson, J.: Immunologic factors and clinical activity in systemic lupus erythematosus. New Engl J Med 278:533-538, 1968.
50. Kirsner, A. B., Diller, J.G., and Sheon, R.P.: Systemic lupus erythematosus with cutaneous ulceration. JAMA 217:821-823, 1971.
51. Vasquez, J.J. and Dixon, F.J.: Immunohistochemical study of lesions in rheumatic fever, systemic lupus erythematosus and rheumatoid arthritis. Lab Invest 6:205-217, 1957.
52. Koffler, D., Schur, P.H., and Kunkel, H.G.: Immunological studies concerning nephritis of systemic lupus erythematosus. J Exp Med 126:607-623, 1967.
53. Das, S.K. and Cassidy, J.T.: Antiheart antibodies in patients with systemic lupus erythematosus. Am J Cardiol 26:630, 1970 (Abstr).
54. Lebowitz, W.B.: The heart in rheumatoid arthritis. Ann Intern Med 58:102-123, 1963.
55. Hollander, J.L., McCarthy, D.J., Astorga, G., and Castro-Murillo, E.: Studies on the pathogenesis of rheumatoid joint inflammation. 1. The "R.A. cell" and a working hypothesis. Ann Intern Med 62:271, 1965.
56. Weissmann, G., Becher, B., Wiedermann, G., and Bernheimer, A.W.: Studies on lysosomes. VII Acute and chronic arthritis produced by intra-articular injections of streptolysins in rabbits. Am J Pathol 46:129, 1965.

E. DOUGLAS WIGLE, M.D.,
CLARENCE H. FELDERHOF, M.D.,
MALCOLM D. SILVER, M.D.,
and ALLAN G. ADELMAN, M.D.

Hypertrophic Obstructive Cardiomyopathy (Muscular or Hypertrophic Subaortic Stenosis)

INTRODUCTION

Cardiomyopathy may be classified clinically as congestive, restrictive, obliterative, or hypertrophic [1]. The hypertrophic variety of cardiomyopathy is characterized by a primary overgrowth of heart muscle involving mainly the left ventricle, especially the ventricular septum, but the right ventricle may also be affected significantly. The hypertrophic left ventricular wall is tremendously thickened and noncompliant, and the left ventricular cavity correspondingly reduced in volume, particularly at end-systole.

In hypertrophic cardiomyopathy, there may be obstruction to left ventricular outflow, in which case the term *hypertrophic obstructive cardiomyopathy* [1] may be applied. In other patients with hypertrophic cardiomyopathy, there is no obstruction to left ventricular outflow which may then be referred to as hypertrophic cardiomyopathy of the nonobstructive variety. The reason one patient with hypertrophic cardiomyopathy develops obstruction to left ventricular outflow and another does not is currently not known. This chapter will deal only with hypertrophic obstructive cardiomyopathy which in North America is usually called muscular [2, 3] or hypertrophic [4, 5] subaortic stenosis. In this chapter, the terms *hypertrophic obstructive cardiomyopathy* and *muscular subaortic stenosis* will be used interchangeably.

Although two nineteenth-century French pathologists [6, 7] and an early twentieth century German pathologist [8] reported postmortem ob-

From the Departments of Medicine and Pathology, University of Toronto, and the Cardiovascular Unit, Toronto General Hospital, Toronto Ontario, Canada.
Supported by the Ontario Heart Foundation.

servations compatible with what we now know of the pathology of obstructive cardiomyopathy, it was Lord Brock who focussed recent attention on the condition in 1957 and again in 1959 when he described "functional obstruction of the left ventricle" from surgical observations [9, 10]. In 1958, Teare's description of asymmetrical hypertrophy of the heart in young adults emphasized the massive degree of ventricular septal hypertrophy that may occur in this condition [11]. Subsequent reports correlated this pathologic picture with the clinical, hemodynamic, electrocardiographic, and angiographic findings in obstructive cardiomyopathy.

Much of the information in this chapter is derived from our own experience with this condition during the past 12 years. Pertinent references to the published literature are made, but there has been no exhaustive attempt to reference the literature. The writings of Braunwald [4, 5] and Goodwin [1, 12] and their collaborators are particularly noteworthy.

From 1960 to 1972, 78 cases of muscular subaortic stenosis have been investigated intensively in the Cardiovascular Unit of the Toronto General Hospital. In referring to our own experience, attention is focussed on the analysis of the first 60 of these cases [13]. Fifty-five of these 60 patients had evidence of obstruction to left ventricular outflow at rest, whereas in 5 the obstruction to left ventricular outflow was latent, in that it was only evident following appropriate pharmacologic stimulation. The ages of these 60 patients when first seen ranged from 11 to 55 years. There were 38 male patients (63 percent) and 22 female patients (37 percent). Twelve patients (20 percent) had a definite family history of the disease, and 11 others (18 percent) had a suspected family history. The condition appeared to be inherited as a Mendelian dominant characteristic.

The Clinical Syndrome

In describing the features of this condition, it is useful to think of the massive ventricular septal and left ventricular free wall hypertrophy that is present, and to picture the pathologic features as causing biventricular inflow and outflow tract obstruction [3]. The obstruction to ventricular inflow results from the hypertrophic muscle rendering the ventricular wall less distensible or compliant than normal [3, 4]. The hypertrophy may be so great that the ventricular cavities are encroached upon. The obstruction to left ventricular outflow, caused by the systolic apposition of the anterior leaflet of the mitral valve and the upper end of the hypertrophic ventricular septum, is not present at the onset of systole but develops during systole. By considering these facts, most of the characteristic features of the condition can be understood.

Table I
Frequency of Symptoms in 60 Patients with Muscular Subaortic Stenosis

Symptom	*No. of Patients*	(%)
Dyspnea	53	88
Angina	43	72
Fatigue	40	66
Palpitations	33	55
Presyncope	33	55
Syncope	11	18
Congestive heart failure	4	7
Supraventricular Arrhythmias	11	18
Total Documented	6	
Atrial fibrillation	2	
Tachycardia	4	
By History	5	

Symptoms

The frequency of various symptoms in 60 hemodynamically proved cases of obstructive cardiomyopathy is shown in Table I. As with other forms of obstruction to left ventricular outflow, dyspnea, angina pectoris, and syncope were prominent, but in addition, fatigue and palpitations were frequently noted. The dyspnea was believed to result mainly from decreased left ventricular compliance with consequent elevation of left ventricular end-diastolic and left atrial pressures. The mitral regurgitation that was invariably present (vide infra) contributed to the elevation of the left atrial pressure, and hence to the presence of dyspnea. Angina pectoris was believed to result from a functional inadequacy of the coronary circulation related to the primary overgrowth of heart muscle and to the presence of obstruction to left ventricular outflow. The coronary arterial tree was usually enlarged and free of atherosclerotic disease, although coronary artery disease may coexist with hypertrophic obstructive cardiomyopathy, especially in the older age groups. Presyncope and syncope on exertion are believed to be related to functional cerebral insufficiency as a result of the obstruction to left ventricular outflow, although some authors favor the occurrence of arrhythmias as the cause of these symptoms.

In 18 percent of these patients, episodes of supraventricular arrhythmia were suspected or documented (Table I). These arrhythmias were accompanied by a marked worsening of the symptoms in most instances, a feature that was believed due to the loss of atrial contraction, which has particularly deleterious effects in patients with noncompliant ventricles. We have observed a systemic embolus with the onset of atrial fibrillation

in one patient and bacterial endocarditis in another. Others have reported a number of instances of both of these complications as well as the fact that pregnancy is well tolerated [12]. We have observed one woman who lost most of the clinical signs of her disease at the seventh month of pregnancy, presumably because of increased blood volume. In our own experience congestive heart failure has been rare (Table I), but others have described a greater incidence [5].

Physical Signs

Decreased right ventricular compliance accounts for the prominent "a" wave in the jugular venous pulse and the fact that the jugular venous pressure usually rises, rather than falls, on inspiration [3]. The occurrence of a right atrial gallop sound can be explained on the same basis. Decreased left ventricular compliance accounts for the prominent left atrial gallop (fourth heart) sound which is not only audible but often palpable, giving rise to a double apex beat (the palpable atrial gallop sound plus the sustained left ventricular heave) [3, 4]. At times 2 *systolic* impulses may be palpable over the left ventricle; the first occurring prior to the outflow tract obstruction and the second after it [14, 15]. In such instances, if the atrial gallop sound is also palpable, a triple impulse may be detected.

The absence of any obstruction at the onset of left ventricular ejection accounts for the fast rising arterial pulse [16, 17]. Careful palpation of the peripheral arterial pulse also reveals a sharp cutoff to the pressure rise at the onset of the obstruction to ventricular outflow. Although the left ventricular impulse is heaving and often displaced to the left, the right ventricular impulse is rarely impressive. On auscultation the first heart sound is normal and the typical murmur, which is located at or just medial to the left ventricular apex, begins after the first heart sound. This crescendo–decrescendo murmur is caused both by the obstruction to left ventricular outflow and the mitral regurgitation. The murmur radiates to the left axilla and also toward the left sternal border and aortic area in diminished intensity, and only rarely is it well heard over the carotid vessels. The mitral regurgitation is believed to account, at least in part, for the frequent occurrence of a left ventricular third heart sound and a diastolic inflow murmur at the apex. A separate systolic murmur is frequently recognizable in the second or third left intercostal spaces, and results from the obstruction to right ventricular outflow that is often present, albeit usually mild in degree [18]. As with other forms of obstruction to left ventricular outflow, left ventricular ejection is prolonged in relation to the severity of the outflow obstruction, resulting in delay of aortic valve closure and consequently a single or paradoxically split second heart sound.

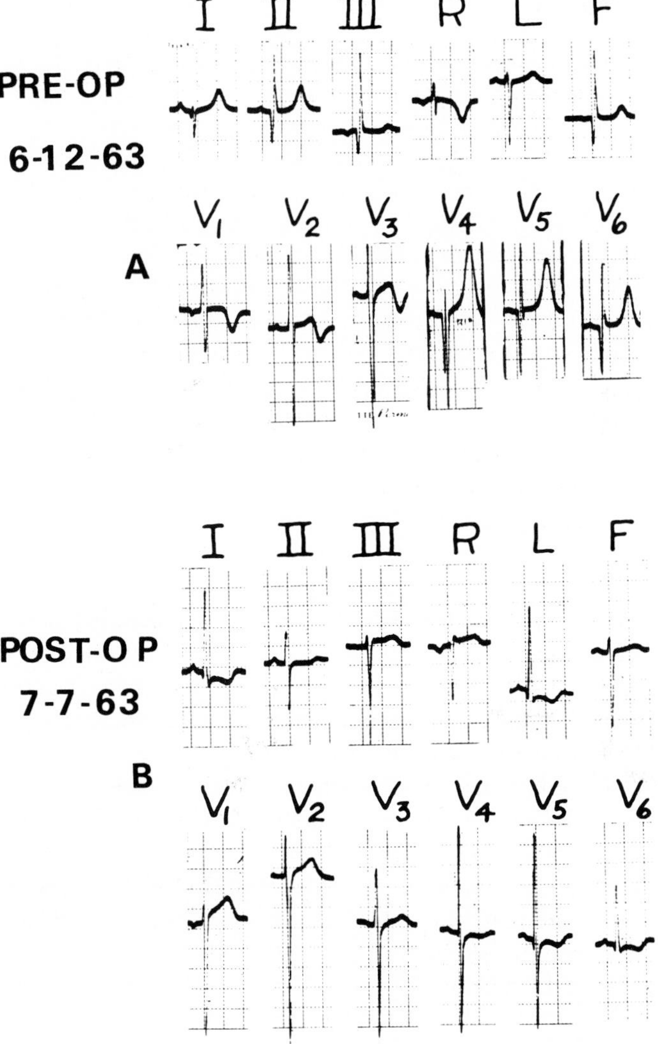

Figure 1. Muscular Subaortic Stenosis. Pre- and postoperative electrocardiograms from a 12-year-old boy with hemodynamically and surgically proved muscular subaortic stenosis. A. Preoperatively, there were prominent Q waves in leads II, III, aVF, and V_4-V_6 as well as tall R waves in the right precordial leads. B. Following the ventriculomyotomy operation, in which the upper anterior ventricular septum was incised, these Q- and R-wave abnormalities disappeared, suggesting that they originated in the ventricular septum (From Wigle, E.D. and Baron, R.H.: Circulation 34:585, 1966, by permission of The American Heart Association, Inc.).

Electrocardiogram

As with clinical signs, the electrocardiogram reflects the underlying pathologic and pathophysiologic abnormalities of the condition. Thus, left ventricular hypertrophy and strain result from the primary muscle overgrowth as well as from the left ventricular outflow obstruction. Left and, less commonly, right atrial hypertrophy develop as a result of decreased compliance of the ventricles. In following-up patients with hypertrophic obstructive cardiomyopathy, the presence or development of left atrial hypertrophy and/or left ventricular hypertrophy and strain, has correlated reasonably well with the severity or progression of clinical symptoms. Similarly, following a successful ventriculomyotomy operation, the electrocardiogram may reveal evidence of decreased left atrial and ventricular hypertrophy [13].

Pathologic "*Q*" waves which, in our experience, occur in about 20 percent of cases, are very helpful diagnostically and are believed to result from the septal hypertrophy that is present, or alternatively from septal fibrosis [19], or from abnormal septal and left ventricular wall activation [20]. The "Q" waves may occur in any leads, but in our experience, have been most common in leads 2, 3, aVF and V_4-V_6. When they have occurred in these leads, they are sometimes accompanied by tall "R" waves in the right precordial leads (Fig. 1). A surgical incision in the anterior end of the ventricular septum (ventriculomyotomy) may not only abolish the "Q" waves but also the tall "R" waves, suggesting that at least in some instances the ventricular septal pathology may explain these ECG abnormalities [19] (Fig. 1). Some authors have referred to these abnormalities as a pseudoinfarction pattern. Selective coronary cineangiograms have been demonstrated to be normal in patients having these abnormal "Q" waves in this condition. A number of authors have drawn attention to the occurrence of delta waves as well as other features of the Wolff-Parkinson-White syndrome [5, 13].

Chest X-ray

The most striking feature of the chest x-ray is usually the prominence of the left ventricle, but severe outflow tract obstruction may be present without any evidence of cardiac enlargement. A bulge along the left heart border, between the region of the left atrial appendage and the left ventricular apex, may indicate enlargement of the anterior end of the ventricular septum [15]. Left and right atrial enlargement are common and result from the decreased ventricular compliance. Typically, the aorta is small

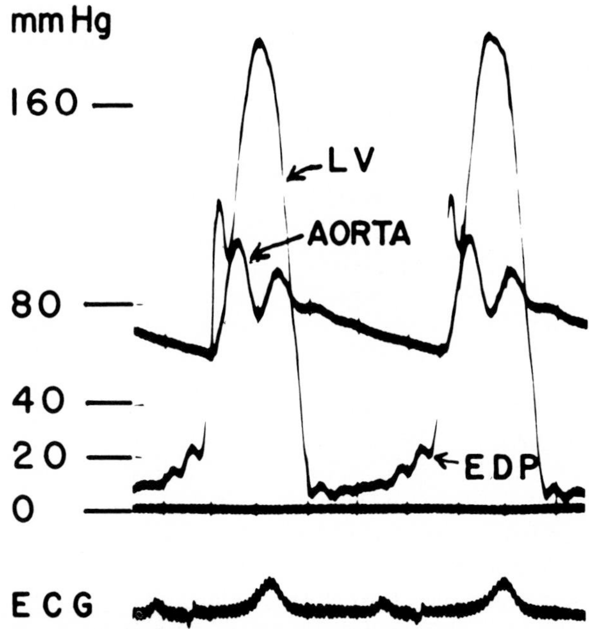

Figure 2. Muscular Subaortic stenosis. Simultaneous left ventricular (LV) and aortic pressure recordings. EDP = left ventricular end-diastolic pressure. See text.

but in the older age group may be dilated for other reasons. Aortic or mitral valve calcification and post-stenotic dilatation of the aorta do not occur unless concommitant aortic or mitral valve disease is present.

Hemodynamics

The pathology and pathophysiology not only account for the clinical features of the condition but also explain the hemodynamic findings. The decreased ventricular compliance accounts for the elevated ventricular end-diastolic pressures (Fig. 2) and the elevated "a" wave and mean pressures in the atria. The mitral regurgitation contributes to the height of the "v" waves and the mean pressure in the left atrium. The hallmark of hypertrophic obstructive cardiomyopathy is the obstruction to left ventricular outflow caused by the systolic apposition of the anterior leaflet of the mitral valve with the hypertrophic ventricular septum. Table II shows the magnitude of the pressure gradient across the left ventricular outflow tract, the left ventricular end-diastolic pressure and the cardiac index in 60 hemodynamically proved cases of obstructive cardiomyopathy arranged accord-

Table II
Left Heart Hemodynamics and Cardiac Indices in 60 Patients with Muscular Subaortic Stenosis

NYHC	No. of Patients	LV-Aortic Gradient (mm. Hg)		LVEDP (mm Hg)		Cardiac Index (liter/min/M^2)	
		Mean	*(Range)*	*Mean*	*(Range)*	*Mean*	*(Range)*
I	4	67.5	(30-80)	12.5	(9-16)	3.9	(2.8-4.5)
II	18	40.5	(0-100)	15.0	(7-33)	3.4	(2.2-4.7)
III-IV	38	67.5	(0-150)	20.0	(7-37)	3.1	(1.4-4.6)

LV = left ventricle; LVEDP = Left ventricular end-diastolic pressure.

ing to the functional status of the patient by the criteria of the New York Heart Classification (NYHC). Aside from the pressure gradients across the outflow tract in the 4 patients in class I (Table II), as patients become more disabled, the severity of the outflow tract obstruction and the degree of elevation of left ventricular end-diastolic pressure increased, while the cardiac index decreased.

Characteristically in obstructive cardiomyopathy, there is a notch on the upstroke of the left ventricular pressure tracing that corresponds to the top of the first (percussion) wave of the aortic pressure tracing (Fig. 2). Following this notch, the left ventricular pressure rises to a peak in mid-to-late systole, whereas the aortic pressure falls from the percussion wave to a low point at midsystole and rises again to the tidal wave in late systole before falling to the dicrotic notch [16]. At the onset of left ventricular ejection, the aortic pressure rises at a rate identical to that in the left ventricle. This sharp rise in arterial pressure contrasts with the characteristically slow-rising arterial pressure in fixed obstruction to left ventricular outflow (supravalvular, valvular or fibrous subvalvular) [17].

The aortic pulse pressure in the post-extrasystolic beat in obstructive cardiomyopathy is smaller than in normal sinus beats, in contradistinction to the finding in the fixed varieties of obstruction to left ventricular outflow, where the aortic pulse pressure in the post-extrasystolic beat is greater than in normal sinus beats [21].

Obstruction to right ventricular outflow is usually mild, and only rarely is it of hemodynamic significance.

Nature of Intraventricular Pressure Differences in Man

As there has been considerable controversy over the nature of intraventricular pressure differences [22] in the past few years, it is perhaps appropriate to discuss here how one can distinguish the intraventricular

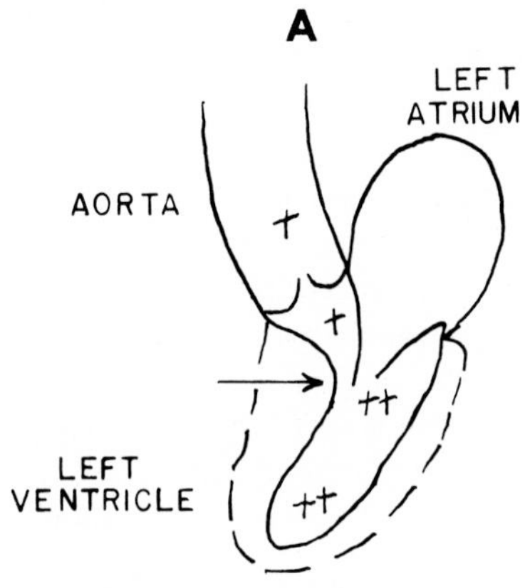

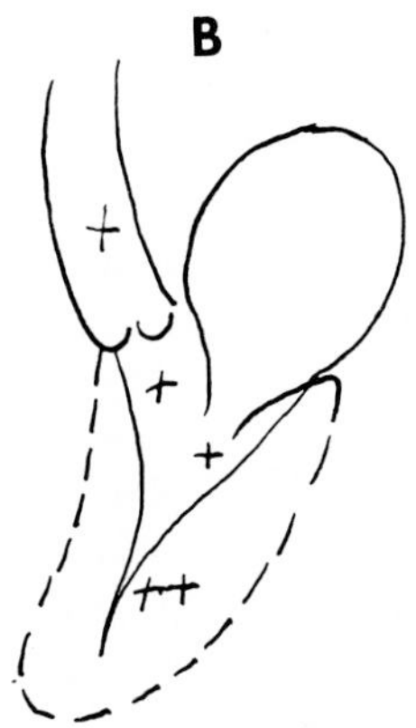

INTRAVENTRICULAR PRESSURE DIFFERENCE DUE TO MUSCULAR SUBAORTIC STENOSIS

INTRAVENTRICULAR PRESSURE DIFFERENCE DUE TO CATHETER ENTRAPMENT IN MYOCARDIUM

Figure 3. Muscular Subaortic Stenosis. A. In this disease, because the obstruction to left ventricular outflow (arrow) is caused by systolic apposition of the ventricular septum and anterior leaflet of the mitral valve, the intraventricular pressure distal to the stenosis (and proximal to the aortic valve) is low (+), whereas all ventricular pressures proximal to the stenosis including the one just inside the mitral valve (the inflow tract pressure) are elevated (++). B. When an intraventricular pressure difference is recorded due to catheter entrapment from cavity obliteration, the elevated ventricular pressure is recorded only in the area of entrapment (++). The intraventricular systolic pressure in all other areas of the left ventricular cavity including that in the inflow tract just inside the mitral valve is low (+) and equal to aortic systolic pressure. The three areas of the left ventricle represented by the +s in each of these diagrams are, from above downward, the outflow tract just below the aortic valve (subaortic region), the inflow tract just inside the mitral valve, and the left ventricular apex. (From Wigle, E.D., Auger, P. and Marquis, Y.: Can Med Assoc J 95:793, 1966, with the permission of the editors.)

pressure gradient that is seen in muscular subaortic stenosis from an intraventricular pressure difference that is the result of catheter entrapment in the myocardium [23-25]. This latter phenomenon is particularly common in hypertrophic cardiomyopathy of the nonobstructive variety because the small end-systolic size and the prominent trabeculation of the left ventricle increase the likelihood of a left ventricular catheter becoming entrapped in the myocardium. Figure 3 demonstrates that in muscular subaortic stenosis, the pressure just inside the mitral valve (the inflow tract pressure) is elevated, as are all intraventricular pressures proximal to the obstruction to left ventricular outflow; whereas in an intraventricular pressure difference due to catheter entrapment in the myocardium, the intraventricular pressure is elevated only in the area of entrapment and the inflow tract systolic pressure is not elevated. It is of paramount importance to be able to distinguish between these two types of intraventricular pressure difference in patients with hypertrophic cardiomyopathy in that the distinction determines whether surgery may be indicated as in hypertrophic *obstructive* cardiomyopathy as opposed to hypertrophic cardiomyopathy without obstruction to left ventricular outflow, in which case, surgery is contraindicated.

The concept of using the inflow tract pressure to distinguish between these two types of intraventricular pressure difference has proved very valuable, especially if one makes the following ancillary observations:

1. When a left ventricular catheter records a high intraventricular pressure in muscular subaortic stenosis, if one opens the proximal end of the catheter, blood shoots out in systole indicating that the distal tip of the catheter is in a high pressure, blood-filled area of the ventricle. In contrast, when a catheter records an elevated intraventricular pressure due to catheter entrapment in the myocardium and the proximal end of the catheter is opened, blood does not shoot out in systole. If one attempts to withdraw blood from such an entrapped catheter, none can be withdrawn in systole because of the catheter tip being entrapped in muscle [25].
2. The elevated intraventricular pressure in muscular subaortic stenosis falls at the time of the dicrotic notch in the aortic pressure, whereas if an intraventricular pressure is elevated from catheter entrapment in the myocardium, this pressure frequently falls after the dicrotic notch in the aortic pressure [25].
3. In muscular subaortic stenosis, the degree of prolongation of left ventricular ejection is proportional to the magnitude of the intraventricular pressure gradient as with other types of left ventricular outflow obstruction. With an intraventricular pressure difference due to catheter entrapment, the length of left ventricular ejection is inversely proportional to the magnitude of the pressure difference [26]. [Catheter entrapment tends to be greater (and the entrapped intraventricular pressure higher) when the left ventricle empties more rapidly (resulting in a shortened ejection time)].

Cineangiographic Observations

In the past 7 years, a number of cineangiographic features of muscular subaortic stenosis have been elucidated. Most of these reports have been concerned with the size and shape of the left ventricle, the appearance of the anterior mitral leaflet in relation to the site of the outflow tract obstruction, and the occurrence of mitral regurgitation [22, 27-31]. In our own studies, there appears to be a definite sequence of events in systole

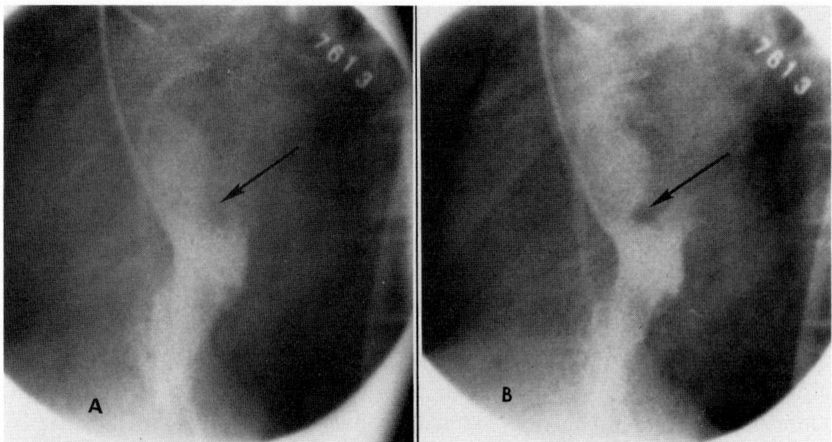

Figure 4. Muscular Subaortic Stenosis. Two systolic frames from a left anterior oblique left ventricular cineangiogram. A. In early systole, the arrow points to the position of the anterior mitral leaflet. B. By midsystole, this leaflet (arrow) has encroached on the left ventricular outflow tract to cause the obstruction to outflow. At the same time the left atrium begins to opacify, indicating the onset of mitral regurgitation. (From Adelman, A.G. et al.: Am J Cardiol 24:689, 1969, with the permission of the editors).

[31]. In early systole there was an extremely rapid ejection into the aorta and the anterior mitral leaflet moved posteriorly out of the outflow tract (Fig. 4A). By mid-systole, the upper ventricular septum appeared to encroach on the outflow tract anteriorly, but perhaps more importantly, the anterior leaflet of the mitral valve was seen to encroach on the posterior aspect of the outflow tract (Fig. 4B). Frequently, there was a radiolucent area in the outflow tract, indicating the site of obstruction to outflow caused by the systolic apposition of the anterior mitral leaflet and the ventricular septum. Mitral regurgitation became evident in mid-systole, coincident with the forward motion of the anterior mitral leaflet and was most evident in the last half of systole. The severity of the mitral regurgitation appeared to account in large measure for the degree of left ventricular emptying in the last half of systole, and hence for the small end-systolic volume of this chamber. At end-systole the 2 hypertrophied papillary muscles were often prominently outlined. Thus, the cineangiographic sequence of events in systole in muscular subaortic stenosis appeared to be "eject-obstruct-leak." Several groups of investigators have now demonstrated that the abnormal systolic anterior movement of the anterior mitral leaflet can also be recognized by ultrasound recordings [32-34].

Pharmacodynamics

Three factors appear to affect the severity of muscular subaortic stenosis in any given case. These are (1) ventricular contractility, (2) ventricular afterload, and (3) ventricular volume. The severity of the obstruction to left ventricular outflow is increased by an increase in ventricular contractility (digitalis glycosides [35], isoproterenol [36-38]) as well as a decrease in ventricular afterload (amyl nitrite (39), nitroglycerin (40), strain of the Valsalva maneuver [40, 41]), or a decrease in ventricular volume (isoproterenol, strain period of the Valsalva maneuver). Conversely, the severity of the obstruction to left ventricular outflow is decreased by a decrease in contractility (beta adrenergic blocking agents [42], as well as an increase in ventricular afterload (methoxamine [36], norepinephrine [43], angiotensin [43], neosynephrine [44]), or an increase in ventricular volume (infusion of blood or plasma [44]).

Isoproterenol is particularly effective in increasing the severity of the outflow tract obstruction because it increases contractility while decreasing ventricular afterload and volume.

Mitral Regurgitation

In addition to studying the occurrence of mitral regurgitation in muscular subaortic stenosis during cineangiography, we have also studied this important facet of the condition using indicator dilution techniques [45]. In these studies, 2 ml indocyanine green dye were injected into the high-pressure area of the left ventricle via a retrograde catheter while blood was simultaneously and continuously withdrawn from the left atrium via a transseptal catheter.

A total of 44 patients with muscular subaortic stenosis have been studied using these techniques. Mitral regurgitation was found in every patient in whom there was evidence of obstruction to left ventricular outflow, at rest [45].

In 20 of the 44 patients studied by dye-dilution techniques, we have infused angiotensin to ameliorate or abolish the outflow tract obstruction in order to assess the relation of the severity of the mitral regurgitation to the severity of the obstruction (Fig. 5). In 16 of these 20 patients the severity of the mitral regurgitation was directly related to the severity of the obstruction to ventricular outflow (Fig. 5) [45]. When angiotensin lessened or abolished the obstruction to ventricular outflow the mitral regurgitation was also lessened or abolished. These preoperative studies allowed us to predict that the surgical relief of the outflow tract obstruction

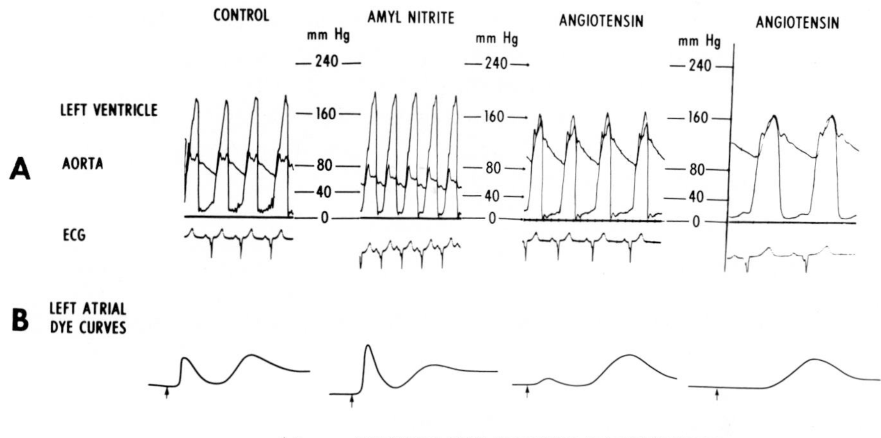

Figure 5. Muscular Subaortic Stenosis. A. Simultaneous left ventricular and aortic pressure recordings. B. Left atrial dye-dilution curves (bottom) inscribed from left to right after left ventricular injection of 2 ml. indocyanine green dye, in control conditions (first panel), after amyl nitrite inhalation (second panel), and during angiotensin infusion (third and fourth panels). The amount of dye leaking back into the left atrium is indicated by the upward deflection of the dye curve occurring immediately to the right of the arrow, which indicates the time of left ventricular injection of the dye. To the right of this regurgitant dye deflection is the recirculation concentration. The intensification of the outflow tract obstruction due to administration of amyl nitrite was accompanied by an increase in the amount of regurgitant dye appearing in the left atrium (second panel). Angiotensin infusion initially reduced (third panel) and eventually abolished (fourth panel) both the outflow tract obstruction and the mitral regurgitation. (From Wigle, E.D. et al.: Am J Cardiol 24:698, 1969, with the permission of the editors).

in these patients would also result in the abolition of the mitral regurgitation. [46].

Of the 20 patients in whom indicator-dilution studies were carried out during pharmacologic intervention, there were 4 in whom angiotensin abolished the outflow tract obstruction but failed to reduce the degree of mitral regurgitation. This suggested to us that in these 4 patients, there was an independent anatomic abnormality of the mitral valve, and that the mitral regurgitation would not vanish after a successful ventriculomyotomy operation. Two of these 4 patients have subsequently come to postmortem examination and both have had congenital mitral valve abnormalities. A third patient has undergone surgery and although the obstruction to left ventricular outflow was completely abolished, the mitral regurgitation remained unchanged postoperatively [46].

In summary, all patients with muscular subaortic stenosis with evidence of obstruction to left ventricular outflow at rest have mitral regurgitation. In roughly 75 percent of these patients the mitral regurgitation was directly related to the severity of the obstruction to left ventricular outflow, whereas in 25 percent the mitral regurgitation was independent of the obstruction to ventricular outflow and was related to an independent anatomic abnormality of the mitral valve.

Natural History

Although early reports suggested that progressive deterioration was characteristic of this condition [47, 48], subsequent reports have suggested a more benign clinical course. Thus, in an excellent review of 98 patients observed for an average of 3 years, Frank and Braunwald [49] found that only 14 patients deteriorated, and 9 died of the disease. Of the remaining 74 patients, 54 remained stable, 14 fluctuated, and 6 improved. In a series of 91 patients observed by Goodwin and his associates for an average of 4 years, 22 improved, 39 remained the same, 12 deteriorated, and 11 died [1]. Parker observed 18 patients for an average of 4 years; there were no deaths, and only 1 of these patients deteriorated [50].

Our own experience with the clinical course in obstructive cardiomyopathy is that it is a condition of progressive deterioration, once symptoms commence [13]. A retrospective and prospective analysis of the clinical course of 60 hemodynamically proved cases revealed that in 41 (68 percent) the murmur was the first evidence of the disease and was noted at an average age of 20 (range 0-46). Fifty-six of the 60 patients (93 percent) developed symptoms (class II, NYHC) an average of 10 years after the murmur was first heard at a mean age of 30 (range 2-50). Forty patients (66 percent) deteriorated to class III-IV, NYHC, an average of 5 years after the onset of symptoms at a mean age of 35 (range 12-56). Of 28 untreated or propranolol-treated patients, 6 (21 percent) died at an average age of 40. Death occurred suddenly, or at the end of years of progressive deterioration.

Patients with a positive family history had a slightly worse prognosis. As previously observed [49], young asymptomatic males with a positive family history were particularly prone to sudden death.

Although others have suggested a more benign clinical course, in our experience hypertrophic obstructive cardiomyopathy is a progressive disorder, once symptoms commence. In attempting to assess the reasons for this difference the following points bear consideration:

1. The analysis of our cases has been both retrospective and prospective, whereas some other series have only been prospective.

2. All of our cases have had evidence of obstruction to left ventricular outflow, whereas other series have included cases without obstruction to left ventricular outflow.
3. Sixty-six percent of our cases reached class III-IV (NYHC) symptomatology, whereas only 25 percent of cases in the 3 series [1, 49, 50] describing a more benign clinical course had such severe symptoms.

It has been recognized for some years now that the decrease in left ventricular compliance is an important feature of this condition [3, 4], and indeed may be more important than the outflow tract obstruction in determining clinical symptoms [3]. Recently, it has been observed that the outflow tract obstruction may disappear in the late stages of the disease at a time when ventricular function and compliance are significantly decreased [12]. This observation has led to the suggestion that the outflow tract obstruction is an incidental finding in this condition [51]. We would not adhere to this latter view. Rather we would subscribe to the view that the outflow tract obstruction would be most significant at a time during the course of the disease when the bizarre muscle fiber hypertrophy was most evident, and prior to the development of significant myocardial fibrosis, at which time it would be reasonable to expect less evidence of outflow tract obstruction and a further decrease in ventricular compliance.

Differential Diagnosis

Most importantly, hypertrophic obstructive cardiomyopathy must be distinguished from hypertrophic cardiomyopathy of the nonobstructive variety, different types of mitral regurgitation, ventricular septal defect, other varieties of obstruction to left ventricular outflow, and coronary artery disease, particularly when associated with papillary muscle dysfunction. Careful clinical examination, including the use of amyl nitrite inhalation and the Valsalva maneuver at the bedside, usually permits an accurate diagnosis of muscular subaortic stenosis to be made. Ultrasonic, hemodynamic, and cineangiographic studies can confirm the clinical impression.

Treatment

The treatment of obstructive cardiomyopathy may consist of doing nothing, avoiding overexertion, the administration of beta-adrenergic blocking agents [42, 52-55], or surgery [56-59]. Propranolol therapy has been frankly disappointing in patients with significant clinical disability [55]. In such patients, any initial improvement on propranolol therapy is usually short-lived and the progressive nature of the myocardial disorder soon overcomes any benefits derived from this treatment. Patients with latent obstruction to ventricular outflow have sometimes done well on propranolol therapy. Patients with mild clinical disability with evidence of outflow obstruction at rest have often had initial improvement, but even in these patients when the period of observation has extended beyond 2 years, the benefits of this therapy have been overcome by progression of the myocardial disorder [55]. It has recently been suggested that the beta-adrenergic blocking agent, practolol, may improve compliance of the left ventricle, but this observation has not yet been confirmed [12]. The results of surgery in obstructive cardiomyopathy have indeed been variable, but at least 3 centers have had good-to-excellent results [57-59]. Using either an ascending aortic approach or this combined with a ventricular approach, the bulging hypertrophic muscle at the anterior end of the ventricular septum is incised or incised and resected. Importance is attached to the depth of the incision into the muscle. Using either of these techniques the operative mortality has been less than 10 percent, and the degree of symptomatic improvement has been very impressive [57-59]. Not only is the outflow tract obstruction abolished in the vast majority of cases but also the mitral regurgitation is relieved if the mitral valve is anatomically normal [46]. It is important in understanding the beneficial affects of this type of surgery to know that this muscle-splitting incision abolishes the abnormal systolic anterior movement of the anterior mitral leaflet [60], which explains why both the obstruction to ventricular outflow and the mitral regurgitation are relieved. The lack of benefit from propranolol therapy in this condition is explicable on the basis that this type of treatment does not abolish the abnormal movement of the anterior mitral leaflet [60], nor does it abolish the obstruction to outflow or the mitral regurgitation. Surgery not only relieves this triad of abnormalities but also usually results in impressive lowering of the left ventricular end-diastolic pressure [57-59]. The underlying primary myocardial disorder, however, is unaffected. Thus, it will be important to study the clinical course of these patients postoperatively in order to assess the effect of surgery on the long-term morbidity and mortality of the condition, which then would presumably reflect on the degree of progression of the primary myocardial disorder.

Current Thoughts on the Nature of the Outflow Tract Obstruction

The fact that a muscle-splitting incision in the anterior end of the hypertrophic ventricular septum in muscular subaortic stenosis abolishes the abnormal anterior movement of the anterior mitral leaflet as well as the obstruction to ventricular outflow and the mitral regurgitation suggests that the myocardial abnormality in this condition is the primary fault. Since it appears that the abnormal systolic movement of the anterior mitral leaflet can account for both the obstruction to outflow and the mitral regurgitation, the question might be asked "How does the apparently primary myocardial fault cause this abnormal systolic movement of the anterior mitral leaflet?" Previous studies of the pathological aspects of this condition have indicated that it is characterized by gross left ventricular hypertrophy, most marked in the ventricular septum. The bizarre nature of the myocardial fiber hypertrophy has been well documented. Recent studies in our laboratory have indicated that the bizarre fiber hypertrophy has centered mainly in the middle layer of the left ventricular wall [46], an area normally occupied by circumferentially arranged muscle fibers [61] which are largely responsible for left ventricular ejection [62].

From the foregoing considerations, the following sequence of events could explain the known pathophysiologic features in this condition. Accelerated contraction of the circumferentially arranged bizarre hypertrophic myocardial fibers in the left ventricular wall could account for the rapid left ventricular ejection in the early nonobstructed phase of systole. This rapid ejection could draw the anterior mitral leaflet into the outflow tract by a Venturi effect, thereby producing obstruction to ventricular outflow and the mitral regurgitation [46]. The possibility of a Venturi effect being operative would be enhanced by the anterior leaflet being closer to the center of the ejection path and/or by the leaflet being less taut in systole than normal. The alteration in left ventricular geometry caused by the ventricular septal hypertrophy is such that these Venturi enhancing mechanisms could be operative. Changes in left ventricular volume, contractility, and afterload which are known to alter the severity of the subaortic stenosis and the mitral regurgitation could do so by affecting the Venturi mechanism, and hence the degree of abnormal movement in systole of the anterior mitral leaflet. [46].

SUMMARY

Hypertrophic obstructive cardiomyopathy (muscular or hypertrophic subaortic stenosis) is a condition in which primary overgrowth of heart muscle, particularly in the ventricular septum, is the primary fault. This myocardial defect renders the ventricular walls nondistensible or noncompliant in diastole and is believed to be the fault that results in the anterior mitral leaflet moving into the outflow tract in systole, thereby causing the obstruction to left ventricular outflow and the mitral regurgitation. Essentially, all aspects of the condition can be understood if the underlying pathology and pathophysiology are kept in mind.

Although some authors have suggested a rather benign clinical course for these patients, our own experience is that once symptoms commence, the clinical course is one of progressive deterioration. There is, however, about a 10-year period of freedom from symptoms between the time the murmur is first noted at an average age of 20 and when symptoms commence at an average age of 30.

A surgical incision into the hypertrophic muscle at the anterior end of the ventricular septum abolishes the abnormal anterior movement of the anterior mitral leaflet, the outflow tract obstruction, the mitral regurgitation, and significantly lowers the left ventricular end-diastolic pressure. Although the symptomatic relief from a successful ventriculomyotomy operation is often striking, the primary myocardial fault remains following this palliative type of surgery. Propranolol therapy has been of greatest value in patients with latent muscular sub-aortic stenosis and in those with mild symptoms. As a rule, this form of therapy has not been of lasting benefit in patients with severe obstruction to left ventricular outflow with disabling symptoms.

ACKNOWLEDGMENT

It is a pleasure to acknowledge the assistance of Dr. Y. Marquis, Dr. P. Auger, Dr. N. Ranganathan, and Dr. G. D. Webb in conducting the studies herein recorded. We wish also to thank Miss Dorothy Goodwin for secretarial assistance and Misses Jean McMeekan and Rose-Marie Cseplo for technical assistance.

REFERENCES

1. Goodwin, J.F.: Congestive and hypertrophic cardiomyopathies. Lancet 1:731, 1970.
2. Brent, L.B., Aburano, A., Fisher, D.L., Morgan, T.J., Myers, J.D., and Taylor, W.J.: Familial muscular subaortic stenosis: An unrecognized form of "idiopathic heart disease" with clinical and autopsy observations. Circulation 21:167, 1960.
3. Wigle, E.D., Heimbecker, R.O., and Gunton, R.W.: Idiopathic ventricular septal hypertrophy causing muscular subaortic stenosis. Circulation 26:325, 1962.
4. Braunwald, E., Morrow, A.G., Cornell, W.P., Aygen, M.M., and Hilbish, T.F.: Idiopathic hypertrophic subaortic stenosis. Am J Med 29:924, 1960.
5. Braunwald, E., Lambrew, C.T., Rockoff, S.D., Ross, J., Jr., and Morrow, A.G.:

Idiopathic hypertrophic subaortic stenosis: I. Description of the disease based upon an analysis of 64 patients. Circulation 29 and 30 (Suppl 4):3, 1964.

6. Liouville, I.: Retrecissement cardiaque sous aortique. Gaz Med (Paris) 24:161, 1869.
7. Hallopeau: Retrecissement ventriculo-aortique. Gaz Med (Paris) 24:683, 1869.
8. Schmincke, A.: Ueber linksseitige muskulose conusstenosen. Dtsch Med Wochschr 11:2082, 1907.
9. Brock, R.C.: Functional obstruction of the left ventricle. Guy's Hosp Rep 106:221, 1957.
10. Brock, R.C.: Functional obstruction of the left ventricle. Guy's Hosp Rep 108:126, 1959.
11. Teare, R.D.: Asymmetrical hypertrophy of the heart in young adults. Br Heart J 20:1, 1958.
12. Swan, D.A., Bell, B., Oakley, C.M., and Goodwin, J.: Analysis of symptomatic course and prognosis and treatment of hypertrophic obstructive cardiomyopathy. Br Heart J 33:671, 1971.
13. Wigle, E.D., Adelman, A.G., Ranganathan, N., Webb, G.D., Silver, M.D., and Bigelow, W.G.: The clinical course in muscular subaortic stenosis. In, Kidd, B.S.L. and Keith, J.D. (Eds.): The Natural History and Progress in Treatment of Congenital Heart Defects. Springfield, Ill. Charles C Thomas, 1971, chap 32, p 245.
14. Cohen, J., Effat, H., Goodwin, J.F., Oakley, C.M., and Steiner, R.E.: Hypertrophic obstructive cardiomyopathy. Br Heart J 26:16, 1964.
15. Wigle, E.D.: Muscular subaortic stenosis: Clinical syndrome with additional evidence of ventricular septal hypertrophy. In, Wolstenholme, G.E.W. and O'Connor, M. (Eds.): Cardiomyopathies. Ciba Found Symp, London, Churchill, 1964, p 49.
16. Brachfeld, N. and Gorlin, R.: Subaortic stenosis: A revised concept of the disease. Medicine 38:415, 1959.
17. Wigle, E.D.: The arterial pressure pulse in muscular subaortic stenosis. Br Heart J 25:97, 1963.
18. Wigle, E.D., Chrysohou, A., and Bigelow, W.G.: Results of ventriculomyotomy in muscular subaortic stenosis. Am J Cardiol 11:572, 1963.
19. Wigle, E.D. and Baron, R.H.: Electrocardiogram in muscular subaortic stenosis. Circulation 34:585, 1966.
20. van Dam, R.T., Roos, J.P., and Durrer, D.: Electrical activation of ventricles and interventricular septum in hypertrophic obstructive cardiomyopathy. Br Heart J 34:100, 1972.
21. Brockenbrough, E.C., Braunwald, E., and Morrow, A.G.: A hemodynamic technic for the detection of hypertrophic subaortic stenosis. Circulation 23:189, 1961.
22. Criley, J.M., Lewis, K.B., White, R.I., and Ross, R.S.: Pressure gradients without obstruction: A new concept of "hypertrophic subaortic stenosis." Circulation 32:881, 1965.
23. Wigle, E.D., Auger, P., and Marquis, Y.: Muscular subaortic stenosis: The initial left ventricular inflow tract pressure as evidence of outflow tract obstruction. Can Med Assoc J 95:793, 1966.
24. Ross, J., Jr., Braunwald, E., Gault, J.H., Mason, D.T., and Morrow, A.G.: Mechanism of the intraventricular pressure gradient in idiopathic hypertrophic subaortic stenosis. Circulation 34:558, 1966.

25. Wigle, E.D., Marquis, Y., and Auger, P.: Muscular subaortic stenosis: Initial left ventricular inflow tract pressure in the assessment of intraventricular pressure differences in man. Circulation 35:1100, 1967.
26. Wigle, E.D., Auger, P., and Marquis, Y.: Muscular subaortic stenosis: The direct relation between the intraventricular pressure difference and left ventricular ejection time. Circulation 36:36, 1967.
27. Klein, M.D., Lane, F.J., and Gorlin, R.: Effect of left ventricular size and shape upon the hemodynamics of subaortic stenosis. Am J Cardiol 15:773, 1965.
28. Dinsmore, R.E., Sanders, C.A., and Harthorne, J.W.: Mitral regurgitation in idiopathic hypertrophic subaortic stenosis. New Engl J Med 275:1225, 1966.
29. Rackley, C.E., Whalen, R.E., and McIntosh, H.D.: Ventricular volume studies in a patient with hypertrophic subaortic stenosis. Circulation 34:579, 1966.
30. Simon, A.L., Ross, J., Jr., and Gault, J.H.: Angiographic anatomy of the left ventricle and mitral valve in idiopathic hypertrophic subaortic stenosis. Circulation 36:852, 1967.
31. Adelman, A.G., McLoughlin, M.J., Marquis, Y., Auger, P., and Wigle, E.D.: Left ventricular cineangiographic observations in muscular subaortic stenosis. Am J Cardiol 24:689, 1969.
32. Shah, P.M., Gramiak, R., and Kramer, D.H.: Ultrasound localization of left ventricular outflow obstruction in hypertrophic obstructive cardiomyopathy. Circulation 40:3, 1969.
33. Popp, R.L. and Harrison, D.C.: Ultrasound in the diagnosis and evaluation of therapy of idiopathic hypertrophic subaortic stenosis. Circulation 40:905, 1969.
34. Pridie, R.B. and Oakley, C.M.: Mechanism of mitral regurgitation in hypertrophic obstructive cardiomyopathy. Br Heart J 32:203, 1970.
35. Braunwald, E., Brockenbrough, E.C., and Frye, R.L.: Studies on digitalis. Comparison of the effects of ouabain on left ventricular dynamics in valvular aortic stenosis and hypertrophic subaortic stenosis. Circulation 26:166, 1962.
36. Braunwald, E. and Ebert, P.A.: Hemodynamic alterations in idiopathic hypertrophic subaortic stenosis induced by sympathomimetic drugs. Am J Cardiol. 10:489, 1962.
37. Krasnow, N., Rolett, E., Hood, W.B., Jr., Yurchak, P.M., and Gorlin, R.: Reversible obstruction of the ventricular outflow tract. Am J Cardiol 11:1, 1963.
38. Whalen, R.E., Cohen, A.I., Sumner, R.G., and McIntosh, H.D.: Demonstration of the dynamic nature of idiopathic hypertrophic subaortic stenosis. Am J Cardiol 11:8, 1963.
39. Wigle, E.D., Lenkei, S.C.M., Chrysohou, A., and Wilson, D.R.: Muscular subaortic stenosis: The effect of peripheral vasodilation. Can Med Assoc J 89:896, 1963.
40. Braunwald, E., Oldham, H.N., Jr., Ross, J., Jr., Linhart, J.W., Mason, D.T., and Fort, L., III.: The circulatory response of patients with idiopathic hypertrophic subaortic stenosis to nitroglycerine and to the Valsalva manoeuver. Circulation 29:422, 1964.
41. Marcus, F.I., Westura, E.E., and Summa, J.: The hemodynamic effect of the Valsalva manoeuver in muscular stenosis. Am Heart J 67:324, 1964.
42. Harrison, D.C., Braunwald, E., Glick, B., Mason, D.T., Chidsey, C.A., and Ross, J., Jr.: Effects of beta adrenergic blockade on the circulation, with particular reference to observations in patients with hypertrophic subaortic stenosis. Circulation 29:84, 1964.
43. Wigle, E.D., David, P.R., Labrosse, C.J., and McMeekan, J.: Muscular sub-

aortic stenosis: Interrelation of wall tension, outflow tract "distending pressure" and orifice radius. Am J Cardiol 15:761, 1965.
44. Goodwin, J.F., Shah, P.M., Oakley, C.M., Cohen, J., Yipintsoi, T., and Pocock, W.: Clinical pharmacology of hypertrophic obstructive cardiomyopathy. In, Wolstenholme, G.E. and O'Connor, M. (Eds): Ciba Found Symp Cardiomyopathies. London, Churchill, 1964, p 189.
45. Wigle, E.D., Adelman, A.G., Auger, P., and Marquis, Y.: Mitral regurgitation in muscular subaortic stenosis. Am J Cardiol 24:698, 1969.
46. Wigle, E.D., Adelman, A.G., and Silver, M.D.: Pathophysiological considerations in muscular subaortic stenosis. In, Wolstenholme, G.E. and O'Connor, M. (Eds.): Ciba Found Study Group No 37. London, Churchill, 1971, p 63.
47. Goodwin, J.F., Gordon, H., Hollman, A., and Bishop, M.B.: Clinical aspects of cardiomyopathy. Br Med J 1:69, 1961.
48. Soulie, P., Joly, F., and Carlotti, J. Les stenoses idiopathiques de la chembre de chasse du ventricule gauche. Acta Cardiol 17:335, 1962.
49. Frank, S. and Braunwald, E.: Idiopathic hypertrophic subaortic stenosis: Clinical analysis of 126 patients with emphasis on the natural history. Circulation 35:759, 1968.
50. Parker, B.M.: The course in idiopathic hypertrophic subaortic stenosis. Ann Intern Med 70:903, 1969.
51. Oakley, C.M.: Hypertrophic obstructive cardiomyopathy—Patterns of progression. Hypertrophic Obstructive Cardiomyopathy. In, Wolstenholme, G.E.W. and O'Connor, M. (Eds.): Ciba Foundation Study Group No. 37. Churchill, London, 1971, p 9.
52. Cherian, G., Brockington, I.F., Shah, P.M., Oakley, C.M., and Goodwin, J.F.: Beta adrenergic blockade in hypertrophic obstructive cardiomyopathy. Br Med J 1:895, 1966.
53. Sloman, G.: Propranolol in management of muscular subaortic stenosis. Br Heart J 29:783, 1967.
54. Flamm. M.D., Harrison, D.C., and Hancock, E.W.: Muscular subaortic stenosis. Prevention of outflow obstruction with propranolol. Circulation 38:846, 1968.
55. Adelman, A.G., Shah, P.M., Gramiak, R., and Wigle, E.D.: Long-term propranolol therapy in muscular subaortic stenosis. Br Heart J 32:864, 1971.
56. Goodwin, J.F., Hollman, A., Cleland, W.P., and Teare, D.: Obstructive cardiomyopathy simulating aortic stenosis. Br Heart J 22:403, 1960.
57. Morrow, A.G., Fogarty, T.J., Hannah, H., III, and Braunwald, E.: Operative treatment in idiopathic hypertrophic subaortic stenosis: Techniques and the results of preoperative and postoperative clinical and hemodynamic assessments. Circulation 37:589, 1968.
58. Bigelow, W.G., Trimble, A.S., Auger, P., Marquis, Y., and Wigle, E.D.: The ventriculomyotomy operation for muscular subaortic stenosis. J Thorac Cardiovasc Surg 52: 514, 1966.
59. Barratt-Boyes, B.G. and O'Brien, K.P.: Surgical treatment of idiopathic hypertrophic subaortic stenosis using a combined left ventricular-aortic approach. Hypertrophic Obstructive Cardiomyopathy. In, Wolstenholme, G.E.W. and O'Connor, M. (Eds.): Ciba Foundation Study Group No. 37. Churchill, London, 1971, p 150.
60. Shah, P.M., Gramiak, R., Adelman, A.G., and Wigle, E.D.: Echocardiographic assessment of the effects of surgery and propranolol on the dynamics of outflow obstruction in hypertrophic subaortic stenosis. Circulation 45:516, 1972.

61. Streeter, D.D., Jr., Spotwitz, H.M., Patel, D.P., Ross, J., Jr., and Sonnenblick, E.H.: Fiber orientation in the canine left ventricle during diastole and systole. Circulation Res 24:339, 1969.
62. Lewis, R. and Sandler, H.: Relationship of ejection fraction and dynamic geometry for the human left ventricle. Circulation 40 (Suppl III): 132, 1969.

JOSEPH K. PERLOFF, M.D.

The Myocardial Disease of Heredofamilial Neuromyopathies

The myocardium is involved in 3 categories of degenerative heredofamilial neuromyopathic diseases, namely, progressive muscular dystrophy, myotonic muscular dystrophy, and Friedreich's ataxia. The following report summarizes current information on the cardiovascular manifestations of these disorders.

PROGRESSIVE MUSCULAR DYSTROPHY

The majority of nonmyotonic progressive muscular dystrophies fall into the following categories:

1. Duchenne's progressive muscular dystrophy
   a. Early onset, rapidly progressive, sex-linked recessive (the classic form of Duchenne's dystrophy)
   b. Early onset, slowly progressive, autosomal recessive
   c. Late onset, slowly progressive, sex-linked recessive (Becker's muscular dystrophy)
2. Limb-girdle dystrophy of Erb
3. Facilscapulohumeral dystrophy of Landouzy-Dejerine

Evidence of cardiovascular disease—subtle or overt—has been found in each of these 3 major categories though with widely varying incidence and severity [1].

From the Hospital of the University of Pennsylvania and the Section of Cardiology (Cardiovascular Pulmonary Division), Department of Medicine, University of Pennsylvania School of Medicine, Philadelphia, Pennsylvania.

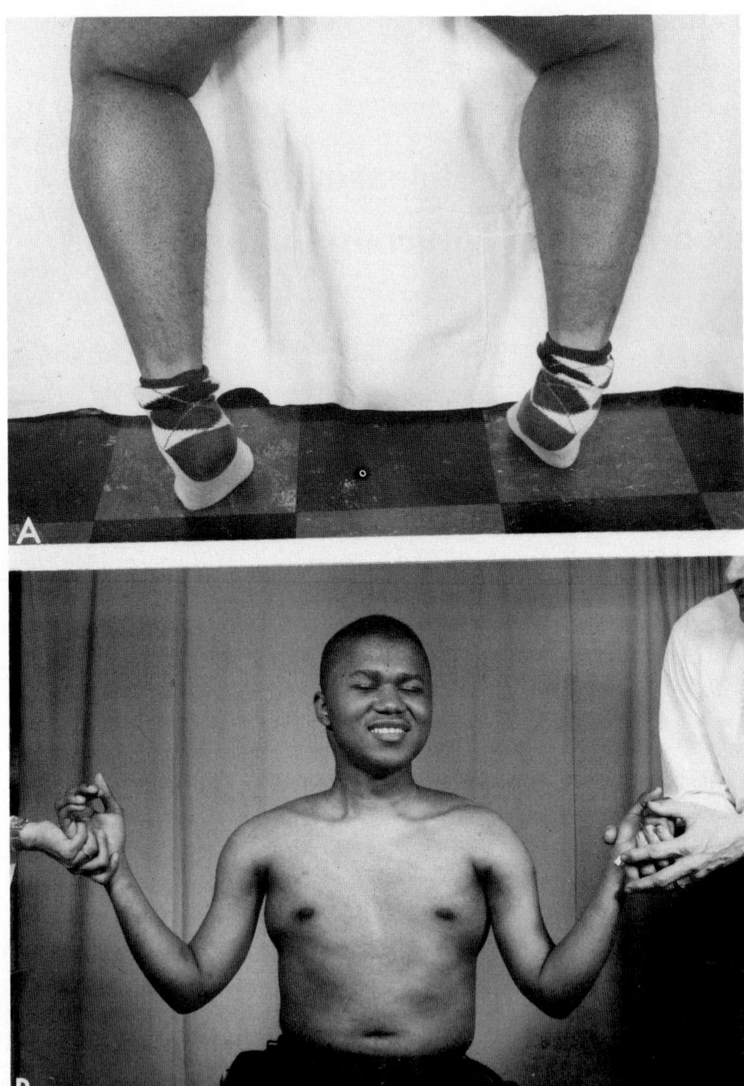

Figure 1. Classic Duchenne's Dystrophy. A. Typical calf pseudohypertrophy. Note that the feet are held in the position of talipes equinovarus. B. The deltoids and pectorals also exhibit pseudohypertrophy.

Duchenne's progressive muscular dystrophy. Classic Duchenne's dystrophy is sex-linked recessive, transmitted by the mother to her sons as *overt* disease, and to 50 percent of her daughters as a *carrier* state. Onset is early in the first decade beginning with weakness of the hip girdle, with subsequent weakness of the shoulders [2]. Pseudohypertrophy of the calves (Fig. 1) is especially marked early in the course of the disease. The gait is clumsy and waddling, and the patient has difficulty climbing stairs and rising from the floor. Weakness and contractures result in talipes equinovarus (Fig. 1), causing patients to walk on their toes, further compromising an already precarious balance. Progressive deterioration generally culminates in a wheel-chair existence by age 12. Dystrophy of chest muscles and diaphragm (Fig. 2) interfere with coughing and breathing. Abrupt episodes of abdominal pain, vomiting, sweating, and palpitations [1, 2] resemble those in Friedreich's ataxia (described in subsequent section). Patients are likely to succumb to pulmonary infection in the second decade although cardiac disease is an important and, at times, dramatic cause of death [1]. Rapidly progressive preterminal heart failure may follow years of circulatory stability during which the only suspicion of cardiac involvement is found in the electrocardiogram. Physical and radiographic examination of the heart are often affected by thoracic deformities and by the high diaphragms of diaphragmatic dystrophy (Fig. 2). A left sternal edge systolic impulse and a loud sound of pulmonary closure are usually due to a decrease in anteroposterior chest dimensions rather than to pulmonary hypertension [1, 3]. An increase in transverse size of the heart may be caused by a high diaphragm rather than ventricular dilatation (Fig. 2). Nevertheless, there appears to be an increased prevalence of both third and fourth heart sounds (quadruple rhythms) and occasionally a patient has mitral regurgitation—not because of heart failure—but because of dystrophic scarring of a papillary muscle and adjacent left ventricular wall [4]. Inappropriate or labile sinus tachycardia [1, 4] is reminiscent of similar rate disturbances in Friedreich's ataxia. It is not known what role, if any, the autonomic nervous system plays in this regard. Our preliminary studies of autonomic regulation of the heart in Duchenne's dystrophy bear on this point. The combination of excessive rate acceleration after atropine followed by effective slowing with propranolol seem to discount the role of the parasympathetic nervous system and implicate augmented sympathetic activity as the cause of resting tachycardia in Duchenne's dystrophy. In addition, a variety of tachyarrhythmias occur, including ectopic atrial and ventricular beats, atrial flutter, paroxysmal ventricular tachycardia, and exaggerated irritability during cardiac catheterization [1]. Necropsy studies have shed at least a little light on the cause of the rhythm disturbances. Although degeneration of neurogenic fibers to the cardiac nodes has not been consistently found [4], occasionally a patient has had occlusive disease of the small coronary arteries to one or both cardiac nodes [4, 5] (Fig. 3).

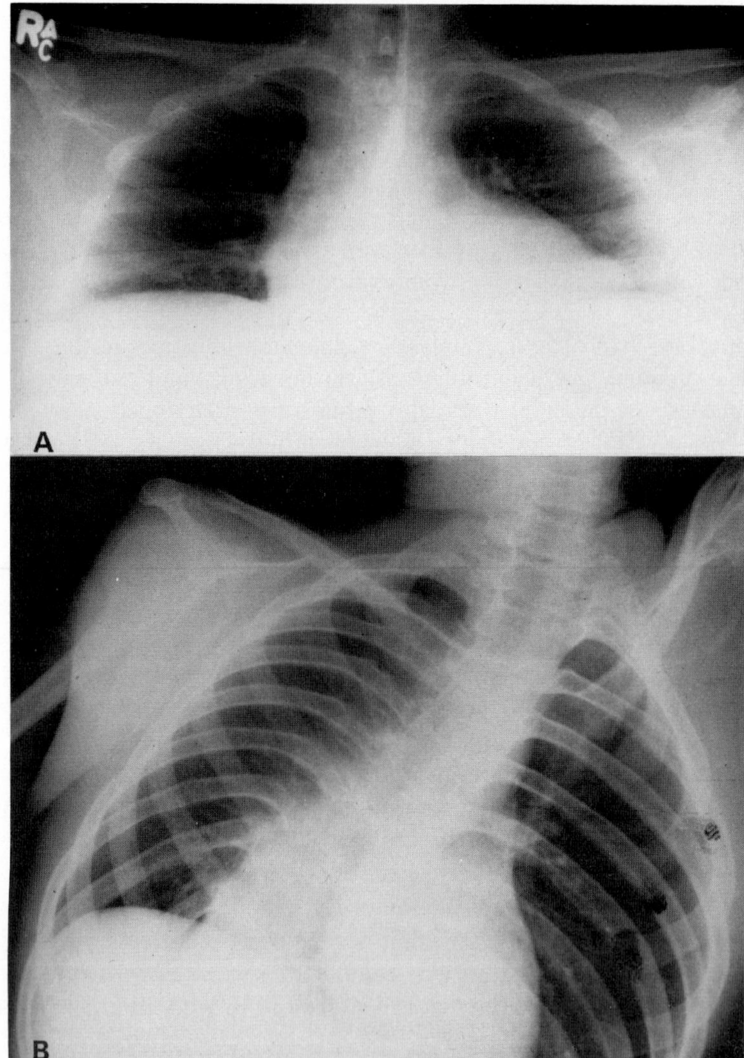

Figure 2. Classic Duchenne's Dystrophy. A. Nine-year-old boy showing distortion of the heart caused by striking symmetrical elevation of the diaphragm. B. Eleven-year-old boy showing distortion of the heart caused by marked scoliosis.

Skeletal muscle enzymes are copiously released into the plasma in Duchenne's dystrophy, but the use of enzyme quantification has not proved useful in detecting myocardial dystrophy [1]. It was hoped that the distinctive profiles of lactic dehydrogenase isozymes might identify active myocardial dystrophy. The isozyme profile in dystrophic skeletal muscle, how-

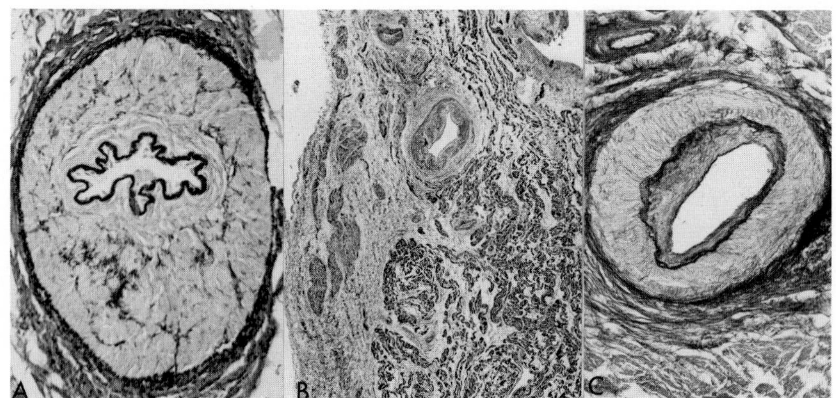

Figure 3. Classic Duchenne's Dystrophy. A. Small intramural coronary artery in the left atrium of an 18-year-old boy who died with Duchenne's dystrophy. There is severe hypertrophy of the media with luminal narrowing. Verhoff Van Gieson elastic tissue stains. B. Section of the right atrium in the region of the sinus node in the same patient as in A. The neurogenic fibers of the sinus node are seen as well as a large intramural coronary artery which has a thick wall and slightly narrowed lumen. Stains for mucopolysaccharides disclosed increased quantities of this material in the vessel. Hematoxylin and eosin stains. C. Right atrial intramural artery from a 12-year-old boy who died with classic Duchenne's muscular dystrophy. The artery exhibits thick medial and intimal walls and a narrowed lumen. This was the only abnormal coronary artery found in the patient. Elastic tissue stain. (Modified from Perloff, J. et al.: Am J Med, 42:179, 1967.)

ever, tends to resemble that of cardiac muscle, thus compromising the specificity of such determinations [2]. Furthermore, coronary sinus catheterization has not convincingly documented myocardial release of enzymes [2].

By far, the most frequent index of suspicion of cardiac involvement is derived from the electrocardiogram [1, 4, 6-8]. A number of the other varieties of heredofamilial neuromyopathic disorders are associated with abnormal electrocardiograms, but only one, the classic sex-linked pseudohypertrophic dystrophy of Duchenne, results in a distinctive uniform electrocardiographic pattern [1, 4, 6-8] (Fig. 4). In addition, the vectorcardiogram has been shown to be a useful supplement to the scalar electrocardiogram [9] (Fig. 4). Tall right precordial R waves with increased R/S amplitude ratios, and deep limb lead and lateral precordial Q waves form a distinctive motif that is related specifically to the classic pseudohypertrophic sex-linked dystrophy of Duchenne (Fig. 4). At times, the deep Q waves coexist with altered shapes of right precordial R waves (RSr′ or polyphasic R waves) [6]. Affected siblings often exhibit identical tracings,

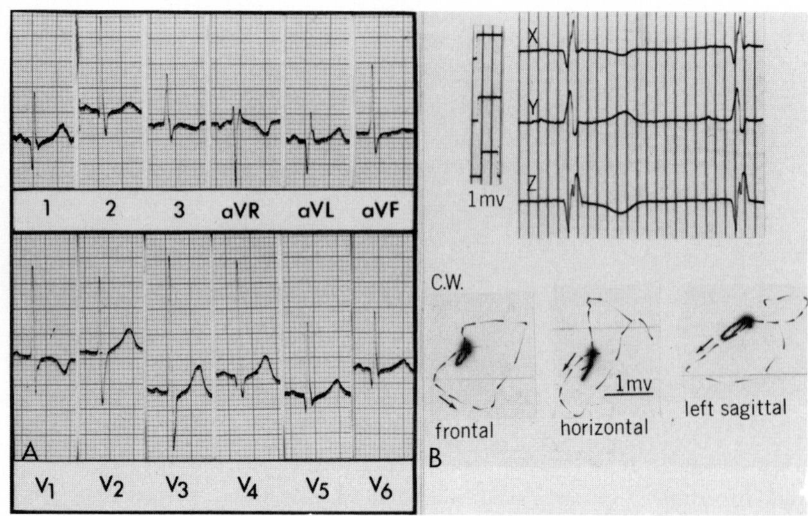

Figure 4. Classic Duchenne's Dystrophy. A. Scalar electrocardiogram in a 14-year-old boy. There is a tall R wave in lead V_1 and deep Q waves in leads I, aVl, and V_{5-6}. B. Scalar and planar Frank vectorcardiogram in a 19-year-old man. The deep Q waves in lead Z (−1.3 mV) and lead X (−0.65 mV) are due to the abnormally prominent early rightward and anterior QRS vector forces. The horizontal and left sagittal planar loops show the accentuation of anterior forces. Time lines are 0.04 second apart. Calibration signal is 1 mV. Dots in the loops are 0.004 second apart. (From Ronan, J.A., Perloff, J.K. et al.: Am Heart J 84:588, 1972.)

and distinctive Duchenne patterns have been found in female carriers who manifest only enzymatic evidence of systemic myopathic disease [6, 8].

The existence of characteristic electrocardiograms in classic Duchenne's dystrophy is no longer debated, but their mechanism is [4, 6]. Studies, thus far, have made it clear that the patterns are not related to thoracic deformity, thoracic muscle atrophy, pulmonary hypertension, hypertrophy of the right ventricle, crista supraventricularis, or interventricular septum, or to abnormalities in right ventricular conduction or to coexisting abnormalities of small intramural coronary arteries [1, 4]. Two theories are current: One, that the electrocardiographic pattern reflects acquired dystrophic myocardial disease, the sites of which are genetically regulated [2], and the other, that the morphology of the electrocardiogram represents a genetically determined persistence of the patterns of infancy and early childhood [6].

Our own observations are not consonant with the idea that the distinctive QRS in Duchenne's dystrophy represents persistence of infantile or childhood patterns [9]. What alternative theories can then be proposed?

It could be argued that the occurrence of identical electrocardiograms in siblings implies a genetic determinant of the distinct electrophysiologic patterns. This genetic determinant might result in either focal anatomic lesions in the heart or electrical alterations without detectable anatomic counterparts. A purely *electrical* explanation is essentially speculative. An *anatomic* basis for the anterior shift of the QRS and deep Q waves would mean that virtually identical zones of myocardium were preselected for dystrophic changes by the genetic determinant. Despite the fanciful nature of this concept, some evidence suggests that it may be so. The prominent anterior forces may represent a relative loss of posterobasal electrical activity as in strictly posterior myocardial infarction [1, 4, 10, 11], and the Q waves may reflect lateral or diaphragmatic extension of the dystrophic zone [4, 10]. One necropsy study lends credence to this theory [4], but proof awaits further electrocardiographic-vectorcardiographic necropsy correlations.

In addition to the release of enzymes into the circulation of dystrophic males [1], the value of creatine phosphokinase quantification has been established as a means of identifying carrier female patients in families with Duchenne's progressive muscular dystrophy. Distinctive Duchenne's electrocardiograms have been found in some female carriers who manifest only enzymatic evidence of systemic myopathic disease [6, 8]. It has been shown that these carrier females, when subjected to quantitative measurements of muscle strength, limb circumference, vital capacity, and physical working capacity may have significantly lower scores than either normal girls or siblings with normal creatine phosphokinase levels [12]. The occurrence of distinctive Duchenne electrocardiograms in female relatives of propositi raises important genetic and clinical questions. Pearson [2] found focal histopathologic changes in skeletal muscle fibers in some asymptomatic female carriers with elevated creatine phosphokinase levels. He postulated that the random nature of muscle involvement was due to X-chromosome mosaicism. If this is so, can mosaicism also play a role in myocardial dystrophy in such patients? Is the same gene responsible for both the systemic and the cardiomyopathic disease? Will female carriers with "dystrophic" electrocardiograms eventually develop overt myocardial disease? Can some cases of "idiopathic cardiomyopathy" be examples of unrecognized myocardial dystrophy? It is interesting in this regard that examination of the family histories of our subjects with classic Duchenne's dystrophy disclosed a mother who died at age 50 with "heart disease of unknown cause."

Slowly progressive muscular dystrophy [13, 14]. Duchenne-type dystrophy may be slowly progressive and either early onset autosomal recessive or late onset sex-linked recessive. When family pedigrees are deficient, it is

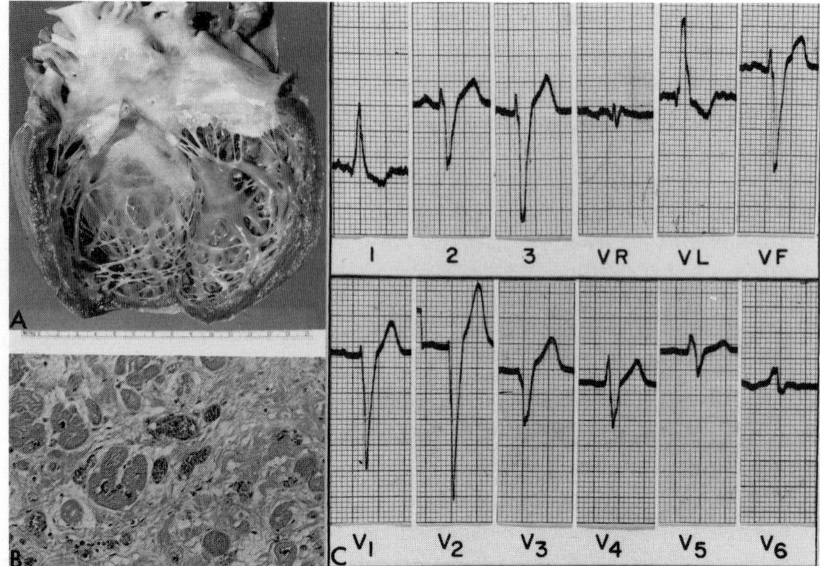

Figure 5. Cardiomyopathy. Gross and histologic photographs of the heart of a 45-year-old man with cardiomyopathy and slowly progressive muscular dystrophy, who died of his cardiomyopathy. A. Photograph shows the dilated flabby left ventricle with focal endocardial thickening. The left atrium is also dilated. B. Microscopic section from the left ventricle shows marked confluent scarring with variations in fiber size. There was no significant coronary artery disease. C. Electrocardiogram from the same patient at age 40 years. The 12-lead tracing shows left axis deviation, QRS prolongation, and small Q waves in leads I and aVl. Four years later the patient developed complete heart block. (modified from Perloff, J. et al.: Circulation 33:625, 1966.)

difficult to distinguish these two subvarieties from each other or from those forms with Erb's limb-girdle dystrophy and calf hypertrophy [2]. Such patients, though comparatively few in number, may not only have serious cardiomyopathy but also stand a good chance of dying from it [1]. The type of cardiac involvement is yet to be thoroughly studied, but it is not the same as in classic Duchenne's dystrophy [1]. One such patient had left bundle branch block, subsequent complete heart block, and at necropsy exhibited widespread dystrophic cardiomyopathy of both ventricles with involvement of the His bundle [1] (Fig. 5).

Limb-girdle dystrophy of Erb. Transmission is typically autosomal recessive with insidious onset in the second decade, but ranging from late first through fourth decades [15]. Dystrophy of the hip girdle usually precedes involvement of the shoulders (Fig. 6). Mild calf pseudohypertrophy occurs

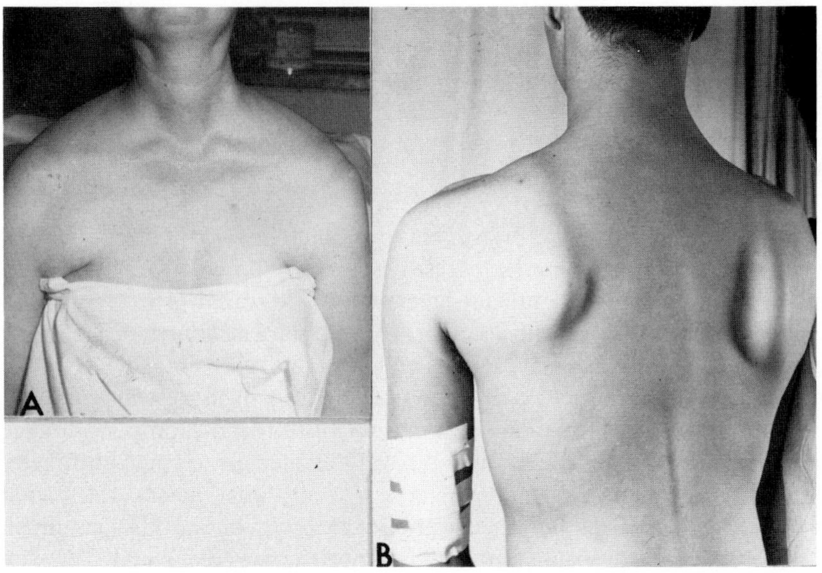

Figure 6. Limb-girdle Dystrophy (Erb). A. Photograph of a woman showing involvement of the shoulder girdle. The pelvic girdle and proximal leg muscles were also involved. The face (not shown) was completely spared. B. Young man with facioscapulohumeral dystrophy (Landouzy-Dejerine). There was involvement of the shoulder girdle, proximal, arm muscles (bandage at biopsy site), and face (not shown).

but rarely [15]. Patients trip easily because the feet are held in plantar flexion. Progression is slow but the majority of affected individuals are incapacitated within 2 decades. Although cardiac involvement is infrequent and seldom severe, it has been known to express itself as (1) disturbances in rhythm and conduction (QRS prolongation, first-degree heart block, right ventricular conduction defects, atrial flutter), (2) abnormal Q waves and minor T wave alterations, (3) third and fourth heart sound quadruple gallop rhythms, and (4) overt heart failure [1]. Symptoms such as dyspnea, cough, and those related to lower respiratory infections may stem from inadequate function of the chest bellows (dystrophy of thoracic and diaphragmatic muscle) and not from cardiac failure.

Facioscapulohumeral dystrophy. Transmission is autosomal dominant with onset from first through fourth decades. Dystrophy begins in the shoulder girdle (scapulohumeral) (Fig. 6) with inevitable subsequent involvement of the face which becomes devoid of lines (thus "facioscapulohumeral"). The hip girdle may be affected years later. Contractures and pseudohypertrophy are exceedingly rare. The course is long and progression insidious with far better prognosis than other forms of muscular dystrophy. Cardiac involvement, if it occurs at all, is rare and clinically unimportant [1].

MYOTONIC DYSTROPHY

Myotonic dystrophy (dystrophia myotonica, myotonia atrophia, myotonia dystrophia, or Steinert's disease) is a slowly progressive degenerative multisystem autosomal dominant heredofamilial disorder [16, 17]. Clinical manifestations characteristically appear in the third or fourth decades [18] although occasional cases are seen in childhood and early infancy. Myotonia (delayed relaxation after contraction) can be provoked by voluntary, mechanical, or electrical stimulation of muscles of the hands, forearms, tongue, and jaw. A myotonic response is typically elicited by tapping the thenar eminence with a percussion hammer, especially after having the patient rapidly open and close the fist. Dystrophy (atrophy or wasting) is initially found in forearms, neck (especially sternocleidomastoid), and face (expressionless myopathic facies) [16, 18] (Fig. 7). There is subsequent disturbance of the extensors of the legs and dorsiflexors of the feet with late involvement of almost any muscle group [18]. Nonmyotonic, nonmyopathic features are of additional interest and include cataracts, gonadal atrophy, frontal baldness or thinning of the hair (Fig. 7), and disease of gastrointestinal muscle [16-18]. Appropriate to this discussion is the cardiac involvement which has been known since the descriptions of Griffith in 1912 [19]. It is important to point out that myotonia congenita (Thomsen's disease) does not involve the heart and is otherwise distinct from myotonic dystrophy [20]. In myotonic dystrophy there is a striking difference between the relative frequency of electrocardiographic alterations and that of clinically overt heart disease [18, 20].

The electrocardiogram is the best indicator of cardiac involvement with abnormalities occurring in approximately two-thirds of cases [18, 20-22], but the overall incidence of overt heart failure is only about 7 percent [20]. As a rule, involvement of the heart is recognized late in the course of myotonic dystrophy, although occasionally cardiac manifestations antedate recognition of the primary disorder [17, 18, 23, 24]. The commonest conduction disturbances are prolongation of the PR interval and the QRS complex, and left bundle branch block [17, 18, 20, 22]. The vectorcardiogram is especially useful in detecting abnormalities of ventricular activation [20, 22]. Left bundle branch block may be intermittent (rate-related) [21], and normal tracings have been observed to progress from sporadic to permanent left bundle branch block [21]. The most fre-

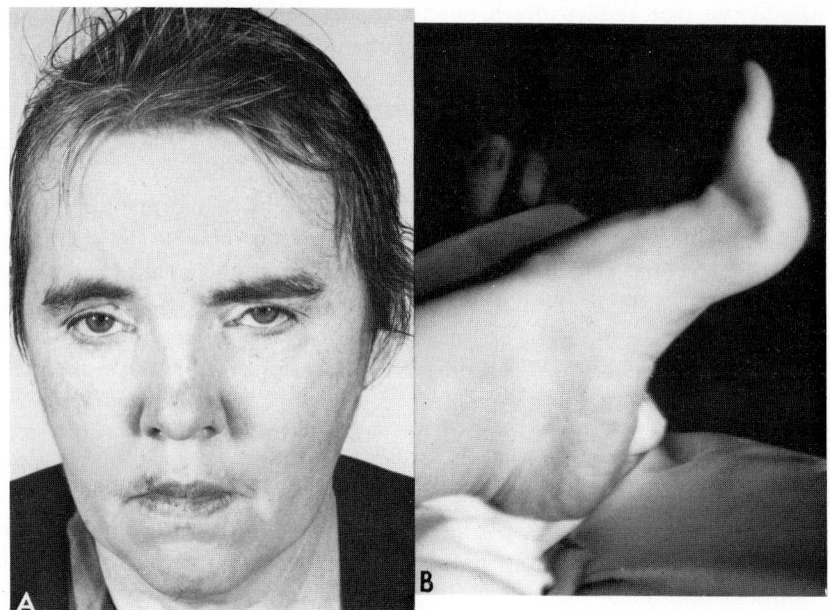

Figure 7. A. Myotonic Muscular Dystrophy. Typical expressionless myopathic facies and thin frontal hair of a 50-year-old woman. B. Friedriech's Ataxia. Typical pes cavus and hammer toe. (From Perloff, J. et al.: Progr. Cardiovasc Dis 12:409, 1970.)

quent rhythm disturbances are sinus bradycardia (in Griffith's original case, the rate ranged from 36 to 50) and atrial fibrillation or flutter [17, 18, 20-23]. Since atrial flutter or fibrillation are usually accompanied by a high-degree atrioventricular block, the ventricular rate is generally well controlled even without digitalis [16]. It should also be pointed out that although sinus bradycardia is a feature of myotonic dystrophy, sinus tachycardia is a feature of Friedreich's ataxia and Duchenne's dystrophy. In addition, low-voltage P waves, ST segment abnormalities, and flattening or inversion of the T waves are common [17, 22]. Occasionally, the tracings exhibit infarct patterns [22], right or left axis deviation [17, 18], complete heart block [18, 24, 25], or ventricular tachycardia or fibrillation [18].

Some patients manifest cardiomegaly without symptoms [18, 21] although the seeming enlargement may be more apparent than real because of the bradycardia. At other times, cardiomegaly accompanies congestive heart failure which can be swift in onset and lethal in degree [21]. There is a tendency for the systemic arterial pressure to be relatively low [20, 23]. Syncope has been ascribed to ventricular fibrillation, complete heart block and severe bradycardia [18, 24]. In view of these comments, it comes as no surprise that sudden death not only occurs [16, 21, 23] but perhaps more frequently than has generally been recognized [22]. In addition to intrinsic heart disease, patients with myotonic dystrophy exhibit cardiopulmonary failure due to disease of the neuromuscular apparatus of respiration [16, 18]. Alveolar hypoventilation results in hypercapnia, hypoxemia, pulmonary hypertension, and right ventricular failure.

Histologically, the heart may be normal. When abnormalities occur, they are neither characteristic [23, 25] nor the same as in skeletal muscle. Light microscopic descriptions include fatty infiltration and replacement, general increase in interstitial connective tissue, marked variation in size of muscle fibers and nuclei, and myofibers that vary from normal to complete destruction [23, 25]. Electron microscopic observations have disclosed vacuoles in the location of sarcoplasmic reticulum and mitochondria [25]. It has been theorized that damage to sarcoplasmic reticulum—a system associated with intracellular impulse transmission—may be responsible for the conduction defects [25]. There is little doubt that the myotonic phenomenon is unrelated to the cardiac disorder since myotonia congenita and myotonic dystrophy are both characterized by myotonia, but heart disease is present only in the latter [20]. It is attractive to relate the changes in both skeletal *and* cardiac muscle to a genetically determined biochemical abnormality [17]. The autonomic nervous system (hyperactivity of the vagus) has been implicated as a cause of the bradycardia and prolonged AV conduction, but not as a cause of intraventricular conduction disturbances. Much may yet be learned from His bundle electrocardiographic studies.

FRIEDREICH'S ATAXIA

A little over a century ago, Friedreich published his account of hereditary ataxia [19, 26]. The disorder chiefly involves the spinocerebellar and pyramidal tracts and the dorsal columns [28], manifesting itself as skeletal deformities, ataxia, and speech disturbances [21]. Onset is in childhood with slowly progressive discoordination of limb movements, ataxia of gait, scanning dysarthria, nystagmus, impairment of deep tendon reflexes and of position and vibratory sense, Babinski's sign, scoliosis, and a distinctive food deformity consisting of pes cavus with hammer toe (Fig. 7) [28-31].

Muscular atrophy increases with disease duration even though Friedreich's ataxia is essentially a neurologic rather than a myopathic disorder. Certain other distinctions should be made. The ataxia in Friedreich's disease is spinal as opposed to the cerebellar ataxia of Marie which is not associated with heart disease [31]. Refsum's disease, an inborn error of lipid metabolism (phytanic acid) [32] involves the heart and is occasionally mistaken for Friedreich's ataxia. Peroneal muscular atrophy (Charcot-Marie-Tooth's disease) is akin to Friedreich's ataxia with both disorders occurring in the same family [31, 33], but peroneal muscular atrophy progresses more slowly than Friedreich's disease, has a better prognosis, is not characterized by ataxia, and—more relevant to this discussion—is not accompanied by heart disease.* Five of Friedreich's original 6 patients had cardiac abnormalities [21], but these abnormalities were considered coincidental, and therefore unrelated to the neurologic disorder [26, 31]. In 1887, Pitt called attention to heart failure as a cause of death in Friedreich's ataxia [31], but the cardiac involvement was generally ignored until Mollaret described the electrocardiographic abnormalities in 1921 [28]. It is now believed that about one-third of patients with Friedreich's ataxia have physical signs or symptoms of heart disease [30, 31], that about 90 percent sooner or later have abnormal electrocardiograms [31, 34], and that at necropsy cardiac involvement approaches 100 percent [30]. In addition to electrocardiographic alterations, clinical manifestations include cardiomegaly without symptoms, congestive heart failure, and disturbances in heart rate, rhythm, and conduction. The severity of the central nervous system disease and the severity of the cardiac involvement do not parallel each other, and the usual pattern is for severe ataxia to exist without clinically overt heart disease [26]. The onset of cardiac manifestations is insidious and difficult to establish [26]. Since the neurological disease curtails physical activity, circulatory demands are reduced and cardiac symptoms may not appear until obvious rhythm disturbances or heart failure supervene [31]. Nevertheless, electrocardiographic abnormalities may be present in young children close to the onset of neurological disease [19], and occasionally signs of heart disease precede the neurologic manifestations [31]. It is of further interest that cardiac abnormalities are sometimes found in neurologically normal siblings [31]. Inappropriate sinus tachycardia is common [26, 28, 31, 34] as in Duchenne's dystrophy. Other rhythm disturbances include supraventricular and ventricular ectopic beats, atrial fibrillation, and paroxysmal atrial tachycardia [26, 28, 31, 34]. The most frequent electrocardiographic alterations are shallow, biphasic, or inverted T waves especially in leads II, III, or aVF [26, 28, 31, 34]. Hypertrophy patterns are of additional interest with left ventricular hypertrophy apparently more common in the slightly to moderately disabled patient, and right ventricular hypertrophy with right axis deviation in the severely handicapped [31].

* *Editorial note:* A recent report has linked peroneal muscular atrophy with familial heart block. [Kay, J.M., Littler, W.A., and Meade, J.B.: Ultrastructure of myocardium in familial heart block and peroneal muscular atrophy. Brit Heart J 34:1081, 1972.]

Occasionally, the P waves are peaked [26] and atrioventricular, or bundle branch block develops [30]. Affected members of a family often exhibit similar electrocardiographic patterns [30]. Abnormalities of the electrocardiogram may appear rapidly and are sometimes reversible [28, 34]. Thus far, there has been no consistent relationship between electrocardiographic and morphologic changes in the heart [31, 34]. The electrocardiogram is the most frequent but not the sole index of cardiac involvement. Congestive heart failure not only occurs but may develop suddenly [26, 28]. Abdominal pain (similar to that in Duchenne's dystrophy) has been related to emboli from mural thrombi, but the cause really remains unknown [28, 31, 34]. Patients sporadically experience chest pain that resembles angina pectoris or cardiac infarction [30, 31, 34], but there is no apparent relationship between chest pain, electrocardiographic patterns, and the coronary arteriopathy of Friedreich's ataxia. Hemodynamic studies have disclosed increased filling pressures in both ventricles with small stroke volumes [31]. Certain physical signs may relate to intrinsic heart disease, but—as in other neuromyopathic disorders—are often influenced by the configuration of the chest (kyphoscoliosis, diminished anteroposterior chest dimensions). A midsystolic murmur and a prominent second heart sound at the left base [31] may relate to the small anteroposterior chest size. Prominent third and fourth sounds [28, 31] may reflect myocardial disease, but must be interpreted with caution in young thin-chested subjects. Similarly, conspicuous precordial impulses may represent ventricular hypertrophy [31] but may also be related to thoracic configuration.

At necropsy, hearts have shown hypertrophy of the ventricles in addition to fiber degeneration and patchy or diffuse interstitial fibrosis [27, 31]. Of special interest is the coronary artery disease of Friedreich's ataxia. Although the coronary arteries may be normal, they may show all stages of intimal proliferation from trivial to complete luminal obliteration [26, 30, 31, 34, 35]. Particular attention has been called to involvement of small coronary arteries [35], but large- and medium-sized branches can also be affected [31]. These vessels exhibit neither thrombi nor atheromatosis [31, 34]. A relationship between the coronary arteriopathy and the diabetes mellitus that tends to occur with Friedreich's ataxia has been speculated upon but remains unproved [31, 34]. Relevant to this point is the absence of vascular disease outside of the heart [34] except in the lungs [35].

Three main theories have been proposed to explain the cardiac involvement in Friedreich's ataxia [26, 28, 30, 31, 34, 35]: (1) The neurological and cardiac diseases both stem from a single genetic defect; (2) The heart disease is at least in part secondary to disease of the nervous system; and (3) The cardiac disease is related to the coronary arteriopathy. Kyphoscoliosis and abnormal rhythmic activity of respiration serve as aggravating but not primary causes of cardiac dysfunction [31]. It is attractive to assume a primary role for the coronary artery disease in producing the rhythm and conduction disturbances, the myocardial fibrosis, and the chest pain [34, 35]. Although no theory can ignore the striking coronary arteriopathy, this mechanism as the sole or prime provoking cause leaves much to be explained. Neither cardiomegaly without symptoms nor inappropriate sinus tachycardia are features of atherosclerotic coronary artery disease. The increased heart rate in Friedreich's ataxia has been considered a compensatory mechanism needed to maintain cardiac output in the presence of reduced stroke volume [31]. However, the autonomic nervous system may play a part in the disturbances of heart rate as well as in the disturbances of rhythm, conduction, and contractility [26, 30, 31, 34]. Both excessive sympathetic activity and deficient parasympathetic function have been considered. Observations in this regard are scanty, but in one pharmacologic investigation, ganglionic blockade tended to normalize inverted T waves [31].

SUMMARY

This report has dealt with the myocardial disease in 3 categories of heredofamilial degenerative neuromyopathic disorders, namely, progressive muscular dystrophy, myotonic muscular dystrophy, and Friedreich's ataxia. In progressive muscular dystrophy, involvement of the heart occurs most frequently and is readily recognized in the early onset, rapidly progressive, sex-linked pseudohypertrophic (classic) dystrophy of Duchenne; cardiac disease may be serious, if not lethal, in the slowly progressive Duchenne-type dystrophy, is uncommon in Erb's limb-girdle dystrophy and occurs rarely, if at all, in facioscapulohumeral dystrophy. In myotonic dystrophy, involvement of the heart occurs frequently (over 50 percent), but is seldom serious. In Friedreich's ataxia, the incidence of cardiac disease is astonishingly high and the disease may be grave.

REFERENCES

1. Perloff, J.K., deLeon, A.C., and O'Doherty, D.: The cardiomyopathy of progressive muscular dystrophy. Circulation 33:625, 1966.
2. Pearson, C.M.: Muscular dystrophy. Am J Med 35:632, 1963.
3. deLeon, A.C., Perloff, J.K., Twigg, H., and Hajd, M.: The straight back syndrome—Clinical cardiovascular manifestations. Circulation 32:193, 1965.
4. Perloff, J.K., Roberts, W.C., deLeon, A.C., and O'Doherty, D.: The distinctive

electrocardiogram of Duchenne's progressive muscular dystrophy. Am J Med 42:179, 1967.

5. James, T.N.: Observations on the cardiovascular involvement including the cardiac conduction system, in progressive muscular dystrophy. Am Heart J 63: 48, 1962.
6. Slucka, C.: The electrocardiogram in Duchenne's progressive muscular dystrophy. Circulation 38:933, 1968.
7. Skyring, A. and McKusick, V.A.: Clinical, genetic and electrocardiographic studies in childhood muscular dystrophy. Am J Med Sci 242:54, 1961.
8. Mann, O., deLeon, A.C., Perloff, J.K., Simanis, J., and Horrigan, F.D.: Duchenne's muscular dystrophy: The electrocardiogram in female relatives. Am J Med Sci 255:376, 1968.
9. Ronan, J.A., Perloff, J.K., Bowen, P.J., and Mann, O.: The vectorcardiogram in Duchenne's progressive muscular dystrophy. Am Heart J 84:588, 1972.
10. Fitch, C.W. and Ainger, L.E.: The frank vectorcardiogram and the electrocardiogram in Duchenne muscular dystrophy. Circulation 35:1124, 1967.
11. Perloff, J.K.: Recognition of strictly posterior myocardial infarction by conventional scalar electrocardiography. Circulation 30:706, 1964.
12. Fowler, W.M., Gardner, G.W., Taylor, R.G., et al.: Quantitative measurements in female siblings and mothers of boys with Duchenne dystrophy. Arch Phys Med 50:301-310, 1969.
13. Mabry, C.C., Roeckel, L.E., Munich, R.L., and Robertson, D.: X-linked pseudohypertrophic muscular dystrophy with a late onset and slow progression. New Engl J Med 273:1062, 1965.
14. Zellweger, H. and Hanson, J.W.: Slowly progressive X-linked recessive muscular dystrophy. Arch Intern Med 120:525, 1967.
15. Jackson, C.E. and Strehler, D.A.: Limb-girdle muscular dystrophy: Clinical manifestations and detection of preclinical disease. Pediatrics 41:495, 1968.
16. Kohn, N.N., Faires, J.S., and Rodman, T.: Unusual manifestations due to involvement of involuntary muscle in dystrophia myotonica. New Engl J Med 271:1179, 1964.
17. Payne, C.A. and Greenfield, J.C.: ECG abnormalities associated with myotonic dystrophy. Am Heart J 65:536, 1963.
18. Church, S.C.: The heart in myotonia atrophica. Arch Intern Med 119:176, 1967.
19. Perloff, J.K., Lindgren, K.M., and Groves, B.M.: Uncommon or commonly unrecognized causes of heart failure. Progr Cardiovasc Dis 12:409, 1970.
20. Orndahl, G., Thulesius, O., Enestrom, S., and Dehlin, O.: The heart in myotonic disease. Acta Med Scand 176:479, 1964.
21. Miller, P.B.: Myotonic muscular dystrophy with electrocardiographic abnormalities. Am Heart J 63:704, 1962.
22. Fearrington, E.L., Gibson, T.C., and Churchill, R.E.: Vectorcardiographic and electrocardiographic findings in myotonia atrophica. Am Heart J 67:599, 1964.
23. Holt, J.M. and Lambert, E.H.N.: Heart disease as presenting features of myotonia atrophica. Br Heart J 26:433, 1964.
24. Petkovich, N.J., Dunn, M., and Reed, W.: Myotonia dystrophica with A-V dissociation and Stokes-Adams attacks. Am Heart J 68:391, 1964.
25. Bulloch, R.T., Davis, J.L., and Hara, M.: Dystrophia myotonica with heart block: A light and electron microscopic study. Arch Pathol 84:130, 1967.
26. Thilenius, O.G. and Gross, B.J.: Friedreich's ataxia with heart disease in children. Pediatrics 27:246, 1961.

27. Hartman, J.M. and Booth, R.W.: Friedreich's ataxia, a neurocardiac disease. Am Heart J 60:713, 1960.
28. Boyer, S.H., Chisholm, A.W., and McKusick, V.A.: Cardiac aspects of Friedreich's ataxia. Circulation 25:493, 1962.
29. Spillane, J.D.: Familial pes cavus and absent ankle jerks. Its relationship with Friedreich's disease and peroneal muscular atrophy. Brain 63:275, 1940.
30. Gauthier, E.J.: Cardiac disease in Friedreich's ataxia. Ann Intern Med 60:892, 1964.
31. Thoren, C.: Cardiomyopathy in Friedreich's ataxia. Acta Pediat (Suppl) 153:1, 1964.
32. Richterich, R., van Mechelen, P., and Rossi, E.: Refsum's disease. Am J Med 29:230, 1965.
33. Roth, M.: Relationship between hereditary ataxia and peroneal muscular atrophy. Brain 71:416, 1948.
34. Ivemark, B. and Thoren, C.: Pathology of the heart in Friedreich's ataxia. Acta Med Scand 175:227, 1964.
35. James, T.N. and Fisch, C.: Observations on the cardiovascular involvement in Friedreich's ataxia. Am Heart J 66:164, 1968.

NOBLE O. FOWLER, M.D.

The Secondary Cardiomyopathies

The secondary cardiomyopathies are those in which myocardial disease is but one manifestation of a systemic illness. The clinical evidence of myocardial involvement, however, may be the principal feature. For example, occasionally in patients with myocardial sarcoidosis, there may be little or no evidence of systemic illness, peripheral lymphadenopathy, skin lesions, parotid or other salivary gland involvement. Mediastinal lymph node enlargement, pulmonary infiltrate, bone disease, hypercalcemia, and hyperglobulinemia may be lacking. Yet the patient may display cardiac enlargement, heart failure, cardiac arrhythmia, or heart block as a result of sarcoidosis. On the other hand, in a different setting, clinical evidence of heart disease may be lacking and myocardial involvement may be discovered at autopsy. For example, leukemia or disseminated lupus erythematosus commonly involve the myocardium without evidence of heart disease during life.

In the classification which we use [1], the idiopathic or primary cardiomyopathies comprise the larger group of patients with myocardial disease; the secondary cardiomyopathies are less common. Segal, Harvey, and Gurel [2] found that the idiopathic myocardial diseases were approximately three times as common as those associated with an identifiable illness. This proportion agrees with our own experience. In the classification that we use, certain of the myocardial diseases are considered to be idiopathic even though there is a suspected association with a specific cause. An example is seen in the patient thought to have postinfectious cardiomyopathy, especially when the infectious agent has not been identified. For example, the picture of idiopathic cardiomyopathy may follow Coxsackie B virus infections of the myocardium [3]. Whether or not the persistent evidence of myocardial involvement is a form of autoimmune disease, or whether it results directly from the original viral invasion of the myocardium is not known. For this reason, we classify patients with persistent evidence of myocardial disease, following presumed viral myocarditis, under the heading of idiopathic cardiomyopathy. Idiopathic nonobstructive cardiomyopathy may be familial [1]. It may be of an obstructive nature as well as either familial or nonfamilial [1]. Thus, familial cardiomyopathy, whether obstructive or nonobstructive, is classified under the idiopathic category. Cardiomyopathy in an alcoholic may or may not be related to the toxic effects of ethanol. When there is doubt, the disease is best classified with the idiopathic group. Alcoholic heart disease is the subject of a separate chapter by Dr. Timothy Regan.

The causes of secondary cardiomyopathies may therefore be classified as follows:

1. Neuromuscular disease [4]
   a. Friedreich's ataxia
   b. Myotonic muscular dystrophy
   c. Duchenne's muscular dystrophy
   d. Facioscapulohumeral muscular dystrophy
   e. Limb-girdle muscular dystrophy
2. Connective tissue diseases
   a. Scleroderma
   b. Dermatomyositis
   c. Rheumatoid heart disease
   d. Rheumatic myocardial disease
   e. Disseminated lupus erythematosus
   f. Ankylosing spondylitis with cardiac involvement
3. Neoplastic heart disease, both primary and metastatic neoplasm, lymphoma, and leukemia
4. Metabolic heart disease
   a. Thyrotoxicosis
   b. Hemochromatosis
   c. Myxedema
   d. Glycogen-storage disease (Pompe's disease)
   e. Infiltrative disease (e.g., Refsum's disease, mucopolysaccharidosis, Hunter's syndrome, Hurler's syndrome, the lipidoses)
   f. Pheochromocytoma
   g. Acromegaly
5. Nutritional disease
   a. Beriberi
   b. Kwashiorkor

6. Myocarditis
   a. Viral: Coxsackie B, Coxsackie A, echovirus, influenza virus, infectious mononucleosis, and others
   b. Parasitic: trichinosis
   c. Protozoal: trypanosomiasis cruzi (Chagas' disease); amebiasis, toxoplasmosis
   d. Bacterial: bacterial endocarditis; septicemia; diphtheria
   e. Unknown or allergic: drug reaction, Loeffler's parietal endocarditis, serum sickness [5]
7. Granulomatous: sarcoidosis
8. Amyloidosis
   a. Primary: senile, familiar, nonfamilial
   b. Secondary
9. Posttraumatic following penetrating or nonpenetrating trauma, or surgical procedures
10. Toxic
    a. Uremia
    b. Alcohol
    c. Carbon monoxide
    d. Thorazine and related drugs
    e. Cobalt
    f. Following radiation therapy
    g. Other drugs and chemical agents

Among 57 patients with a specific etiology of myocardopathy (secondary myocardial disease), Harvey and associates found connective tissue diseases the most common (17 patients) [6]. Seven had bacterial myocarditis; 7, uremia; 6 had hyperthyroidism; 4, rheumatoid arthritis; 3 each had malignant disease, sarcoidosis, or toxic cardiomyopathy. Two had amyloid disease; 2 had hemochromatosis; the remaining 3 were in the miscellaneous category.

Presenting features of the secondary myocardial diseases. The clinical findings in patients with secondary myocardial diseases are usually similar to those demonstrated by patients who have idiopathic myocardial disease with the addition that clinical evidence of the underlying illness is usually present. Since the clinical features of the myocardial diseases are described elsewhere in this book, we will only summarize them here.

The majority of patients with myocardial disease, whether of the idiopathic or secondary variety, seek medical attention because of the symptoms of heart failure. As a rule, the heart failure is biventricular, but at times involvement of one ventricle may dominate the clinical picture. Usually the symptoms of left ventricular failure predominate over those of right ventricular failure. Hence, effort dyspnea, nocturnal dyspnea, cough, expectoration, orthopnea, and weakness may occur either alone as evidence of left ventricular failure or in combination with the usual signs of right ventricular failure: dependent edema, hepatic engorgement, and evidence of systemic venous congestion. At times, evidence of right heart failure may dominate the clinical picture, and signs of left ventricular enlargement and dysfunction must be sought with care. In such instances, the clinical picture of idiopathic (primary) pulmonary hypertension may be simulated. Other clinical features which may suggest myocardial disease are somewhat less common. Among these are cardiac arrhythmias, especially ventricular premature beats, atrioventricular block, or atrial fibrillation. Syncope which results from heart block, tachyarrhythmia, or cerebral embolism may be the first sign of cardiomyopathy. Sudden death may be the ultimate expression of this feature of the illness. At other times, either systemic arterial embolism or pulmonary embolism initiate the clinical symptoms. At times, myocardial disease is unrecognized until previously unknown cardiac enlargement is found by means of a routine physical examination, a survey chest radiograph, or an electrocardiogram.

Myocardial disease may occur at any age. Coxsackie B myocarditis may occur in the neonatal period as the result of Coxsackie B infection in the mother. Although middle life is the most fertile period for the myocardial diseases, cardiomyopathy is common in patients in their seventies and eighties. The idiopathic myocardial diseases seem to be somewhat more common in men and in Negroes.

Criteria for the diagnosis of the myocardial diseases. The following are our criteria for the clinical diagnosis:

A. Positive features
   1. Cardiac enlargement, with or without cardiac decompensation
   2. Evidence of left ventricular enlargement although clinical evidence of right ventricular enlargement may predominate
   3. Abnormal electrocardiogram
   4. Usually, a third or fourth sound gallop, or both, especially if there is congestive heart failure

B. Negative features
   1. Absence of sustained systemic arterial hypertension
   2. Absence of constrictive pericarditis or cardiac tamponade
   3. Absence of rheumatic or other valvular heart disease
   4. Absence of sufficient pulmonary dysfunction to cause cor pulmonale
   5. Absence of angina pectoris

It must be recognized that patients with myocardopathy may have murmurs of tricuspid insufficiency, mitral insufficiency and, rarely, aortic insufficiency. These presumably result from dilation of the respective valvular ring and, in the case of AV valves, at times from dysfunction of right or left ventricular papillary muscles.

Physical findings. The physical findings related to the cardiovascular system are not specific for myocardial disease but may be strongly suggestive of that possibility. When there is evidence of a systemic illness known to involve the myocardium in a patient with unexplained heart disease, the probability of myocardial disease is suggested. For example, the skin may show evidence of sarcoidosis, scleroderma, dermatomyositis, lupus erythematosus, or hemochromatosis. On physical examination, there may be evidence of a neuromuscular disease or of a lymphoma or a neoplasm of the lung or breast. The examination of the cardiovascular system is important since signs of aortic valve disease and mitral stenosis are ordinarily absent in patients with cardiomyopathy; on the other hand, cardiac enlargement, gallop rhythm, and mitral or tricuspid insufficiency are common. Hence, jugular vein engorgement, dependent pitting edema, hepatic engorgement, or pleural effusion may be found as evidence of right heart failure, and there is often a left parasternal systolic lifting impulse related to right ventricular enlargement. Tachypnea, fine pulmonary basilar rales, cough, and labored breathing are commonly present as evidence of left ventricular decompensation. Tachycardia is common in patients with cardiac decompensation. Ordinarily, there is evidence of left ventricular enlargement. The cardiac apex impulse thus is usually displaced laterally and downward beyond the fifth left intercostal space and the midclavicular line. In addition, the apical impulse is characteristically diffuse and heaving, and covers an area the size of a half-dollar or more. The systemic arterial blood pressure is often normal, but the pulse pressure may be narrow, and the diastolic pressure may be temporarily elevated during heart failure. Pulsus alternans is common, and may be brought out by having the patient sit or stand.

Cardiac auscultation. Cardiac murmurs may be entirely absent, or they may be present and even conspicuous. The commonest murmur is an apical systolic murmur which may be either pansystolic or of the delayed variety, associated with papillary muscle dysfunction. These murmurs may raise the question of primary mitral valve disease. As a rule, they diminish or disappear when the patient improves, whereas those caused by rheumatic fever may become more obvious as the patient improves. Cardiac fluoroscopy may or may not be helpful in separating rheumatic mitral disease from cardiomyopathy. Calcification within the mitral valve usually indicates rheumatic disease, but left atrial enlargement may be prominent in cardiomyopathy as well as in rheumatic mitral disease. The second commonest murmur is that of tricuspid insufficiency. It is most likely to be found in the cardiomyopathy patient who has both right and left ventricular decompensation and is ordinarily associated with considerable right ventricular enlargement. The murmur is pansystolic and loudest at the left lower sternal edge. It is often increased on inspiration and may be associated with prominent regurgitant CV waves in both deep and external jugular venous pulses. These signs of tricuspid regurgitation, like those of mitral regurgitation, usually recede when the patient responds to treatment for his cardiac decompensation. Other murmurs are relatively uncommon. Occasionally, the murmur of aortic valve insufficiency is found, and a few patients with cardiomyopathy display the systemic signs of an increased arterial pulse pressure with aortic insufficiency. Shabetai described an apical delayed diastolic murmur like that of mitral stenosis in patients with idiopathic cardiomyopathy [7]. This murmur was attributed to obstruction of the left ventricular inflow tract. Atrial and ventricular diastolic gallops may simulate a short middiastolic murmur and thus incorrectly suggest mitral stenosis.

Gallop rhythm is extremely common in myocardial disease, and the diagnosis of cardiomyopathy should be held in question if gallop rhythm is not heard, especially if there is no gallop during periods of heart failure or when the heart is greatly dilated. Both presystolic and diastolic apical left ventricular gallops are extremely common. Their impulses are usually palpable as well as audible, especially when the patient is examined in the left lateral decubitus position. At times, there is a summation gallop. There are often additional gallop sounds along the lower left sternal edge which are accentuated during inspiration. These diastolic sounds may be of right ventricular origin.

Electrocardiogram

The electrocardiogram is almost always abnormal in patients with cardiomyopathy.

Rhythm. Cardiac arrhythmias are very common. Atrial fibrillation was found in almost one-third of one group of patients with cardiomyopathy [8]. Atrial flutter has been observed in a number of instances in our patients. Premature ventricular beats are common. Paroxysmal ventricular tachycardia is found occasionally. Both complete and partial AV block have been especially common in patients with sarcoidosis.

Ventricular complexes. The pattern of left ventricular hypertrophy is perhaps the commonest single ECG feature among cardiomyopathy patients.

Left bundle branch block is often found. Abnormal Q waves or QS patterns suggesting myocardial infarction or necrosis are frequently observed in our patients. Abnormal left axis deviation with left anterior fascicular block is very common. The Wolff-Parkinson-White syndrome is more often seen in obstructive than in nonobstructive cardiomyopathy but may occur in the latter.

The T waves may display a variety of changes and at times mimic those due to myocardial ischemia.

P Waves. Frequently, there are broad notched P waves in the limb leads—at times with a large late negative component in lead V_1. These findings suggest left atrial involvement. At times the P waves display high voltage in leads II, III, aVF, and V_1, suggesting right atrial involvement.

SPECIFIC VARIETIES OF SECONDARY CARDIOMYOPATHY

The neuromuscular diseases which affect the myocardium are discussed in the chapter by Dr. Joseph Perloff and will not be discussed here.

Connective Tissue Diseases

Scleroderma. This disease may affect the heart in one of several ways. It may produce the variety of scleroderma heart disease, described by Weiss [9], which is accompanied by myocardial degeneration, acute and chronic inflammation, and myocardial fibrosis [10]. Myocardial fibrosis, a nonspecific pathologic finding, was observed in 81 percent of 58 autopsies in patients with scleroderma, and was significantly more common than in controls [11]. Scleroderma may affect the heart by invading the pericardium, but pericarditis is often related to accompanying uremia. Scleroderma may affect either the mitral or tricuspid valve. It may produce cor pulmonale through pulmonary fibrosis accompanied by pulmonary vascular involvement. It may produce systemic arterial hypertension through renal involvement. Scleroderma may involve the coronary arteries and lead to myocardial infarction [10]; however, large areas of myocardial necrosis are exceptional. The intimal thickening of scleroderma is usually limited to the intramyocardial coronary arteries. The possibility of scleroderma myocardial disease, or scleroderma heart disease, should be considered in the patient who has heart disease accompanied by the signs suggesting scleroderma, including shiny inelastic skin over the face and the upper extremities (Fig. 1), Raynaud's syndrome, dilatation of the esophagus with loss of peristalsis,

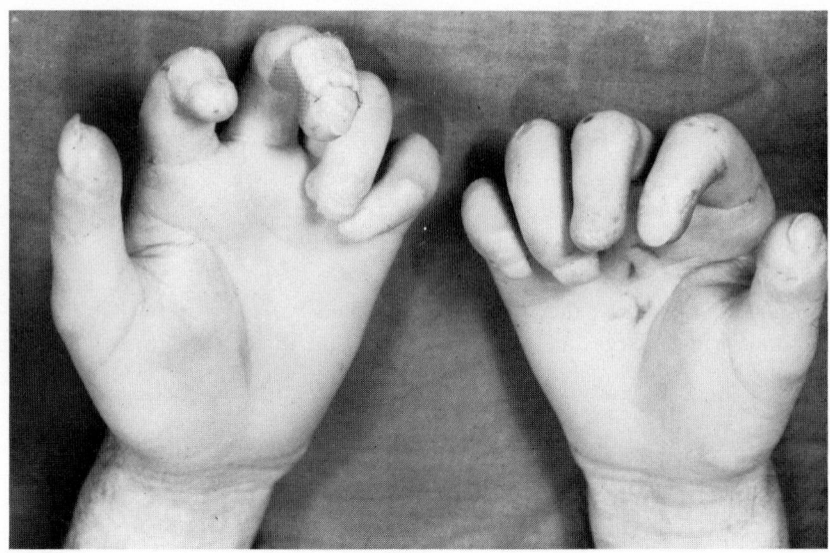

Figure 1. Sclerodactylia. From a patient with scleroderma. (Courtesy of Dr. E.A. Gall.)

and unexplained pulmonary fibrosis demonstrated by the chest radiography. Uremia may result from necrotizing renal vasculitis.

Dermatomyositis. Patients with dermatomyositis may have cardiac involvement. Cardiac enlargement was found, however, in only 5 of 40 patients in one series [12]. In another study of 8 autopsies in children, the myocardium was normal in 4 and showed small foci of inflammatory cells in 4 [13]. In many centers, dermatomyositis is considered a variety of polymyositis [14]. The diagnosis is suggested by the presence of fever, edema, and erythema of the skin, tenderness and weakness of the skeletal muscles, especially of the shoulder girdle, pelvic girdle, and extremities. Dysphagia may occur. Raynaud's syndrome is common. There may be periorbital edema and heliotrope pigmentation with a butterfly rash across the cheeks. Electromyography may prove useful in the diagnosis. A skin biopsy may confirm the diagnosis. In many instances, there is an underlying malignant tumor. Uncommonly, patients with polymyositis develop myocarditis. In this disease, inflammation of the His bundle and bundle branches may cause complete AV block [15, 16].

Rheumatoid heart disease, including ankylosing spondylitis. With systemic rheumatoid arthritis, there may be involvement of the myocardium as well as aortic or mitral valve disease, or pericarditis [17]. Ankylosing spondylitis is generally considered to be a different disease. Ninety-five percent of the patients with the latter are men. Patients who have ankylosing spondylitis may develop complete heart block [18] or aortic insufficiency [19]. As a rule, aortic insufficiency occurs in only 5 to 10 percent of those with the disease and in those who have been ill for 10 years, or more.

Rheumatic fever. Isolated myocardial disease caused by rheumatic fever occurs but is very uncommon in the absence of rheumatic valvular disease. The writer has observed only a very few patients who had Aschoff bodies in the myocardium without distinctive rheumatic valvular disease. Some such patients present the clinical picture of protracted heart failure without arthritis, fever, or pancarditis.

Disseminated lupus erythematosus. Lupus erythematosus is believed to involve the myocardium quite commonly [20]. In some studies, it was reported to involve the heart in as many as 40 to 50 percent of patients. The possibility should be considered in the patient who has evidence of myocardial involvement and who has the characteristic features of lupus erythematosus which include fever, skin rash, arthritis, Raynaud's phenomenon, occasional splenomegaly, pleuritis, or pericarditis. The foregoing findings are especially suggestive when they occur in a young woman in the menstruating age group. The patient may also have hypertension and the nephrotic syndrome. The joint lesions may resemble those of rheumatoid arthritis.

Laboratory data tend to show pancytopenia, hemolytic anemia, and biologically false-positive tests for syphilis. The urine may show evidence of lupus nephritis. Serum complement levels are usually decreased when there is active lupus nephritis. The antinuclear antibody tests are usually positive and of the diffuse variety. The LE cell test is usually positive.

Drug-induced lupus-like syndromes. A clinical syndrome of pleurisy, fever, arthritis, pericarditis, and arteritis may follow the use of certain drugs. Myocardial involvement probably accompanies this illness. The drugs most likely to cause this syndrome are procainamide, hydralazine, isoniazide, and diphenylhydantoin, but other drugs may be responsible [21]. Prospective studies have shown that prolonged use of procainamide may be followed by serologic and hematologic abnormalities in as many as 50 percent of patients [22]. LE cells and antinuclear antibodies commonly appear. The drug-induced lupus-like syndromes differ from spontaneous lupus erythematosus in that skin rash and nephritis are usually absent; the syndrome is ordinarily reversible on withdrawal of the offending agent, but death may occur.

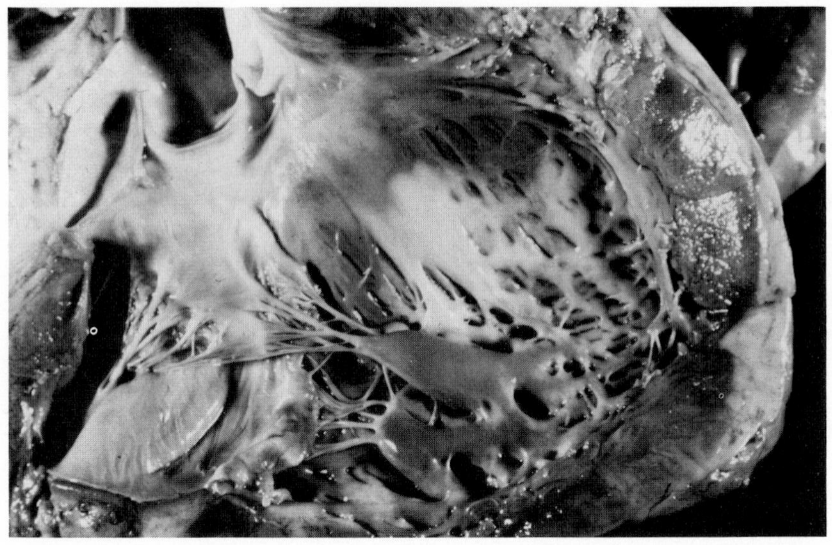

Figure 2. Cardiac invasion by lymphoma.

Neoplastic Heart Involvement

Primary myocardial involvement by neoplasm is very uncommon. Rhabdomyoma may be found in patients who have tuberous sclerosis with the characteristic skin lesions of adenoma sebaceum. When a patient is known to have a neoplasm and the cardiac examination shows evidence of pericarditis, arrhythmia or congestive heart failure, the possibility of neoplastic involvement of the heart should be strongly considered. In some autopsy studies of patients who died of malignant tumor, the heart was reported to be involved by neoplasm in as many as 20 to 30 percent [23]. Patients who had leukemia, lymphoma, or myeloma were found to have heart involvement at autopsy in 36 percent of instances [23]. Cardiac involvement is especially common in leukemia, but this seldom reaches the level of clinical expression. Carcinoma of the breast in women and carcinoma of the lung in men are perhaps the commonest neoplasms that involve the heart. However, in our experience (Fig. 2), lymphoma is a neoplasm which commonly leads to clinical evidence of involvement of the heart. Malignant melanoma, although not a common neoplasm, is said to be especially prone to involve the heart. In 1 of our patients, complete heart block with syncope was the presenting feature of carcinoma of the lung which had metastasized to the heart in a man in his forties.

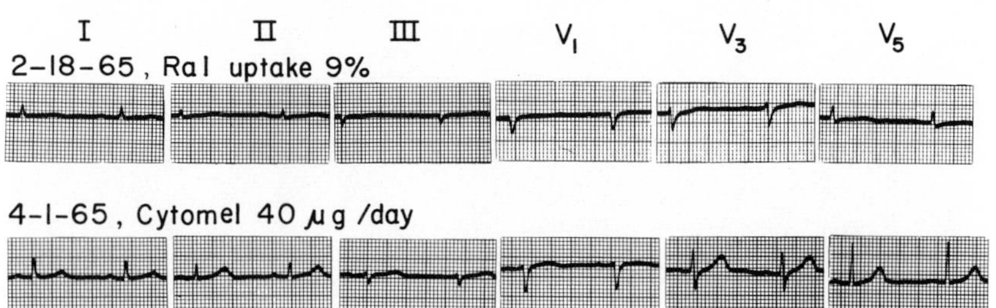

Figure 3. Myxedema. Electrocardiogram showing low-voltage QRS complexes and response to treatment. (From Fowler, N.O.: *Cardiac Diagnosis*, Courtesy of Harper & Row, New York, 1968.

Metabolic Diseases

Thyrotoxicosis may be followed by cardiomyopathy and by persistent cardiac enlargement with gallop rhythm and cardiac failure, even in the absence of other heart disease [24]). Circulating thyroid hormone is believed to have a direct effect on the myocardium [25].

Myxedema commonly produces pericardial effusion and is often associated with coronary artery disease or hypertension. Myxedema may cause myocardial disease [26] although this concept is not universally accepted. Myxedema is suggested by the physical findings of apathy, puffy features, hoarseness, a low-pitched voice, cold intolerance, hair loss, especially involving the scalp hair and the outer third of the eyebrows, diminished sweating, slow pulse, hypothermia, somnolence, delayed relaxation phase of the deep tendon reflexes, evidence of serious effusions, and the demonstration of low-voltage electrocardiographic complexes (Fig. 3). The diagnosis can be confirmed by measurement of serum T_4 levels, or study of the thyroid uptake of radioactive iodine.

Hemochromatosis should be considered as a possibility in the patient who has myocardial disease, diabetes, evidence of skin bronzing or grayish discoloration, and evidence of liver cirrhosis (Fig. 4). Iron may be deposited in the AV node, leading to heart block and arrhythmias [27]. At times, the skin pigmentation is inconspicuous. The possibility of myocardial hemochromatosis is especially to be considered in patients who have been exposed to secondary iron overload caused by transfusion as well as in those who have the idiopathic disease. Patients with long-standing anemia, such as sickle cell anemia, thalassemia, or aplastic anemia, are prone to develop hemochromatosis, especially if they have received 100 transfusions or more. Patients who drink a good deal of red wine also may develop

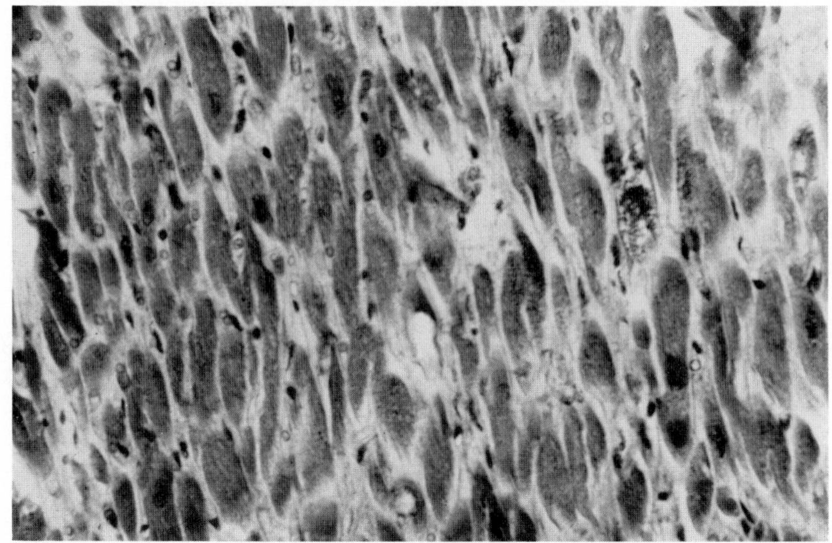

Figure 4. Myocardial hemochromatosis. Hematoxylin and eosin stain.

hemochromatosis. Patients with nutritional cirrhosis may develop hemochromatosis following a portocaval shunt performed for bleeding esophageal varices. A good screening test for this disease is to determine the plasma iron level. When this value exceeds 150 μg/100 ml, or 50 percent of transferrin capacity, the possibility of the disease is increased. In one study of symptomatic patients with hemochromatosis, the plasma iron was above 150 μg/100 ml in 31 of 32 patients [28]. In only 4 of 100 normal subjects did plasma iron exceed this value and then not consistently. The diagnosis of hemochromatosis can be established by liver biopsy.

Patients with pheochromocytoma may develop myocardial damage with fibrosis and collections of inflammatory cells within the myocardium [29]. Fatal arrhythmia or pulmonary edema may ensue. Paroxysmal hypertension, weight loss, palpitation, and increased basal metabolic rate with elevated fasting blood sugar may suggest the diagnosis,, which can be confirmed by urinalysis for catecholamines, vanilmandelic acid (VMA), or normetanephrines.

Acromegaly may be associated with heart disease [30, 31]. Glycogen-storage disease (Pompe's disease) is an unusual cause of myocardial disease and generally is found only in infants [32]. Dr. George Hug of the Children's Hospital in Cincinnati, Ohio has specialized in the study of this unusual disease.

Uncommon diseases which may infiltrate the myocardium include:

Refsum's disease [33], Fabry's disease [34], the various mucopolysaccharidoses such as Hunter's syndrome, Hurler's syndrome [35], and also the various lipidoses [36].

Nutritional Disease

Beriberi may involve the myocardium and produce a variety of high-output heart failure with gallop rhythm, elevated systemic venous pressure, and tachycardia [37]. Blankenhorn laid down the criteria for the diagnosis of beriberi heart disease, and these included insufficient evidence of other etiology, evidence of thiamine deficient diet for 3 months or more, presence of elevated systemic venous pressure, dependent edema, enlarged heart with sinus rhythm, minor electrocardiographic changes, physical signs consistent with either pellagra or beriberi, and either a therapeutic response to thiamine, or death, with autopsy findings consistent with the diagnosis [38]. Beriberi has also been reported to be followed by a low-output variety of heart failure [39]. This is apparently uncommon.

Kwashiorkor, a dietary disease associated with protein deficiency, especially common in Africans, may be followed by a form of heart failure and may be considered a variety of cardiomyopathy [40].

Myocarditis

There are several varieties of myocarditis. Viral myocarditis may result from Coxsackie B virus, Coxsackie A virus, echovirus, influenza virus, infectious mononucleosis, poliovirus, mumps, measles, German measles, infectious hepatitis, chickenpox, smallpox, vaccinia, epidemic hemorrhagic fever, arbor viruses, yellow fever, psittacosis, lymphopathia venereum, herpes simplex, and lymphocytic choriomeningitis. Reiter's syndrome, rabies and cytomegalovirus also may involve the myocardium [41].

In a report by Smith [41], of 42 patients with Coxsackie B myocarditis or pericarditis, 20 had pericarditis. Six of the 22 with myocarditis did not recover completely and eventually died. Coxsackie B myocarditis may be followed by a clinical picture similar to that commonly seen in idiopathic cardiomyopathy. In this case the patient no longer has tachycardia and fever, except as related to heart failure or its complications. As a rule, patients with Coxsackie B myocarditis recover completely if they survive [42]. The subject of viral myocarditis is analyzed by Dr. Abelmann in a separate chapter, and therefore it will not be discussed further in this chapter.

Myocarditis also may result from trichinosis [43] which may be suggested by a history of ingestion of insufficiently cooked pork and the observations of periorbital swelling, fever, tender muscles, cardiac enlargement, gallop rhythm, and eosinophilia. The trichinosis skin test is positive, and circulating IgE may be increased [44]. The diagnosis may be confirmed by skeletal muscle biopsy. Protozoal disease, such as trypanosomiasis cruzi, syphilis, or toxoplasmosis, may produce myocarditis. Myocardial disease caused by Chagas' disease (trypanosomiasis cruzi) is usually believed to be limited to South America. Two cases, however, have been reported in Texas, and there is serologic evidence of its existence in man in the southeastern United States [45].

Toxoplasmosis. The clinical features of toxoplasmosis are fever, adenopathy, muscle pain, and skin rash. There may be a history of eating insufficiently cooked meat or of association with cats. Meningitis may occur [46]. Myocarditis and pneumonitis may develop. The treatment of leukemia with adrenal steroids and folic acid antagonists may activate toxoplasmosis and cause fatal myocarditis [47]. The Sabin-Feldman dye test is useful in the diagnosis.

Myocarditis may occur as a complication of bacterial infections [48], for example, septicemia, including that which results from bacterial endocarditis. Myocarditis may follow pneumonia [49]. Myocarditis also may be of unknown cause or of the allergic variety, occurring with reactions to drugs and to smallpox vaccination. Löffler's parietal endocarditis may be associated with endomyocardial disease and eosinophilia; the peripheral blood leukocyte counts may be as high as 81,000 per cubic mm with as much as 98 percent eosinophils. Thrombi may occur over the endocardium, in the coronary arteries, and in the pulmonary arteries [50, 51]. Myocarditis has been descriped in patients with amebiasis [52]. Myocardial involvement may follow radiation for thoracic tumors [53]. In rabbits, a single dose of 2,000 rads of radiation caused acute radiation pancarditis within 6 to 48 hours, followed by a latent period of 2 to 70 days. The late stage is characterized by myocardial fibrosis, pericardial fibrosis, and pericardial effusion [54]. Ethiopian louse-borne relapsing fever caused by the Spirochete *Borrelia recurrentis* may be complicated by interstitial myocarditis and heart failure [55].

Diphtheritic Myocarditis

Diphtheritic myocarditis is produced by the action of the diphtheria exotoxin on the myocardium. It is a common cause of death in diphtheria and may be associated with peripheral neuropathy. Clinical evidence of myocardial involvement may appear at the end of the first week or the beginning of the second week of the illness. Electrocardiographic S-T segment and T-wave abnormalities are common; AV block and intra-

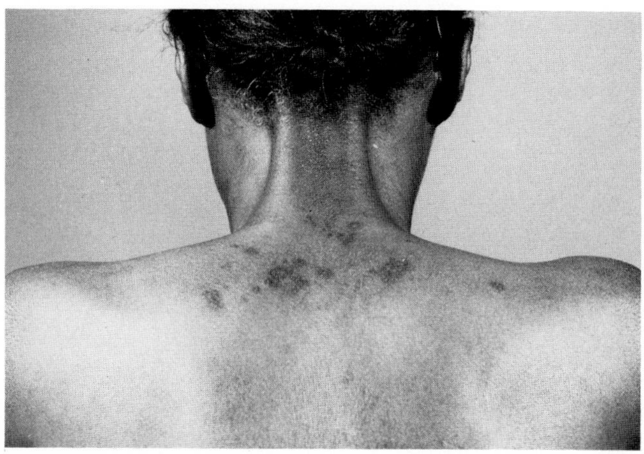

Figure 5. Myocardial Sarcoidosis. Skin lesions of sarcoidosis in a Negro woman. (From Fowler, N.O.: *Physical Diagnosis of Heart Disease*, Courtesy of the MacMillan Company, New York, 1962.)

ventricular conduction disturbances may appear [56, 57]. In a study of 46 children with diphtheria, evidence of myocardial involvement was found in 46 percent [57].

Sarcoidosis

Sarcoidosis may involve the heart and circulation in one of several ways. It may produce cor pulmonale through pulmonary involvement. Sarcoidosis may produce myocardial involvement leading to heart block [58], cardiac tachyarrhythmia [58], heart failure and sudden death. Ventricular aneurysm may occur [58]. Cardiac sarcoidosis rarely may involve the pericardium [59]. Valvular involvement is extremely rare. Sarcoidosis is a disease of unknown cause. It is no longer thought to be related to tuberculosis or to exposure to pine pollens. The majority of patients with sarcoidosis are Negroes. Myocardial involvement is said to occur in perhaps 13 to 20 percent of patients [60]. Clinical evidence of myocardial involvement is said to be much less common than this figure would suggest [61]. Most patients with sarcoid involvement of the heart have other manifestations of the disease, including cervical and mediastinal adenopathy, ocular involvement, pulmonary infiltration, increased serum calcium levels, hyperglobulinemia, or skin lesions (Fig. 5). The diagnosis may be established by biopsy of the skin, lymph node, or liver. We have, however, observed several patients with sarcoidosis of the myocardium in whom the other features were not conspicuous. We have now observed 5 patients who have had either complete heart block or sudden death from cardiac

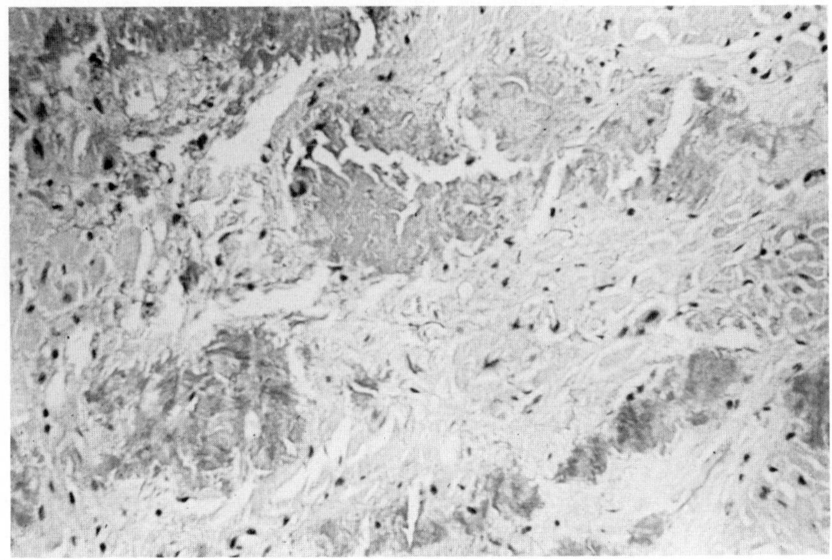

Figure 6. Cardiac Amyloidosis. Congo red stain.

arrhythmias as the manifestation of myocardial sarcoidosis. The Kveim intradermal test may prove useful in the diagnosis, but this is a debated issue.

Amyloidosis of the Heart

Cardiac amyloidosis is one of the less common varieties of cardiomyopathy, but we have observed at autopsy several such patients each year. The possibility of cardiac amyloidosis should be considered under one of the following circumstances:

1. Appearance of cardiomyopathy in a patient of 70 years or more (senile cardiac amyloidosis [62]. Amyloid deposits are largely restricted to the heart and blood vessels in this group of patients but also are found in the brain and pancreas [63]. Cardiac failure may occur.
2. Appearance of cardiomyopathy in a patient over the age of 60 who has any of the following.
   a. Low-voltage QRS on electrocardiogram
   b. QS pattern on electrocardiogram suggestive of myocardial infarction without a history of chest pain (Fig. 6 and 7)
   c. Heart failure intractable to medical management
   d. Hemodynamic pattern suggestive of constrictive pericarditis (restrictive or constrictive cardiomyopathy)
3. Family history of amyloid disease, in which instances the heart disease may

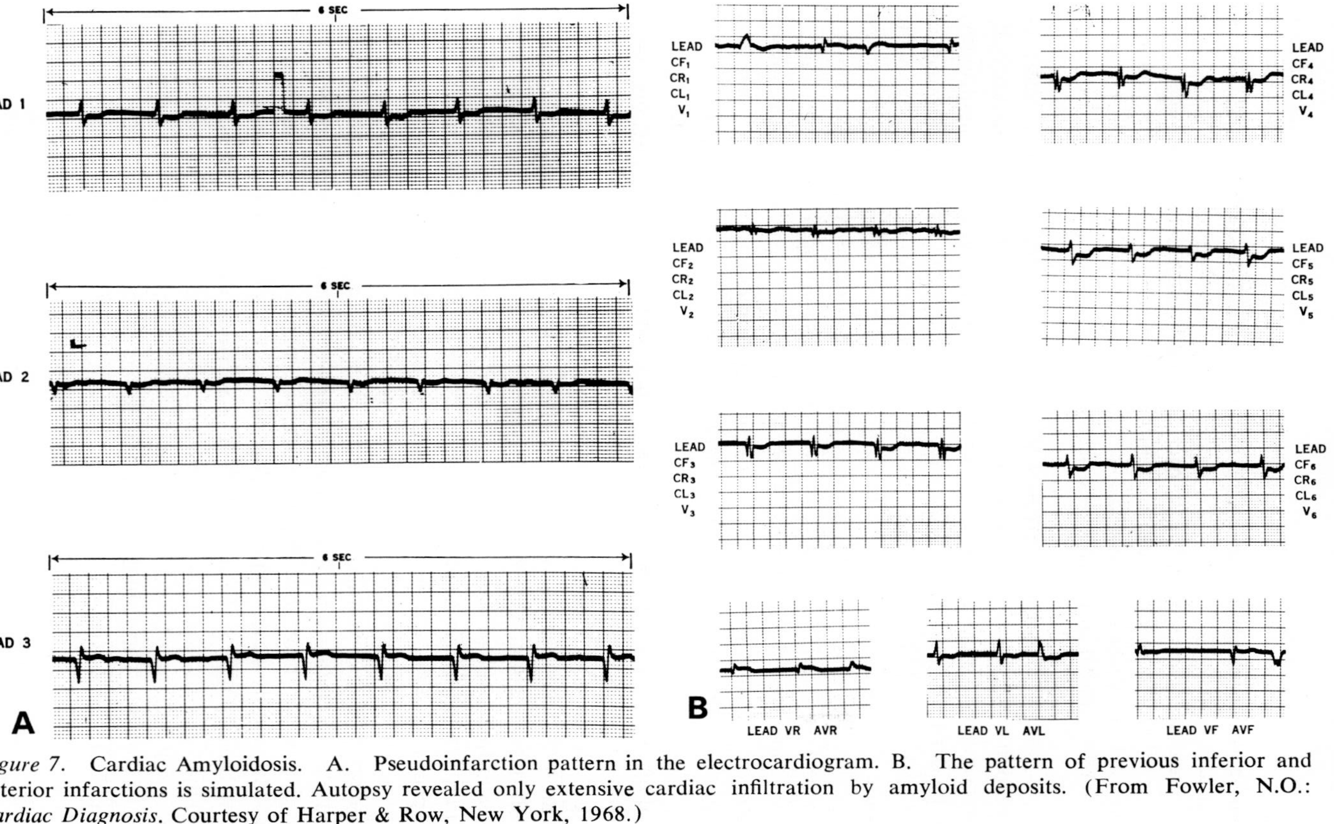

Figure 7. Cardiac Amyloidosis. A. Pseudoinfarction pattern in the electrocardiogram. B. The pattern of previous inferior and anterior infarctions is simulated. Autopsy revealed only extensive cardiac infiltration by amyloid deposits. (From Fowler, N.O.: *Cardiac Diagnosis*. Courtesy of Harper & Row, New York, 1968.)

appear earlier than in the preceding varieties and at times in the third or fourth decades of life.

4. Presence of disease known to cause secondary amyloidosis: chronic ulcerative colitis, rheumatoid arthritis, chronic suppuration, tuberculosis, multiple myeloma, neoplasm, or ankylosing spondylitis. Cardic involvement is often minimal or absent in patients with secondary amyloidosis [64].

Clinical findings compatible with secondary amyloidosis suggest the possibility of secondary cardiac amyloidosis. These include hepatomegaly, splenomegaly, evidence of a nephrotic syndrome, peripheral neuropathy, or evidence of adrenal insufficiency. Other physical findings may suggest the possibility of primary amyloid disease in a patient with cardiomyopathy. These include enlargement of the tongue, skin hemorrhages, and waxy skin deposits. The diagnosis of amyloidosis may be confirmed by the Congo Red test or by biopsy. If there is obvious involvement of the tongue, skin, or liver, that area should be biopsied. When primary cardiac amyloidosis is suspected, biopsy of the gums or of the rectal mucosa may disclose amyloid deposits in the walls of the blood vessels, on microscopic examination.

A recent report by Buja and associates [65] reviewed postmortem findings of 15 patients with clinically significant amyloidosis of the heart. Twelve of these patients had heart failure lasting from 1 day to 13 months before death. In 13, the cardiac involvement was primary. In 2, the involvement was secondary to multiple myeloma. The patients did not improve with digitalization. One had hemodynamic findings suggesting constrictive pericarditis; 4 had large tongues; 4 had peripheral neuropathy; 4 had familial amyloidosis, and they were 21, 31, 35, and 74 years of age, respectively. One of the patients with primary amyloidosis was only 38; another was 48, and the others were over 50 years of age. Thirteen of the patients had low-voltage QRS complexes on electrocardiograms, and 9 had electrocardiograms that simulated old myocardial infarction. Amyloid disease of the heart has been reported to cause valvular dysfunction but did not in this series. Amyloid deposits were limited to the heart in only 2 of these patients. Each patient had valvular deposits but no apparent valvular dysfunction; 13 had splenic involvement, 12 had kidney involvement, and 11 had bowel involvement. The pancreas, skin, and lungs were also involved. Three had angina which was associated only with amyloid involvement of the coronary arteries. Intimal deposits narrowed the intraluminal coronary arteries in 6 patients.

Trauma

Myocardial disease may also follow trauma of either penetrating or nonpenetrating nature. The clinical picture may be similar to that of the postmyocardial-infarction syndrome [66] and the postcardiotomy syndrome

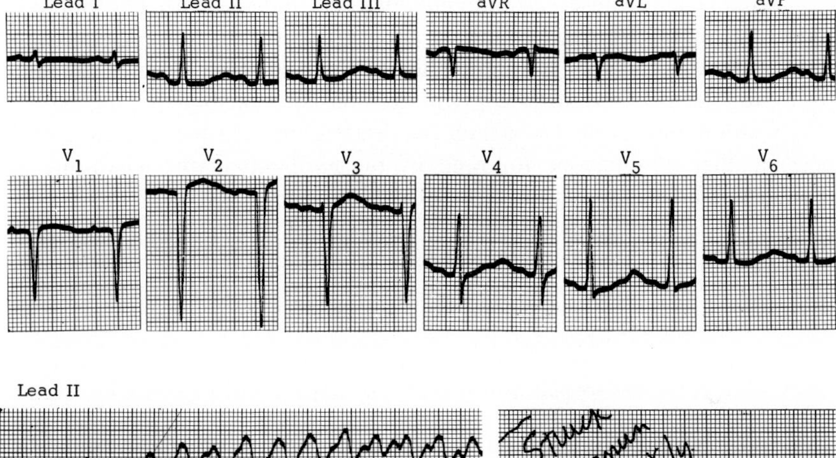

Figure 8. Toxic Cardiomyopathy. Electrocardiogram showing large U waves, followed by ventricular tachycardia and fibrillation which responded to a precordial blow ("thump-version"). The patient was a 35-year-old mental patient with no clinical evidence of previous heart disease who was receiving Mellaril, 1200 mg daily and Thorazine 300 mg daily. Following his sudden death, autopsy showed no anatomic evidence of heart disease. (Courtesy of Te-Chuan Chou, M.D.)

[67]. There is a latent period of 2 weeks or more following the original insult; this is followed by both pericardial and myocardial involvement with fever and a tendency to recurrence. The illness is often responsive to adrenal steroid therapy.

Toxic Cardiomyopathy

In addition to alcoholism, exposure to certain drugs has been suspected of damaging the myocardium and at times of producing clinical signs of heart muscle disease. The ingestion of cobalt in beer has been believed to be responsible for some instances of beer-drinker's myocardosis, reported in Omaha, Minneapolis, Quebec, and Leuven, Belgium [68]. In guinea pigs, larger doses of cobalt were found to produce myocardial, endocardial, and pericardial disease [69]. Chlorpromazine hydrochloride, thioridazine hydrochloride, imipramine, and amitryptiline are suspected of causing myocardial damage, arrhythmia, and heart failure [70] (Fig. 8). Numerous other drugs have been suspected of causing myocardial damage and even cardiac decompensation [30].

Uremia may cause cardiomyopathy [71], and this may contribute to the heart failure which is found in about 50 percent of uremic patients. Other important factors leading to heart failure in these patients are fluid overload, electrolyte imbalance, hypertension, and anemia.

Carbon monoxide poisoning can lead to myocardial necrosis. It is possible that this may be followed by the cardiomyopathy syndrome although this association is not firmly established.

REFERENCES

1. Fowler, N.O.: Differential diagnosis of cardiomyopathies. Progr Cardiovasc Dis 14:113, 1971.
2. Segal, J.P., Harvey, W.P., and Gurel, T.: Diagnosis and treatment of primary myocardial disease. Circulation 32:837, 1965.
3. Sainani, G.S., Krompotic, E., and Slodki, S.J.: Adult heart disease due to the Coxsackie virus B infection. Medicine 47: 133, 1968.
4. Perloff, J.K., deLeon, A.C., Jr., and O'Doherty, D.: The cardiomyopathy of progressive muscular dystrophy. Circulation 33:625, 1966.
5. Neustadt, D.H.: Transient electrocardiographic changes simulating an acute myocarditis in serum sickness. Ann Intern Med 39:126, 1953.
6. Harvey, W.P., Segal, J.P., and Gurel, T.: The clinical spectrum of primary myocardial disease. Progr Cardiovasc Dis 7:17, 1964.
7. Shabetai, R. and Davidson, S.: Hypertrophic obstructive subvalvular mitral stenosis. Ann Intern Med 72:783, 1970.
8. Fowler, N.O., Gueron, M., and Rowlands, D.T., Jr.: Primary myocardial disease. Circulation 23:498, 1961.
9. Weiss, S., Stead, E.A., Jr., Warren, J.V., and Bailey, O.T.: Scleroderma heart disease with consideration of certain other visceral manifestations of scleroderma. Arch Intern Med (Chicago) 71:738, 1943.
10. Sackner, M.A., Heinz, E.R., and Steinberg, A.J.: The heart in scleroderma. Am J Cardiol 17:542, 1966.
11. D'Angelo, W.A., Fries, J.F., Masi, A.T., and Shulman, L.E.: Pathologic observations in systemic sclerosis (scleroderma). Am J Med 46:428, 1969.
12. O'Leary, P.A. and Waisman, M.: Dermatomyositis: A study of forty cases. Arch Dermatol Symp 41:1001, 1940.
13. Banker, B.Q. and Victor, M.: Dermatomyositis (systemic angiopathy) of childhood. Medicine 45:261, 1966.
14. Barwick, D.D. and Walton, N.J.: Polymyositis. Am J Med 35:646, 1963.
15. Schaumburg, H.: Brief recording. Heart block and polymyositis. New Engl J Med 284:480, 1971.
16. Lynch, P.G.: Cardiac involvement in chronic polymyositis. Br Heart J 33:416, 1971.
17. Weintraub, A.M. and Zvaifler, N.J.: The occurrences of valvular and myocardial disease in patients with chronic joint deformity. Am J Med 35:145, 1963.
18. Hoffman, G.D. and Leight, L.: Complete atrioventricular block associated with rheumatoid disease. Am J Cardiol 16:585, 1965.

19. Clark, W.S., Kulka, J.P., and Bauer, W.: Rheumatoid aortitis with aortic regurgitation. Am J Med 22:580, 1957.
20. Harvey, A.M., Shulman, L.E., Tumulty, P.A., Conley, C.L., and Schoenrick, E.H.: Systemic lupus erythematosus: Review of the literature and clinical analysis of 138 cases. Medicine 33:291, 1954.
21. Alarcon-Segovia, D.: Drug-induced lupus syndromes. Mayo Clin Proc 44:664, 1969.
22. Taylor, J., Kosowsky, B., and Lown, B.: Complications of procaine amide in a prospective anti-arrhythmic study. Circulation 44 (Supp. II): 43, 1971.
23. Hanfling, S.M.: Metastatic cancer to the heart: Review of the literature and report of 127 cases. Circulation 22:474, 1960.
24. Graettinger, J.S., Muenster, J.J., Selverstone, L.A., and Campbell, J.A.: A correlation of clinical and hemodynamic studies in patients with hyperthyroidism with and without congestive heart failure. J Clin Invest 38:1316, 1959.
25. Buccino, R.A., Spann, J.F., Jr., Pool, P.E., Sonnenblick, E.H., and Braunwald, E.: Influence of the thyroid state on the intrinsic contractile properties and energy stores of the myocardium. J Clin Invest. 46: 1669, 1967.
26. Graettinger, J.S., Muenster, J.J., Checchia, C.S., Grissom, R.L., and Campbell, J.A.: A correlation of clinical and hemodynamic studies in patients with hypothyroidism. J Clin Invest 37:502, 1958.
27. James, T.N.: Pathology of the cardiac conduction system in hemochromatosis. New Engl J Med 271:92, 1964.
28. Finch, S.C. and Finch, C.A.: Idiopathic hemochromatosis, an iron storage disease. Medicine 34:381, 1955.
29. Van Vliet, P.D., Burchell, H.B., and Titus, J.L.: Focal myocarditis associated with pheochromocytoma. New Engl. J Med 274:1102, 1966.
30. Perloff, J.K., Lindgren, K.M., and Groves, B.M.: Uncommon or commonly unrecognized causes of heart failure. Progr Cardiov Dis 12:409, 1970.
31. Pepine, C.J. and Aloia, J.: Heart muscle disease in acromegaly. Am J Med 48:530, 1970.
32. McArdle, B.: Metabolic myopathies. Am J Med 35:661, 1963.
33. Richterich, R., van Mechelen, P., and Rossi, E.: Refsum's disease (heredopathia atactica polyneuritiformis): An inborn error of lipid metabolism with storage of 3, 7, 11, 15-Tetramethyl hexadecanoic acid. I. Report of a case. Am J Med 39:230, 1965.
34. Ferrans, V.J., Hibbs, R.G., and Burda, C.D.: The heart in Fabry's disease. Am J Cardiol 24:95, 1969.
35. McKusick, V.: Heritable Diseases of Connective Tissue, 3rd Ed. St. Louis, Mosby, 1966.
36. Brady, R.O., Johnson, W.G., and Uhlendorf, B.W.: Identification of heterozygous lipid storage diseases. Current status and clinical applications. Am J Med 51:423, 1971.
37. Akbarian, M., Yankopoulos, N.A., and Abelmann, W.H.: Hemodynamic studies in beriberi heart disease. Am J Med 41:197, 1966.
38. Blankenhorn, M.A., Vilter, C.F., Scheinker, I.M., and Austin, R.S.: Occidental beriberi heart disease. JAMA 131:717, 1946.
39. Robin, E. and Goldschlager, N.: Persistence of low cardiac output after relief of high output by thiamine in a case of alcoholic beriberi and cardiac myopathy. Am Heart J 80:103, 1970.

40. Higginson, J., Gillanders, A.D., and Murray, J.F.: The heart in chronic malnutrition. Br Heart J 14:213, 1952.
41. Smith, W. G.: Coxsackie B myopericarditis in adults. Am Heart J 80:34, 1970.
42. Helin, M., Savola, J., and Lepinleimu, K.: Cardiac manifestations during Coxsackie B5 epidemic. Br Med J 3:97, 1968.
43. Segar, L.F., Kashtan, H.A., and Miller, P.B.: Trichinosis with myocarditis: Report of a case treated with ACTH. New Engl J Med 252:397, 1955.
44. Rosenberg, E.B., Polmar, S.H., and Whalen, G.E.: Increased circulating IgE in trichinosis. Ann Intern Med 75:575, 1971.
45. Farrar, W.E., Jr., Kagan, I.G., Everton, F.D., and Sellers, T.F., Jr.: Serologic evidence of human infections with Trypanosoma Cruzi in Georgia. Am J Hyg 78:166, 1963.
46. Feldman, H.A.: Toxoplasmosis. New Engl J Med 279:1370 and 1431, 1968.
47. Wertlake, P.T. and Winter, T.S.: Fatal toxoplasma myocarditis in an adult patient with acute lymphocytic leukemia. New Engl J Med 273:438, 1965.
48. Blankenhorn, M.A. and Gall, E.A.: Myocarditis and myocardosis. Circulation 13:217, 1956.
49. Saphir, O. and Amromin, G.D.: Myocarditis in instances of pneumonia. Ann Intern Med 28:963, 1948.
50. Brink, A.J. and Weber, H.W.: Fibroplastic parietal endocarditis with eosinophilia; Löffler's endocarditis. Am J Med 34:52, 1963.
51. Castleman, B. and McNeely, B.U.: Case Records of Massachusetts General Hospital. Presentation of a case: 36-1970. New Engl J Med 283:476, 1970.
52. Duma, R.J., Ferrell, H.W., Nelson, E.C., and Jones, M.M.: Primary amebic meningoencephalitis. New Engl J Med 281:1315, 1969.
53. Fajardo, L.F., Stewart, J.R., and Cohn, K.E.: Morphology of radiation-induced heart disease. Arch Pathol 86:512, 1968.
54. Fajardo, L.F. and Stewart, J.F.: Experimental radiation-induced heart disease. Am J Pathol 59:299, 1970.
55. Parry, E.H., Warrell, D.A., Perine, P.L., Vukotich, D., and Bryceson, A.D.M.: Some effects of louse-borne relapsing fever on the function of the heart. Am J Med 49:472, 1970.
56. Gore, I.: Myocardial changes in fatal diphtheria. Am J Med Sci 215:257, 1948.
57. Tajermoa. A.C.: Electrocardiographic abnormalities and serum transaminase levels in diphtheritic myocarditis. J Pediat 75:1008, 1969.
58. Duvernoy, W.F.C. and Garcia, R.: Sarcoidosis of the heart presenting with ventricular tachycardia and atrioventricular block. Am J Cardiol 28:348, 1971.
59. Gozo, E.G., Coxnow, I., Cohen, H.C., and Okun, L.: The heart in sarcoidosis. Chest 60:379, 1971.
60. Mayock, R.L., Bertrand, P., Morrison, C.E., and Scott, J.H.: Manifestations of sarcoidosis. Analysis of 145 patients with a review of nine series selected from the literature. Am J Med 35:67, 1963.
61. Scadding, J.G.: Sarcoidosis. Eyre and Spottiswoode, London, 1967, p. 291.
62. Buerger, L. and Braunstein, H.: Senile cardiac amyloidosis. Am J Med 28:357, 1960.
63. Wright, J.R., Calkins, E., Brum, W.J., Stolte, G., and Schultz, R.T.: Relation of amyloid to aging. Medicine 48:39, 1969.
64. Dahlin, D.C.: Classification and general aspects of amyloidosis. Med Clin N Am 34:1107, 1950.

65. Buja, L.M., Khoi N.B., and Roberts, W.C.: Clinically significant cardiac amyloidosis. Clinicopathologic findings in 15 patients. Am J Cardiol 26:394, 1970.
66. Dressler, W.: The post-myocardial-infarction syndrome: A report on forty-four cases. Arch Intern Med 103:28, 1959.
67. Engle, M.A., and Ito, T.: The post-pericardiotomy syndrome. Am J Cardiol 7:73, 1961.
68. Sullivan, J.F., George, R., Bluvas, R., and Egan, J.D.: Myocardiopathy of beer drinkers: Subsequent course. Ann Intern Med 70:277, 1969.
69. Mohiuddin, S.M., Taskar, P.K., Rheault, M., Roy, P-E., Chenard, J., and Morin, Y.: Experimental cobalt cardiomyopathy. Am Heart J 80:532, 1970.
70. Alexander, C.S. and Nino, A.: Cardiovascular complications in young patients taking psychotrophic drugs. A preliminary report. Am Heart J 78:757, 1969.
71. Comty, C.M., Cohen, S.L., and Shapiro, F.L.: Pericarditis in chronic uremia and its sequels. Ann Intern Med 75:173, 1971.

NOBLE O. FOWLER, M.D.

The Treatment of Myocardial Diseases

The treatment of the myocardial diseases may be discussed conveniently by dividing myocardial diseases into 3 large groups. These include

1. The obstructive cardiomyopathies
2. The idiopathic cardiomyopathies
3. The cardiomyopathies which are secondary to some systemic illness

The treatment of the obstructive cardiomyopathies is included in Dr. Wigle's chapter on that subject and will not be considered here. We shall begin our discussion with a consideration of the treatment of the second group: the idiopathic cardiomyopathies.

Diagnostic Classification

An effective approach to the management of patients with myocardial disease should begin with a proper diagnostic classification. It is essential to be certain that the patient does not have a variety of heart disease other than myocardial disease. It is important to exclude coronary artery disease, systemic hypertensive disease, valvular disease, pericardial disease, lung disease, or congenital heart disease. Then, it is necessary to determine the background of the myocardial disease and to identify predisposing factors if they exist. Patients with idiopathic myocardopathy, also called primary myocardopathy, comprise the largest group of those with myocardial disease. In the experience of Segal, Harvey, and Gurel with over 200 patients with myocardial disease at Georgetown University, patients with idiopathic cardiomyopathy were observed three times as often as those with a systemic illness involving the myocardium (secondary myocardopathy) [1]. In patients with no evidence of a systemic disease that might involve the myocardium, a history of alcoholism may suggest a cause and also an approach to the treatment of a patient with myocardial disease. A family history of myocardopathy may shed light on the background of the illness and also may give some clues as to prognosis. We have observed that members of a family with this disease often die at approximately the same age. Factors which may contribute to cardiac dysfunction should be identified; for example, coexisting systemic hypertension, cardiac arrhythmias, and systemic or pulmonary embolism are common complications in myocardial disease. Patients with myocardial disease may suffer from additional heart disease. We have studied patients with both valvular disease and myocardial disease. We have observed patients in whom myocardial disease began with acute myopericarditis; hence, acute inflammatory pericardial disease and myocardial disease may coexist. In this setting patients may have both cardiac tamponade or constrictive pericarditis and underlying cardiomyopathy. Patients whose illness begins with myopericarditis may in time develop constrictive pericarditis. Patients with myocardial disease should be carefully studied for evidence of a systemic illness such as lupus erythematosus, amyloid disease, or anemia that may cause or aggravate heart disease. Uncommonly, myocardial biopsy is to be considered when there is a possibility of detecting a specific cause for which, there is a precise form of treatment. After proper diagnostic classification and appropriate treatment, patients with myocardial disease who have responded satisfactorily to therapy should be reevaluated periodically for evidence of relapse.

Identification of Therapeutic Targets in Myocardial Disease

Once the diagnosis and proper classification have been made, it may then be possible to identify specific therapeutic targets in patients with cardiomyopathy. For example, does the patient have a ventricular arrhythmia and is there danger of cardiac arrest and sudden death? Does the patient have advanced atrioventricular block which might respond to adrenal steroid therapy or may he need an implanted electronic endocardial or epicardial pacemaker? Does the patient have congestive heart failure which may require prolonged bed rest in addition to digitalis glycosides, diuretics, and a low sodium diet? Does the patient show evidence of progressive cardiac enlargement which suggests the need for bed rest? Does the patient have systemic or pulmonary embolism which indicate a need for anticoagulant therapy? Should anticoagulant therapy be used prophylactically in the absence of embolism, especially when the patient is at bed rest, or when there is heart failure or atrial fibrillation? Is there accompanying pericarditis which may suggest that the patient should be treated with adrenal steroids, or should pericardial fluid be aspirated to relieve tamponade or for further diagnostic study? Does the patient have angina pectoris and syncope? In our experience with patients who have myocardial disease angina pectoris is very rare unless there is obstructive cardiomyopathy. Syncope may suggest cardiac arrhythmia or obstructive cardiomyopathy, with treatment directed toward those specific targets.

Specific therapy in the myocardial diseases may be considered under several headings depending on the presenting features and background of the illness.

The Etiologic Background of the Myocardial Disease

In most patients with idiopathic myocardial disease, a specific cause has not been identified although several possibilities have been suggested. Alcohol is commonly suggested as an etiologic factor in idiopathic cardiomyopathy [2], and by some it is thought to be the principal cause [3]. In our published studies, only one-third of the patients with an autopsy-confirmed diagnosis of myocardiopathy had a history of alcoholism [4]. When there is a history of alcoholism, withdrawal of alcohol is essential [5]. Abstinence from alcohol may be followed by improvement in cardiac arrhythmias, improvement of abnormal electrocardiographic T waves, decrease in cardiac size, and perhaps relief of congestive heart failure. Burch and associates recently completed a study of 37 patients with advanced alcoholic cardiomyopathy treated by means of prolonged bed rest [6, 7]. Most of these patients had a history of excessive alcohol consumption for 6 years or more, and the great majority had a history of inadequate diet. Twenty-one of these patients lost all symptoms, and the heart size returned to normal. Withdrawal of alcohol might be an important contributor to the improvement of these patients. Only 5 patients in this group had little or no benefit from prolonged bed rest. Beer drinkers who have consumed large quantities of beer containing a cobalt additive may improve when their beer consumption is terminated [8]. Phenothiazines and related drugs have been suspected of causing cardiomyopathy, cardiac arrhythmia, and sudden death [9]. Withdrawal of drugs, which may cause myocardial damage, is essential to proper management. If the patient has fever and other findings suggestive of antecedent viral disease, such as a history of an upper respiratory infection, a history of pericarditis, or a history of enteritis, or when there are considerable tachycardia with gallop rhythm and cardiac failure suggesting active myocarditis, then adrenal steroids may be useful in management.

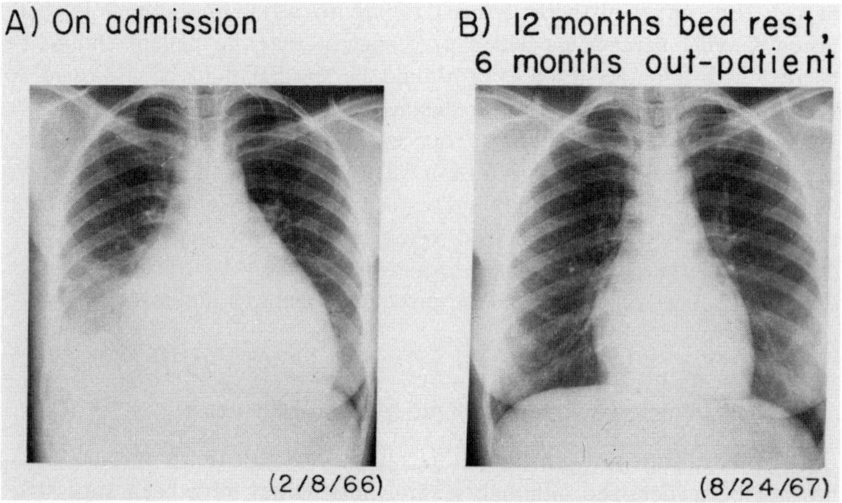

A) On admission

B) 12 months bed rest, 6 months out-patient

(2/8/66)

(8/24/67)

Figure 1. Postpartal Cardiomyopathy. Improvement in cardiac function and heart size in a patient treated with prolonged bed rest. (From Burch, G.E. et al.: The effect of prolonged bed rest on postpartal cardiomyopathy. Am Heart J 81:186, 1971, by permission.)

Bed Rest

Congestive heart failure or pronounced cardiac dilatation indicate a need for rest, digitalis, diuretics, and sodium restriction. Occasionally, prolonged bed rest is required, although many of our patients respond with loss of the symptoms and signs of congestive heart failure after only a few weeks of bed rest when this treatment is supplemented by digitalis, diuretic therapy, and the proper diet with sodium restriction. The patient should be restricted to bed as long as the enlarged heart continues to decrease in size. Maximum improvement usually requires 4 weeks to 3 months; infrequently, a longer period of bed rest is needed. Bed rest in cardiac patients offers the advantage of decreasing heart rate, stroke volume, blood pressure, and the vigor of contraction, thus tending to reduce heart size [6]. Burch and associates described their treatment of more than 50 patients with idiopathic cardiomyopathy. These workers observed 37 patients with cardiomyopathy who were hospitalized and treated with prolonged bed rest: Patients were permitted to feed themselves and to use a bedside commode but engaged in no other activity. There was an approximate average of 50 percent decrease in cardiac diameter after 12 months of bed rest (Fig. 1). In perhaps 50 percent of these patients whose hearts decreased in size, the improvement was maintained [10, 11]. In a later report, McDonald and coworkers found that the heart size returned to normal in 10 of 25 patients with idiopathic cardiomyopathy who cooperated in a program of prolonged bed rest [11a]. Because of economic factors which limit the period of hospitalization, and because most of our patients with cardiomyopathy and heart failure demonstrate an adequate response to shorter periods of bed rest, we have seldom used this measure in treatment of our own patients. In 4 patients with advanced heart failure, we prescribed 6 months or more of bed rest. In 3 of them, there were satisfactory results. In the remaining patient, a 19-year-old mother of twins who had postpartum myocardiopathy, there was no improvement of cardiac enlargement or cardiac decompensation after 1 year of bed rest.

Digitalis

It is generally agreed that digitalis should be used in the treatment of congestive heart failure associated with cardiomyopathy [12]. In a symposium edited by Harvey in 1965, a preference was expressed for digoxin over other digitalis preparations [12]. Recent reports suggest that there are important differences in the completeness of absorption of various brands of digoxin when given orally [13]. It has been suggested, although not proved, that patients with cardiomyopathy may be more sensitive to digitalis than many other cardiac patients. It was recommended that somewhat less than average doses be used. In a study of serum glycoside levels, Killip and associates did not confirm the impression that patients with cardiomyopathy were more sensitive to digitalis than other cardiac patients [13a]. For initial digitalization we ordinarily use digoxin 0.25 mg every 6 hours orally for 6 doses and then a daily maintenance dosage of 0.25 to 0.5 mg, orally. The choice of dosage is guided by the therapeutic response or signs of toxicity. If there is no urgency, an even safer method of digitalization may be used. Marcus and associates demonstrated that satisfactory blood levels of digoxin are attained when the patient is given a maintenance dosage of digoxin for 1 week [14]. They showed that the blood level of digoxin was the same after 1 week of treatment with 0.5 mg digoxin orally each day, whether or not a loading dose was used. Hence, one may give the patient 0.25 to 0.5 mg digoxin by mouth each day in anticipation that the patient will be digitalized in 1 week. The dosage of 0.5 mg digoxin daily will be excessive as a maintenance dose for many patients; hence, we prefer an oral dose of either 0.25 mg once a day or 0.25 mg each morning and 0.125 mg each evening. In patients with advanced heart disease, or in those over 50, the maintenance dose of digoxin is often as little as 0.125 mg daily. In the treatment of congestive heart failure, the usual management was recommended in Harvey's symposium. In addition to digitalis, sodium restriction and diuretics, including thiazides and mercurial diuretics were found useful. Today, ethacrynic acid, 50 mg orally after meals or furosemide 40 mg 1 to 4 times daily may be considered for use in place of, or in addition to, the mercurial diuretics and spironolactones recommended in the 1965 Symposium. The merit or sodium restriction was emphasized in the Symposium. A 500-mg per day sodium dietary intake may be needed initially in patients hospitalized for congestive failure. Although a more generous intake of sodium was permitted after improvement, patients were advised to avoid salty foods even after they were fully compensated.

Anticoagulants

Anticoagulants are recommended in patients with cardiomyopathy when their course is complicated by systemic or pulmonary embolism. In making a recommendation for anticoagulant therapy, it is assumed that there are none of the usual contraindications to anticoagulants such as severe hypertension, severe liver disease, hemorrhagic diathesis, bleeding peptic ulcer or other gastroenteric bleeding, or recent operation on the nervous system. The Symposium in Circulation also recommended the prophylactic use of anticoagulants in patients who had cardiac decompensation even in the absence of demonstrated thromboembolism [12]. It is well known that thromboembolism is very common in these patients [11a]. In our group of patients with cardiomyopathy who came to autopsy either pulmonary or systemic thromboemboli were found in over one-third [4] and over half had cardiac mural thrombi [4]. Patients with alcoholic cardiomyopathy are said to be at very high risk of thromboembolism [5]. However, in treating 48 patients with alcoholic cardiomyopathy by means of prolonged bed rest, anticoagulants were used by McDonald and associates [7] only when embolism had already occurred.

Cardiac Arrhythmias

Frequently ventricular premature contractions and ventricular tachycardia occur commonly in patients with myocardial disease. In one report 54 percent of 46 Jamaican patients with cardiomyopathy died suddenly, an event though related to a ventricular arrhythmia [15]. Atrioventricular block with Stokes-Adams episodes is frequent in patients with myocardial disease. Atrial fibrillation is especially common and was found prior to death in approximately one-third of our autopsied patients. The arrhythmias are treated in the same manner as in patients with other varieties of heart disease. McDonald and associates used D.C. electric cardioversion in 2 patients with atrial fibrillation complicating idiopathic cardiomyopathy [11a]. In complete heart block, especially if related to sarcoidosis, one might wish to administer adrenal steroids. An electronic cardiac pacemaker is indicated when complete atrioventricular block has been accompanied by symptoms of syncope, weakness, cerebral dysfunction, exertional dyspnea, congestive heart failure, or renal failure. Ventricular premature beats and ventricular tachycardia may prove difficult to suppress. Patients with ventricular premature beats may be treated with procainamide 250 to 500 mg orally every 6 hours, although Koch-Weser presented evidence that plasma concentration fluctuations are minimized by giving this drug every 3 hours [16]. Long-term procainamide therapy may be complicated by a lupus-like syndrome. Alternatively, one may use quinidine, 200 to 400 mg every 6 hours orally for the treatment of ventricular premature contractions. Quinidine may cause syncope or sudden death owing to ventricular fibrillation. Bretylium tosylate, 200 to 400 mg orally every 6 hours may be used but its absorption may be erratic when given orally. Ventricular tachycardia can usually be reverted to sinus rhythm with Lidocaine 50 to 100 mg intravenously or with D.C. shock but recurrences may be a problem. In patients with ventricular tachycardia which is refractory to drug therapy, electronic pacing of the right ventricle at a rate of 100 to 120 beats per minute may be required to prevent recurrences. Ventricular pacing may be combined with procainamide or quinidine therapy.

Adrenal Steroid Therapy

The use of adrenal steroids is considered in patients with idiopathic cardiomyopathy especially when there is evidence of an active inflammatory process. Burch and coworkers found that adrenal steroids did no harm but were not particularly useful in the treatment of cardiomyopathy [11]. With regard to specific indications for steroids, patients with myocardial disease who have complete heart block, sarcoid cardiomyopathy, fever, and pericarditis suggesting an acute process or intractable heart failure may be considered as candidates for adrenal steroid therapy. Segal and associates [18] recommended a trial of adrenal steroids for patients with atrial, AV junctional, and ventricular arrhythmias. We use an initial dosage of 15 mg prednisone orally every 6 hours. When there is a favorable response, the dose is gradually reduced after 1 to 3 weeks. An attempt is made to dis-

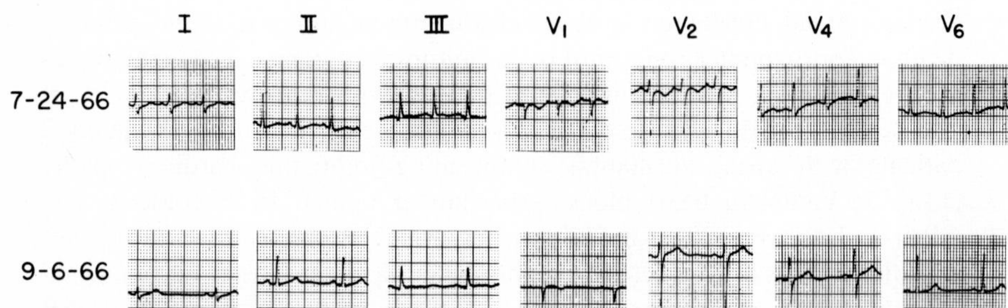

Figure 2. Febrile Myopericarditis. Electrocardiograms of a 25-year-old woman with acute febrile myopericarditis occurring in the third trimester of her first pregnancy (record of 7/24/66). Heart size and electrocardiogram returned to normal (record of 9/6/66) and have remained so following treatment with Prednisone, 120 mg daily.

continue the adrenal steroid after 6 to 9 weeks. We have observed favorable responses of patients with congestive heart failure, pericarditis, and tachycardia but only in febrile patients. In 1 pregnant woman with febrile myopericarditis, heart failure did not improve with digitalis, bed rest, sodium restriction, or diuretics. It was necessary to increase the dose of prednisone to 120 mg per day to control heart failure and tachycardia (Fig. 2). Despite the possible danger of aggravating a viral infection, steroids seem useful in some patients with myocarditis [19]. Patients who are receiving adrenal steroid therapy are watched closely for hypokalemia, sodium and water retention, osteoporosis, hypertension, opportunistic infection, hyperglycemia, and gastroenteric bleeding.

Management of Patients Who Have Improved or Apparently Recovered from Cardiomyopathy

In some patients with acute febrile myopericarditis and congestive heart failure, recovery is apparently complete after subsidence of the acute episode. However, in most patients who have developed heart failure with considerable cardiac dilatation, although striking improvement may occur, the danger of relapse is ever present. Other patients with cardiomyopathy display chronic, very slowly progressive cardiac enlargement for a period of a decade or more without developing congestive failure. The patient should be observed as an outpatient at intervals of 6 weeks to 6 months depending on the degree of recovery and the persisting symptomatology. Physical effort should be restricted to that which does not produce symptoms. Most of these patients are able to work. The patient should avoid activities which may compromise cardiac function. Alcoholism is an especially common danger. We advise against pregnancy especially in patients who have developed heart failure during or shortly after pregnancy. In one study, the risk of pregnancy after peripartal cardiomyopathy had developed appeared greatly increased when the heart size had not returned to normal [17].

TREATMENT OF THE SECONDARY CARDIOMYOPATHIES

In patients who have one of the secondary cardiomyopathies, the prognosis is greatly affected by the nature of the systemic illness which is responsible for the cardiomyopathy. Segal and associates studied 57 patients with an identified cause of secondary cardiomyopathy [18]. Collagen disease was responsible in 30 percent; bacterial disease, in 12 percent; uremia, in 12 percent; hyperthyroidism, in 11 percent; rheumatoid disease in 7 percent; malignant disease in 5 percent; sarcoidosis, in 5 percent; amyloid disease, in 4 percent; and hemochromatosis, in 4 percent. As already emphasized, proper diagnostic classification is important. Myocardial biopsy is seldom needed to achieve this end. Patients with myocardopathy without apparent cause should be carefully evaluated for hypercalcemia, hyperglobulinemia, hilar lymph node involvement, cervical lymph node involvement, skin lesions and liver involvement which may reflect sarcoidosis [20]. Adrenal steroid therapy may be useful in myocardial sarcoidosis, but the results of such treatment may be difficult to evaluate. Complete heart block caused by sarcoidosis may respond to steroid therapy [21]. We have observed 3 young women with myocardial sarcoidosis in whom there was no clinical evidence of sarcoidosis elsewhere. Two of these women had complete heart block complicated by syncope and sudden death; the third also died suddenly, probably of a cardiac arrhythmia. At autopsy, sarcoidosis was apparently limited to the heart muscle in 2. Hence, occasionally, the physician might wish to obtain a cardiac muscle biopsy in order to arrive at a specific diagnosis. It is possible to obtain a closed-chest myocardial biopsy in one of two ways. A small biopsy forceps at the end of a right heart catheter (Bioptome) may be used to biopsy the right ventricular aspect of the interventricular septum [22]. Percutaneous needle biopsy of the right or left ventricle may be obtained by means of a Terry [23] or Silverman [23a] needle. Because of the dangers of cardiac arrhythmia, coronary artery perforation, or cardiac tamponade [23a], the possible therapeutic advantage of such a procedure must be weighed carefully against its hazards. In a recent study of 198 patients, cardiac tamponade followed myocardial biopsy in 8, but there were no deaths. Important changes in therapy resulted in only 8 of 198 patients [23a]. When myocardial biopsy is deemed essential, an open thoracotomy might be a safer means of carrying out this procedure.

Myocarditis

With regard to viral myocarditis, one must consider the possibilities of Coxsackie B virus, Coxsackie A virus, echovirus, poliomyelitis virus, mumps, measles, infectious hepatitis, vaccinia, infectious mononucleosis, or chicken pox [24]. We can suggest no specific therapy for patients with viral myocarditis other than bed rest and careful observation for possible complications, but the possibility of adrenal steroid therapy might be considered if the patient is not doing well. When cardiac arrhythmias are a complication, it may be desirable to observe the patient in a cardiac monitoring unit. Rheumatic myocarditis, in the absence of valvular disease, is extremely uncommon. Perhaps occasionally, a patient has this problem and may respond to adrenal steroids. Septic myocarditis should be treated by identifying the cause of septicemia, and then using the appropriate antibiotics. Uremic myocardopathy can be treated by peritoneal dialysis or, if the renal disease is irreversible, by hemodialysis or, perhaps renal transplantation. In toxoplasma myocardopathy, the administration of sulfadiazine and pyrimethamine together is to be considered [25]. Adrenal steroid therapy may prove beneficial in patients with heart failure caused by trichinosis. In polymyositis, myocardial involvement is believed to be uncommon. Myocarditis may occur, however, and when the His bundle or bundle branches are involved, complete AV block may ensue. In one such instance, electronic pacing of the ventricles was used [26]. Adrenal steroid therapy may prove useful.

In patients with such connective tissue diseases as rheumatoid disease, dermatomyositis, scleroderma or disseminated lupus erythematosus, the possibility of adrenal steroid therapy may merit serious consideration. There is apparently little that adrenal steroid therapy can accomplish in scleroderma, but it might accomplish much more in patients with the other connective tissue diseases. When there is secondary cardiomyopathy related to amyloid disease or metastatic tumor, we have little to offer most patients, therapeutically. One of the more common neoplastic diseases which invades the myocardium is lymphoma. As many as 24 percent of patients with lymphoma have cardiac involvement at the time of death [27]. Only 5 of 48 patients, however, had clinical signs of their cardiac involvement. In lymphomatous myocardopathy, nitrogen mustards and adrenal steroids may be useful. Beriberi, now extremely rare in the United States, which may be a cause of high-output heart failure with gallop rhythm, dependent edema, and high venous pressure is usually associated with either pellagra or peripheral neuropathy [28]. The patient may respond to large doses of thiamine, administered parenterally. On the other hand, some patients with beriberi reach an irreversible state and do not respond to thiamine [29]. The value of digitalis in acute beriberi heart disease is in question, and some writers have described beneficial effects in occasional patients with beriberi, but not in all [29, 30].

Thyroid Disease

In patients with hyperthyroidism, cardiomyopathy may be a problem. There are a number of ways in which hyperthyroidism may affect cardiac function. There may be uncoupling of oxidative phosphorylation; further, the thyroid hormone has a direct effect on the heart muscle. In addition, there may be evidence of increased sympathetic activity. Because of the latter, beta adrenergic blocking agents such as propranolol are often used in patients with thyrotoxicosis, whether or not cardiac enlargement and decompensation are present. There is uncertainty, however, that the ensuing slowing of the heart rate actually improves myocardial function. There is some risk that large doses of propranolol may precipitate heart failure [31]. The patient with thyrotoxicosis usually responds well to treatment of the thyrotoxicosis either with methimazole, with radioactive iodine, or to a subtotal thyroidectomy. With myxedema, there is some doubt as to the existence of independent cardiomyopathy. Many myxedematous patients have coronary disease, and pericardial effusion is common. In the treatment of myxedema, thyroid hormone must be used cautiously because of the danger of provoking or aggravating angina pectoris. Thyroid extract is usually started at an oral dosage of 16 mg a day, and gradually increased to 90 to 180 mg daily. Increments in dosage are usually made at intervals of 2 weeks. The patient should be observed carefully for the development or aggravation of angina pectoris, since coronary artery disease is common in older patients with myxedema.

It is important to evaluate the possibility of hemochromatosis in patients with cardiomyopathy. This diagnosis should be considered when there is evidence of liver disease, pigmentation of the skin, and diabetes mellitus. It should also be considered in patients with prolonged refractory anemias, especially those who have received many blood transfusions. The pigmentation of the skin may not be conspicuous. The determination of plasma iron levels may be a useful screening test for hemochromatosis; in a study of 32 patients with symptomatic hemochromatosis, 31 had plasma iron values above 150 μg per 100 ml blood [32]. The same authors found that only 4 of 100 normal subjects had serum iron values above 150 μg per 100 ml and then not consistently. The plasma iron-binding globulin is usually saturated above 50 percent of capacity in patients with hemochromatosis (25 of 25 patients with idiopathic hemochromatosis studied by Finch and Finch [32]). In those without this disease, the saturation is usually below this value. In patients with hemochromatosis and heart disease, there is evidence that bleeding 1 unit of blood every week or so decreases iron stores and may lead to an improvement of congestive heart failure [33, 33a].

Catecholamine-induced cardiomyopathy may occur in patients with pheochromocytoma [34]. The diagnosis may be suspected from the clinical features of paroxysmal attacks of headache and tachycardia often accompanied by excessive sweating. Hypertension may be paroxysmal or sustained and may be accompanied by orthostatic hypotension. Chest pain and blurring of vision may accompany these attacks and weight loss is common. Fasting hyperglycemia may be present. Analyses of 24-hour urine samples usually show an increased content of VMA and catecholamines. The electrocardiogram may show left ventricular hypertrophy, premature ventricular contractions, and very abnormal T waves suggestive of ischemia. Sinus tachycardia is common. Occasionally, myocardial infarction is simulated or may, in fact, be a complication. Catecholamine synthesis may be partially blocked by alpha-methyl-para-tyrosine [35], and the cardiac effects of catecholamines may be reduced by treatment with the beta adrenergic blocking agent, propranolol. The latter may be desirable in preparation for surgical removal of the tumor; this operation is occasionally complicated by alarming and even fatal ventricular arrhythmia. The hypertensive effects of the pheochromocytoma may be treated with phenoxybenzamine.

Cardiac Transplants

In patients with cardiomyopathy whose heart failure does not respond to other methods of treatment, the question of cardiac transplant may arise. Such treatment is more likely to be considered for a young or middle-aged adult who is otherwise in good health.

Cardiac transplant is much less commonly carried out now than a few years ago because of the universal problem of host rejection of the transplanted heart. Gail has recently raised the legitimate question as to whether or not cardiac transplant does prolong life [36]. Das and coworkers have demonstrated bound immunoglobulin and complement in the hearts of patients with cardiomyopathy who underwent cardiac transplant [37]. It is our opinion that until the immunologic problems can be resolved, cardiac transplant must be regarded as an experimental procedure which should probably be restricted to medical centers that are carrying out promising immunologic investigations.

REFERENCES

1. Segal, J.P., Harvey, W.P., and Gurel, T.: Diagnosis and treatment of primary myocardial disease. Circulation 32:837, 1965.
2. Burch, G.E. and DePasquale, N.: Alcoholic cardiomyopathy. A review. Am J Cardiol 23:723, 1969.
3. Alexander, C.S.: Idiopathic heart disease. I. Analysis of 100 cases with special reference to chronic alcoholism. Am J Med 41:213, 1966.
4. Fowler, N.O., Gueron, M., and Rowlands, D.T., Jr.: Primary myocardial disease. Circulation 23:498, 1961.
5. Regan, T.J.: Ethyl alcohol and the heart. Circulation 44:957, 1971.
6. Burch, G.E. and Giles, T.D.: Alcoholic cardiomyopathy. Concept of the disease and its treatment. Am J Med 50:141, 1971.
7. McDonald, C.D., Burch, G.E., and Walsh, J.J.: Alcoholic cardiomyopathy managed with prolonged bed rest. Ann Intern Med 74:681, 1971.
8. Kesteloot, H., Roelandt, J., Willems, J., Claes, J.H., and Joossens, J.V.: An enquiry into the role of cobalt in the heart disease of chronic beer drinkers. Circulation 37:854, 1968.
9. Alexander, C.S. and Nino, A.: Cardiovascular complications in young patients taking psychotropic drugs. Am Heart J 78:757, 1969.
10. Burch, G.E., Walsh, J.J., and Black, W.C.: Value of prolonged bed rest in management of cardiomegaly. JAMA 183:81, 1963.
11. Burch, G.E., Walsh, J.J., Ferrans, V.J., and Hibbs, R.: Prolonged bed rest in the treatment of the dilated heart. Circulation 32:852, 1965.

11a. McDonald, C.D., Burch, G.E., and Walsh, J.J.: Prolonged bed rest in the treatment of idiopathic cardiomyopathy. Am J Med 52:41, 1972.

12. Harvey, W.P.: Comments on Symposium. Circulation 32:857, 1965.
13. Lindenbaum, J., Mellow, M.H., Blackstone, M.O., and Butler, V.P., Jr. Variation in biologic availability of digoxin from four preparations. New Engl J Med 285:1344, 1971.

13a. Killip, T., Donnelly, W., and Morrison, J.: Digitalis and cardiomyopathy. Circulation 46 (Suppl. II): 175, 1972.

14. Marcus, R.I., Burkhalter, L., Cuccia, C., Pavlovich, J., and Kapadia, G.G.: Administration of tritiated digoxin with and without a loading dose. A metabolic study. Circulation 34:865, 1966.
15. Miller, B.R., Moseley, H.S., DaCosta, L.R., Sandison, J.W., and Stuart, K.L.: The prognosis in idiopathic cardiomyopathy in Jamaica. Pathol Microbiol (Basil) 35:49, 1970.
16. Koch-Weser, J., Klein, S.W., Foo-Canto, L.L., Kastor, J.A., and DeSanctis, R.W.: Antiarrhythmia prophylaxis with procainamide in acute myocardial infarction. New Engl J Med 281:1253, 1969.
17. Demakis, J.G., Rahimtoola, S.H., Sutton, G.C., Meadows, W.R., Szanto, P.B., Tobin, J.R., and Gunnar, R.M.: Natural course of peripartum cardiomyopathy. Circulation 44:1053, 1971.

18. Segal, J. P., Harvey, W.P., and Gurel, T.: Diagnosis and treatment of primary myocardial disease. Circulation 32:837, 1965.
19. Perloff, J.K.: The cardiomyopathies—current perspectives. Circulation 44:942, 1971.
20. Porter, G.H.: Sarcoid heart disease. New Engl J Med 263:1350, 1960.
21. Scadding, J.G.: Sarcoidosis. London, Eyre and Spottiswoode, 1967, p. 301.
22. Konno, S. and Sakakibara, S.: Endo-myocardial biopsy. Dis Chest 44:345, 1963.
23. Sutton, D.C. and Sutton, G.C.: Needle biopsy of the human ventricular myocardium: Review of 54 consecutive cases. Am Heart J 60:364, 1960.
23a. Shirey, E.K., Hawk, W.A., Mukerji, D., and Effler, D.B.: Percutaneous myocardial biopsy of the left ventricle. Experience in 198 patients. Circulation 66:112, 1972.
24. Smith, W. G.: Coxsackie B myopericarditis in adults. Am Heart J 80:34, 1970.
25. Feldman, H.A.: Toxoplasmosis. New Engl J Med 279:1370; 1431, 1968.
26. Schaumburg, H.H., Nielsen, S.L., and Yurchak, P.M.: Brief recording. Heart block in polymyositis. New Engl J Med 284:480, 1971.
27. Roberts, W.C., Glancy, D.L., and DeVita, V.T., Jr.: Heart in malignant lymphoma (Hodgkin's disease, lymphosarcoma, reticulum cell sarcoma and mycosis fungoides): A study of 196 autopsy cases. Am J Cardiol 22:85, 1968.
28. Blankenhorn, M.A.: Effect of vitamin deficiency on the heart and circulation. Circulation 11:288, 1955.
29. Akbarian, M., Yankopoulos, N.A., and Abelmann, W.H.: Hemodynamic studies in beriberi heart disease. Am J Med 41:197, 1966.
30. Blankenhorn, M.A., Vilter, C.F., Scheinker, I.M., and Austin, R.S.: Occidental beriberi heart disease. JAMA 131:717, 1946.
31. Leonard, J.J. and DeGroot, W.J.: The thyroid state and the cardiovascular system. Mod Conc Cardiovasc Dis 38:23, 1969.
32. Finch, S.C. and Finch, C.A.: Idiopathic hemochromatosis, an iron storage disease. Medicine 34:381, 1955.
33. Williams, R., Smith, P.M., Spicer, E.J.F., Barry, M., and Sherlock, S.: Venesection therapy in idiopathic haemochromatosis. An analysis of 40 treated and 18 untreated patients. Quart J Med 38:1, 1969.
33a. Easley, R.M. Jr., Schreiner, B.F. Jr., and Yu, P.N. Brief recordings: reversible cardiomyopathy associated with hemochromatosis. New Engl J Med 287:866, 1972.
34. Van Vliet, P.D., Burchell, H.B., and Titus, J.L.: Focal myocarditis associated with pheochromocytoma. New Engl J Med 274:1102, 1966.
35. Sjoerdsma, A., Engelman, K., Waldmann, T.A., Cooperman, L.H., and Hammond, W.G.: Pheochromocytoma: Current concepts of diagnosis and treatment. Ann Intern Med 65:1302, 1966.
36. Gail, M.H.: Does cardiac transplantation prolong life? Ann Intern Med 76:815, 1972.
37. Das, S.K., Callen, J.P., Dodson, V.D., and Cassidy, J.T.: Immunoglobulin binding in cardiomyopathic hearts. Circulation 44:612, 1971.

Index

Acromegaly, and myocardial disease, 108
  electrocardiogram, 201, 202
Adenosine diphosphate, 134, 136, 137, 143
Adenosine triphosphate, 134, 136, 137, 138, 139, 141, 142, 146, 147
Adenovirus myocarditis, 258
Adrenal steroids. *See* Steroids, adrenal
Afterload, ventricular, 125, 126, 128
Alcohol
  experimental cardiomyopathy
    intraventricular conduction times, 243, 244
    structural abnormalities, 245
  hemodynamic effects of, 237, 238, 241, 242, 243
Alcoholic myocardial disease (alcoholic cardiomyopathy), 9, 33–34, 158–159, 233–249, 363
  angiotensin load test, 237
  arrhythmias, 248
  electrocardiogram, 248
  myocardial O_2 consumption, 124
  nutritional aspects, 236
  skeletal muscle in, 247
  treatment, 248
Aldolase, 135
Amyl nitrite, in obstructive cardiomyopathy, 156
Amyloidosis, 90, 91–92, 269, 352–353
  electrocardiogram, 200
Anemia, and myocardial disease, 109
Angina, in myocardial disease, 49–50
Angiotensin, in alcoholic cardiomyopathy, 237
Ankylosing spondylitis, myocardial disease, 344–345
Antibody, heart reactive (HRF), 282, 283, 285
  after cardiac surgery, 288, 289
  with idiopathic pericarditis, 289
  after myocardial infarction, 289
  in rheumatic fever, 283, 285
  in rheumatoid arthritis, 292
  in systemic lupus erythematosus, 292
Anticoagulants, in myocardial diseases, 366

Arrhythmias, in myocardial diseases, 366–367
Arteriosclerotic heart disease (coronary artery disease), 50, 51
Ataxia, Friedreich's. *See* Friedreich's ataxia

Bed rest in treatment, 363, 364
Beriberi, 9, 109, 159, 178, 268, 349
  treatment, 370–371
  electrocardiogram, 199–200
Beta adrenergic blockade, in obstructive cardiomyopathy, 157
Biopsy, myocardial, 369–370

Calcification, of myocardium, 100, 101
Calcium, in myocardial contraction, 140, 141
Cardiac output, in congestive cardiomyopathy, 147–151
  in obstructive cardiomyopathy, 152–153
Cardiomyopathy. *See* myocardium, diseases of
Chagas' disease, 106, 107, 350
  electrocardiogram, 201
Charcot-Marie-Tooth disease, 331
Citric acid cycle, 138, 139, 140
Cobalt cardiomyopathy, 110, 111, 363
Collagen disease, 106
Complement, in myocardium
  in rheumatic fever, 284
Coronary artery disease. *See also* Arteriosclerotic heart disease
  oxygen consumption of myocardium, 124
Coxsackie virus myocarditis, 260–262
Creatine phosphate, 146, 147
Cushing's syndrome, myocardium in, 108
Cytomegalus virus myocarditis, 259

Daunorubicin, causing cardiomyopathy, 110
Dermatomyositis, 344
  electrocardiogram in, 199
Diabetes mellitus, myocardial metabolism in, 132
Digitalis, in viral myocarditis, 272–273
  in obstructive cardiomyopathy, 155
  in myocardial disease, 365
Diphtheritic cardiomyopathy, 161–162, 350–351
Diuretics, in viral myocarditis, 273
  in myocardial disease, 365

Duchenne's muscular dystrophy, 320–326
  coronary disease in, 323
  electrocardiogram, 199, 323–325
  heritable aspects, 228, 325
Dystrophy, muscular. *See* Muscular dystrophy

Embden-Meyerhof pathway, 134–135
Embolism, in myocardial disease, 47–48
Endocardial fibroelastosis, 30, 31, 32
Endomyocardial fibrosis, 32, 84–89
  hemodynamics, 151
  immune mechanisms, 287
Eosinophilia, in endomyocardial disease, 84–89
Erb's limb-girdle dystrophy, 326

Fabry's disease
  electrocardiogram, 201
Facioscapulohumeral dystrophy, 327, 328
Fatty acid uptake, by myocardium, 132–133
Fenn effect, 128
Fibroelastosis, endocardial, 30–32, 269
Flavine adenine dinucleotide, 137, 139
Frank-Starling effect, 145, 151
Friedreich's ataxia, 330–333
  coronary disease, 332
  electrocardiogram, 199, 331–332
  familial aspects, 216–217
Fructose-6-phosphate, 135

Gallop rhythm, 43, 44, 342
  in obstructive cardiomyopathy, 300
Gamma globulin (immunoglobulin)
  in myocardium in rheumatic fever, 283
  in idiopathic cardiomyopathy, 286
  after cardiac transplant, 291
Glucose, utilization by myocardium, 131
Glucose-6-phosphate, 135
Glycogen storage disease, 102–103, 178, 269
Glycolysis, myocardial, 134–135

Heart transplantation, immunology of, 290–291
Hemochromatosis, 100–102, 268–269, 347–348
  treatment, 371–372
Hemodynamics
  in congestive cardiomyopathy, 147–151

in obstructive cardiomyopathy, 152–157
Hexokinase, 135
Hypertensive heart disease, 54, 55, 70
Hypertrophic cardiomyopathy (obstructive cardiomyopathy, idiopathic hypertrophic subaortic stenosis, muscular subaortic stenosis), 13–15, 30, 45, 71–84, 152–158, 297–314
amyl nitrite, 156, 308
angiography, 174–177, 306–307
beta adrenergic blockade, 157, 308, 312, 314
cardiac output in, 152–153
catheter entrapment, 305–306
diagnosis, 311
digitalis in, 155, 308
electrocardiogram, 183, 184, 185, 186, 187, 188, 189, 190, 191, 194, 195, 301, 302
exercise, 156
familial aspects, 215–220, 227
hemodynamics, 303–306
isoproterenol, 155, 308
mitral insufficiency in, 82, 308–309
methoxamine, 155
natural history, 310
nitroglycerine, 155, 308
phenylephrine, 155, 308
radiology of, 171–177, 302–303
signs, 300
surgical operation, 311–314
symptoms, 298–300
systolic pressure gradient in, 154, 304–306
treatment, 311–314
Valsalva maneuver, 156, 308
vectorcardiogram, 194, 197
Hypokaliemia, and myocardial disease, 109

Idiopathic hypertrophic subaortic stenosis. *See* Hypertrophic cardiomyopathy
Immunoglobulin. *See* Gamma globulin
Infectious mononucleosis myocarditis, 257
Influenza myocarditis, 258–259
Iron, deposits in myocardium, 100–102
Isoproterenol, in obstructive cardiomyopathy, 155

Ketone body, myocardial utilization, 133
Krebs' cycle, 138, 139, 140
Kwashiorkor, 109, 349

Lactate uptake of myocardium, 131–132
Leukemia, 99
Löffler's endocarditis, 86–88, 350
Lupus erythematosus, 345
immunologic studies, 291–292
Lymphoma, of heart, 98, 99, 346
treatment, 370

Melanoma, 97, 99
Mellaril, and cardiomyopathy, 355
Methoxamine, in obstructive cardiomyopathy, 155
Mitral regurgitation
in obstructive cardiomyopathy, 82, 306, 308–310
in myocardial disease, 341
Mumps, of heart, 105, 257
Murmur, in myocardial disease, 45, 341–342
Muscular dystrophy, 319–328
Duchenne's dystrophy, 320–326
Erb's limb-girdle dystrophy, 326
facioscapulohumeral dystrophy, 327–328
myotonic dystrophy, 328–330
Myocarditis, 3, 4, 5, 6, 7, 12
chronic, 6
Coxsackie, 12, 104, 349
diphtheritic, 3, 161–162
Fiedler's, 4
giant cell, 92–96
influenzal, 12
mumps, 105
non-viral, 266
rheumatic, 5, 267
treatment, 370
tuberculous, 267
viral, 104–106, 253–275. *See* Viral myocarditis
Myocardium, diseases of (cardiomyopathy). *See also* Myocarditis
arrhythmia, 46
classification, 26–28, 39, 60–61, 338–339
coronary, 16, 34
diagnosis, 50, 51, 340–341
familial, 214, 220–228
heart failure, 40
idiopathic, 61–71
angiography, 171

Myocardium *(continued)*
electrocardiogram, 182–197, 342–343
radiology of, 167–171
vectorcardiogram, 193, 197
infiltrative, 89–92
obstructive (hypertrophic), 13, 14, 15, 30, 45, 71–84, 152–158
primary, 18
restrictive, 30, 150, 158
secondary, 33, 337–356
radiology, 177–178
treatment, 361–373
Myocardium, oxygen consumption, 119–130
fatty acid uptake, 132–133
glucose uptake, 131
ketone body uptake, 133
lactate uptake, 131–132
respiratory quotient, 129–130
Myocardosis, 7–8
Myxedema, 347
treatment, 371

Neoplasm, of heart, 346
Nicotinamide adenine dinucleotide, 135, 136, 137, 139
Nitroglycerine, in obstructive cardiomyopathy, 155

Obstructive cardiomyopathy. *See* Hypertrophic cardiomyopathy

Pericardial disease, 51, 52, 178, 267
Peroneal muscular atrophy, 331
Phenothiazine drugs, and cardiomyopathy, 355, 363
Phenylephrine, in obstructive cardiomyopathy, 155
Pheochromocytoma, treatment, 372
Phosphohexokinase, 135
Pompe's disease, 102–103
Postpartal heart disease (peripartal heart disease), 8, 29
Pregnancy, myocardial disease of, 8, 29
risk in myocardial disease, 228
Preload, ventricular, 125, 127
Propranolol, in obstructive cardiomyopathy, 311, 312, 314
Psittacosis myocarditis, 259

Radiation-induced cardiomyopathy, 350
Rest, prolonged, in treatment, 363, 364
Restrictive cardiomyopathy, 150, 158
Rheumatic heart disease, 52, 53
Rheumatic myocarditis, 267, 283–286
bound gamma globulin, 283
complement deposits, 284
heart reactive antibody, 283, 285
immunologic studies, 283–286
Rheumatoid arthritis, immunologic studies, 292
myocardial disease, 344–345
Rubella myocarditis, 256
Rubeola myocarditis, 255

Sarcoidosis, 94–96, 270, 337, 351–352, 369
electrocardiogram, 200
Sarcomeres, 140, 141, 142, 143, 144
Sarcoplasmic reticulum, 141
Scleroderma, 343–344
electrocardiogram in, 199
Secondary cardiomyopathies, 33, 337–356
radiology, 177–178
Septum, ventricular
in hypertrophic cardiomyopathy, 80–81
Starling curve, 144, 145
Steroids, adrenal, in treatment, 363, 367–368, 370
in viral myocarditis, 273
Subaortic stenosis. *See* Hypertrophic cardiomyopathy

Thyrotoxic cardiomyopathy, 108, 160–161, 178, 347
treatment, 371
Toxic cardiomyopathy, 355
Toxoplasmosis, 350
treatment, 370
Transplant, of heart, 372–373
Trauma, and cardiomyopathy, 354–355
Trichinosis, 349–350
Trypanosoma Cruzi, in Chagas' disease, 106, 350
Tuberculous myocarditis, 267

Ubiquinone, 137
Uremia, and cardiomyopathy, 356
treatment, 370

Valsalva maneuver, in obstructive cardiomyopathy, 156
Varicella myocarditis, 257
Variola myocarditis, 256
Vectorcardiogram
in nonobstructive cardiomyopathy, 193, 197

in obstructive cardiomyopathy, 194, 197
Viral hepatitis, and myocarditis, 257–258
Viral myocarditis
adenovirus, 258
clinical features, 263–265
Coxsackie virus, 260–262, 349
cytomegalovirus, 259
diagnosis, 265–271
histology, 254
incidence, 254–255
infectious mononucleosis, 257
influenza, 258–259
mumps, 257
poliomyelitis virus, 260
prevention, 273
prognosis, 274
psittacosis, and ornithosis, 259
rubella, 256
rubeola, 255
treatment, 271–273
varicella, 256–257
variola, 256
viral hepatitis, 257–258
Vmax, 124, 126

Wolff-Parkinson-White syndrome
in cardiomyopathy, 194

Z bands, 140

3 a
4 b
5 c
6 d
7 e
8 f
9 g
0 h
1 i
8 2 j